60 Years of Survival Outcomes at The University of Texas MD Anderson Cancer Center

M. Alma Rodriguez • Ronald S. Walters
Thomas W. Burke
Editors

60 Years of Survival Outcomes at The University of Texas MD Anderson Cancer Center

Springer

Editors
M. Alma Rodriguez, MD
Department of Lymphoma and Myeloma
The University of Texas MD Anderson Cancer Center
Houston, TX, USA

Ronald S. Walters, MD
Department of Breast Medical Oncology
The University of Texas MD Anderson Cancer Center
Houston, TX, USA

Thomas W. Burke, MD
Department of Gynecologic Oncology
The University of Texas MD Anderson Cancer Center
Houston, TX, USA

ISBN 978-1-4614-5196-9 ISBN 978-1-4614-5197-6 (eBook)
DOI 10.1007/978-1-4614-5197-6
Springer New York Heidelberg Dordrecht London

Library of Congress Control Number: 2012951619

Printed on acid-free paper

Springer is part of Springer Science+Business Media (www.springer.com)

Contents

1 **Introduction** ... 1
M. Alma Rodriguez

2 **History of MD Anderson's Tumor Registry** ... 5
Sarah H. Taylor

3 **Statistical Methods** ... 13
Geoffrey G. Giacco, Sarah H. Taylor, and Kenneth R. Hess

4 **Breast Cancer** ... 19
Aman U. Buzdar, Thomas A. Buchholz, Sarah H. Taylor, Gabriel N. Hortobagyi, and Kelly K. Hunt

5 **Prostate Cancer** ... 35
Deborah A. Kuban, Karen E. Hoffman, Paul Corn, and Curtis Pettaway

6 **Non–Small Cell Lung Cancer** ... 45
Ritsuko Komaki, Anne S. Tsao, and Reza J. Mehran

7 **Small Cell Lung Cancer** ... 63
Frank V. Fossella

8 **Colon Cancer** ... 77
Cathy Eng, Patrick Lynch, and John Skibber

9 **Ovarian Cancer** ... 85
Robert L. Coleman and David M. Gershenson

10 **Cervical Cancer** ... 97
Patricia J. Eifel and Charles Levenback

11 **Endometrial Cancer** 109
Thomas Burke, Anuja Jhingran, Karen Lu, and Russell Broaddus

12 **Pancreatic Cancer (Exocrine)** 119
Jason Fleming, Matthew Katz, Rosa Hwang, and Gauri Varadhachary

13 **Kidney Cancer** 133
Scott E. Delacroix Jr., Surena F. Matin, John Araujo, and Christopher G. Wood

14 **Bladder Cancer** 143
Robert S. Svatek, Ashish M. Kamat, Arlene Siefker-Radtke, and Colin P.N. Dinney

15 **Cutaneous Melanoma** 153
Jeffrey E. Gershenwald, Geoffrey G. Giacco, and Jeffrey E. Lee

16 **Liver Cancer** 167
Evan S. Glazer and Steven A. Curley

17 **Esophageal Cancer** 177
Linus Ho, Wayne Hofstetter, Ritsuko Komaki, and Steven Hsesheng Lin

18 **Gastric Cancer** 189
Alexandria T. Phan and Paul F. Mansfield

19 **Acute Myeloid Leukemia** 205
Emil J. Freireich

20 **Chronic Lymphocytic Leukemia/Small Lymphocytic Lymphoma** 211
Apostolia-Maria Tsimberidou and Michael J. Keating

21 **Hodgkin Lymphoma** 225
Michelle Fanale, Bouthaina Dabaja, Uday Popat, Paolo Anderlini, and Anas Younes

22 **Non-Hodgkin Indolent B-Cell Lymphoma** 241
Sattva S. Neelapu

23 **Non-Hodgkin Aggressive B-Cell Lymphoma** 251
M. Alma Rodriguez

24 **Multiple Myeloma** 263
Donna Weber and Raymond Alexanian

25 **Head and Neck Cancer** 271
Ehab Hanna, Bonnie Glisson, Kian Ang, and Randal Weber

26 Thyroid Cancer 295
Steven I. Sherman, Nancy Perrier, and Gary L. Clayman

27 Soft Tissue Sarcomas 311
Vinod Ravi, Raphael Pollock, and Shreyaskumar R. Patel

28 Sarcomas of Bone 319
Valerae Lewis

Index 337

Contributors

Raymond Alexanian Department of Lymphoma and Myeloma, The University of Texas MD Anderson Cancer Center, Houston, TX, USA

Paolo Anderlini Department of Stem Cell Transplantation and Cellular Therapy, The University of Texas MD Anderson Cancer Center, Houston, TX, USA

Kian Ang Department of Radiation Oncology, The University of Texas MD Anderson Cancer Center, Houston, TX, USA

John Araujo Department of Genitourinary Medical Oncology, The University of Texas MD Anderson Cancer Center, Houston, TX, USA

Russell Broaddus Department of Pathology, The University of Texas MD Anderson Cancer Center, Houston, TX, USA

Thomas A. Buchholz Department of Radiation Oncology, The University of Texas MD Anderson Cancer Center, Houston, TX, USA

Thomas W. Burke Department of Gynecologic Oncology, The University of Texas MD Anderson Cancer Center, Houston, TX, USA

Aman U. Buzdar Department of Breast Medical Oncology, The University of Texas MD Anderson Cancer Center, Houston, TX, USA

Gary L. Clayman Department of Head and Neck Surgery, The University of Texas MD Anderson Cancer Center, Houston, TX, USA

Robert L. Coleman Department of Gynecologic Oncology and Reproductive Medicine, The University of Texas MD Anderson Cancer Center, Houston, TX, USA

Paul Corn Department of GU Medical Oncology, The University of Texas MD Anderson Cancer Center, Houston, TX, USA

Steven A. Curley Department of Surgical Oncology, The University of Texas MD Anderson Cancer Center, Houston, TX, USA

Bouthaina Dabaja Department of Radiation Oncology, The University of Texas MD Anderson Cancer Center, Houston, TX, USA

Scott E. Delacroix Department of Urology, The University of Texas MD Anderson Cancer Center, Houston, TX, USA

Colin P.N. Dinney Department of Urology, The University of Texas MD Anderson Cancer Center, Houston, TX, USA

Patricia J. Eifel Department of Radiation Oncology, The University of Texas MD Anderson Cancer Center, Houston, TX, USA

Cathy Eng Department of Gastrointestinal Medical Oncology, The University of Texas MD Anderson Cancer Center, Houston, TX, USA

Michelle Fanale Department of Lymphoma and Myeloma, The University of Texas MD Anderson Cancer Center, Houston, TX, USA

Jason Fleming Department of Surgical Oncology, The University of Texas MD Anderson Cancer Center, Houston, TX, USA

Frank V. Fossella Department of Thoracic/Head and Neck Medical Oncology, The University of Texas MD Anderson Cancer Center, Houston, TX, USA

Emil J. Freireich Department of Special Medical Education, Leukemia, The University of Texas MD Anderson Cancer Center, Houston, TX, USA

David M. Gershenson Department of Gynecologic Oncology and Reproductive Medicine, The University of Texas MD Anderson Cancer Center, Houston, TX, USA

Jeffrey E. Gershenwald Department of Surgical Oncology, The University of Texas MD Anderson Cancer Center, Houston, TX, USA

Geoffrey G. Giacco Department of Tumor Registry, The University of Texas MD Anderson Cancer Center, Houston, TX, USA

Evan S. Glazer Department of Surgery, The University of Arizona Medical Center, Tucson, AZ, USA

Bonnie Glisson Department of Thoracic Head and Neck Oncology, The University of Texas MD Anderson Cancer Center, Houston, TX, USA

Ehab Hanna Department of Head and Neck Surgery, The University of Texas MD Anderson Cancer Center, Houston, TX, USA

Kenneth R. Hess Department of Biostatistics, The University of Texas MD Anderson Cancer Center, Houston, TX, USA

Linus Ho Department of Gastrointestinal Medical Oncology, The University of Texas MD Anderson Cancer Center, Houston, TX, USA

Karen E. Hoffman Department of Radiation Oncology, The University of Texas MD Anderson Cancer Center, Houston, TX, USA

Gabriel N. Hortobagyi Department of Breast Medical Oncology, The University of Texas MD Anderson Cancer Center, Houston, TX, USA

Kelly K. Hunt Department of Surgical Oncology, The University of Texas MD Anderson Cancer Center, Houston, TX, USA

Rosa Hwang Department of Surgical Oncology, The University of Texas MD Anderson Cancer Center, Houston, TX, USA

Anuja Jhingran Department of Radiation Oncology, The University of Texas MD Anderson Cancer Center, Houston, TX, USA

Ashish M. Kamat Department of Urology, The University of Texas MD Anderson Cancer Center, Houston, TX, USA

Matthew Katz Department of Surgical Oncology, The University of Texas MD Anderson Cancer Center, Houston, TX, USA

Michael J. Keating Department of Leukemia, The University of Texas MD Anderson Cancer Center, Houston, TX, USA

Ritsuko Komaki Department of Radiation Oncology, The University of Texas MD Anderson Cancer Center, Houston, TX, USA

Deborah A. Kuban Department of Radiation Oncology, The University of Texas MD Anderson Cancer Center, Houston, TX, USA

Jeffrey E. Lee Department of Surgical Oncology, The University of Texas MD Anderson Cancer Center, Houston, TX, USA

Charles Levenback Department of Gynecologic and Reproductive Medicine, The University of Texas MD Anderson Cancer Center, Houston, TX, USA

Valerae Lewis Department of Orthopaedic Oncology, The University of Texas MD Anderson Cancer Center, Houston, TX, USA

Steven Hsesheng Lin Department of Radiation Oncology, The University of Texas MD Anderson Cancer Center, Houston, TX, USA

Karen Lu Department of Gynecologic Oncology and Reproductive Medicine, The University of Texas MD Anderson Cancer Center, Houston, TX, USA

Patrick Lynch Department of Gastroenterology, Hepatology, & Nutrition, The University of Texas MD Anderson Cancer Center, Houston, TX, USA

Paul F. Mansfield Department of Surgical Oncology, The University of Texas MD Anderson Cancer Center, Houston, TX, USA

Surena F. Matin Department of Urology, The University of Texas MD Anderson Cancer Center, Houston, TX, USA

Reza J. Mehran Department of Thoracic and Cardiovascular Surgery, The University of Texas MD Anderson Cancer Center, Houston, TX, USA

Sattva S. Neelapu Department of Lymphoma and Myeloma, The University of Texas MD Anderson Cancer Center, Houston, TX, USA

Shreyaskumar R. Patel Department of Sarcoma Medical Oncology, The University of Texas MD Anderson Cancer Center, Houston, TX, USA

Alexandria T. Phan Department of GI Medical Oncology, The University of Texas MD Anderson Cancer Center, Houston, TX, USA

Nancy Perrier Department of Surgical Oncology, The University of Texas MD Anderson Cancer Center, Houston, TX, USA

Curtis Pettaway Department of Urology, The University of Texas MD Anderson Cancer Center, Houston, TX, USA

Raphael Pollock Department of Surgical Oncology, The University of Texas MD Anderson Cancer Center, Houston, TX, USA

Uday Popat Department of Stem Cell Transplantation and Cellular Therapy, The University of Texas MD Anderson Cancer Center, Houston, TX, USA

Vinod Ravi Department of Sarcoma Medical Oncology, The University of Texas MD Anderson Cancer Center, Houston, TX, USA

M. Alma Rodriguez Department of Lymphoma and Myeloma, The University of Texas MD Anderson Cancer Center, Houston, TX, USA

Steven I. Sherman Department of Endocrine Neoplasia and Hormonal Disorders, The University of Texas MD Anderson Cancer Center, Houston, TX, USA

Arlene Siefker-Radtke Department of Genitourinary Medical Oncology, The University of Texas MD Anderson Cancer Center, Houston, TX, USA

John Skibber Department of Surgical Oncology, The University of Texas MD Anderson Cancer Center, Houston, TX, USA

Robert S. Svatek Department of Urology, The University of Texas Health Science Center, San Antonio, TX, USA

Sarah H. Taylor Department of Tumor Registry, The University of Texas MD Anderson Cancer Center, Houston, TX, USA

Anne S. Tsao Department of Thoracic Head and Neck Oncology, The University of Texas MD Anderson Cancer Center, Houston, TX, USA

Apostolia-Maria Tsimberidou Department of Investigational Cancer Therapeutics, The University of Texas MD Anderson Cancer Center, Houston, TX, USA

Gauri Varadhachary Department of GI Medical Oncology, The University of Texas MD Anderson Cancer Center, Houston, TX, USA

Donna Weber Department of Lymphoma and Myeloma, The University of Texas MD Anderson Cancer Center, Houston, TX, USA

Randal Weber Department of Head and Neck Surgery, The University of Texas MD Anderson Cancer Center, Houston, TX, USA

Christopher G. Wood Department of Urology, The University of Texas MD Anderson Cancer Center, Houston, TX, USA

Anas Younes Department of Lymphoma and Myeloma, The University of Texas MD Anderson Cancer Center, Houston, TX, USA

Chapter 1
Introduction

M. Alma Rodriguez

The University of Texas MD Anderson Cancer Center, which began operations in 1944, was designated one of the first three comprehensive cancer centers in 1971 under the National Cancer Act and has kept that designation ever since. The first leader of the institution, Dr. Randolph Lee Clark, was a visionary who, from the onset of planning the institution, understood the importance of having an integral record of the many cancer patients treated at the institution and of their survival outcomes. He therefore included, as part of the institution's operational plan, a tumor registry that since 1944 has continuously captured the story of the treatment and outcome of every patient who has walked through the doors of the institution. This uninterrupted data repository, unique in its consistency throughout the institution's history, permits us to retrospectively analyze the changes in survival outcome made within the setting of our cancer-specific care-delivery system over the past 60 years. This monograph is the result of a retrospective review of our Tumor Registry data across six decades and presents a snapshot of the parallel history of cancer care at the institution.

As you will see, survival outcomes, in general, have significantly improved for cancer patients across nearly all disease sites during those 60 years. In some disease categories, this change has been dramatic even for disseminated stages of the disease, whereas in others, such as lung cancer, relatively a little has changed over the course of more than half a century. In the major solid tumors, such as breast and prostate cancers, as well as in gastrointestinal malignancies, very significant

M.A. Rodriguez
Department of Lymphoma and Myeloma, The University of Texas MD Anderson Cancer Center, 1515 Holcombe Blvd, Unit 1485, Houston, TX 77030, USA
e-mail: marodriguez@mdanderson.org

M.A. Rodriguez et al. (eds.), *60 Years of Survival Outcomes at The University of Texas MD Anderson Cancer Center*, DOI 10.1007/978-1-4614-5197-6_1,

improvements in outcome have been seen for locally invasive presentations. These improvements can be attributed to multiple factors, but we believe a key element is our disease-based model of care, which integrates multidisciplinary planning and management focused on each specific cancer. Hence, the significant improvements in breast malignancies, for example, can be attributed to concurrent application and improvements in multiple disciplines: progressively better and more accurate diagnostic imaging tools, increasingly effective adjuvant chemotherapy, progressively refined surgical interventions, and progressively advancing radiotherapeutic technologies. All of these modalities and processes have been integrated into algorithms of care for each disease category and are updated as new evidence arises that requires change in disease management. A sample algorithm is illustrated in Fig. 1.1.

Another very important and critical part of the care-delivery design at MD Anderson has been the inclusion of clinical research. Applying the advances made in research to the bedside care of patients, a process summarized in this monograph, has been a driving force at our institution. In situations where clinical investigation is a priority, our clinical care algorithms integrate this recommendation.

The improvements made in cancer outcome across six decades have been incremental and stepwise and do not rely on any single strategy. These improvements have been achieved by integrating the efforts of multiple disciplines. Furthermore, increasing public awareness of the importance of cancer screening and making these screening methods more readily accessible have led to the detection and management of cancer at earlier stages, which can make an enormous difference in terms of survival outcome.

The Tumor Registry is not just a history of cancer care at MD Anderson. It has been a cornerstone for outcomes research and has been instrumental to our clinicians publishing many articles that have influenced cancer care practices. We believe that the Tumor Registry will lead to even bigger contributions to cancer care as information technologies develop. The continually evolving electronic medical records technologies, we hope, will lead to structured documents that standardize clinical terminology and data capture. This would result in more consistent information that would be comparable not only within but across institutions. Furthermore, it is critical to have centralized data that continuously and consistently capture meaningful clinical outcomes. Tumor registries in the future should be increasingly integrated with medical records to ensure more timely and complete data capture.

The value of any care-delivery system is ultimately defined by incremental improvements and consistently sustained good results. We believe that health care delivery that focuses on a group of diseases, self-reflects, self-corrects, and integrates research in all aspects of the management of illness, in a continuum and with consistency, can result in sustained outcome improvement.

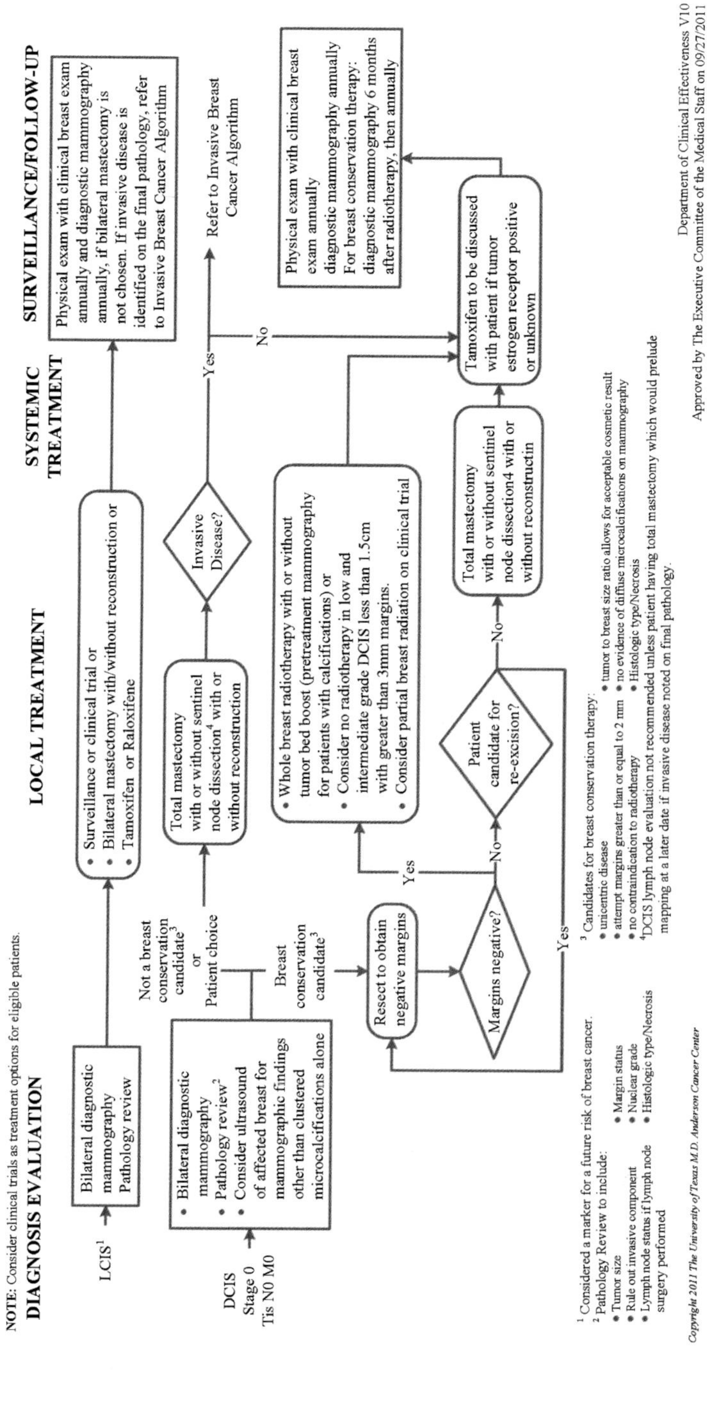

Fig. 1.1 Sample algorithm. Used with permission from MD Anderson Cancer Center.

Chapter 2
History of MD Anderson's Tumor Registry

Sarah H. Taylor

The Tumor Registry Department at The University of Texas MD Anderson Cancer Center is responsible for a database that contains demographic and disease information for all patients assigned a medical record number at MD Anderson, starting with the first patient registered on March 1, 1944. In its function as a hospital registry, the Tumor Registry database contains information about every patient seen at the institution, regardless of the patient's final diagnosis. The institution has always focused on cancer, and every patient has come to the institution because of a cancer-related issue: some with a malignancy, some with a benign or nonneoplastic condition, and some to rule out cancer. Because of this, each patient's information is of value to the hospital.

The institution, originally named the Texas State Cancer Hospital and the Division of Cancer Research in 1941 and then renamed to MD Anderson Hospital for Cancer Research of The University of Texas in 1942, had two purposes from its beginning—to conduct cancer research and to provide care for cancer patients. The registry database was initially established in September 1948 and was housed in the Department of Epidemiology. Eleanor Macdonald was appointed as Professor of Epidemiology and department head.

Miss Macdonald is known as the first cancer epidemiologist. Before coming to MD Anderson, she worked for the Massachusetts Department of Public Health, where she was the first to precisely determine incidence rates for cancer, and for the Connecticut State Health Department, where she developed the first population-based cancer registry and conducted the first vital status follow-up for cancer patients [1].

By the time Miss Macdonald arrived at MD Anderson in 1948, a total of 2,857 patients had come to the hospital. Under Miss Macdonald's leadership, a

S.H. Taylor (✉)
Department of Tumor Registry, The University of Texas MD Anderson Cancer Center, 1400 Pressler Street, Unit 1442, Houston, TX 77030, USA
e-mail: shtaylor@mdanderson.org

M.A. Rodriguez et al. (eds.), *60 Years of Survival Outcomes at The University of Texas MD Anderson Cancer Center*, DOI 10.1007/978-1-4614-5197-6_2,

multifunctional department was established, and its responsibilities included abstraction of data, patient vital status follow-up, epidemiological research, and consultative services for basic and clinical researchers ([2], p. 41). In this new department, Dr. R. Lee Clark, MD Anderson's first president, established a section of information and statistics. Miss Macdonald developed a code of 200 pertinent items applicable to each patient that were designed in anticipation of requests for information for administrative, clinical, and research areas ([2], p. 107). The department also developed and maintained an IBM data processing unit to facilitate access and use of data. Information was stored on punch cards for each case and then stored in indices for "easy recall" ([2], p. 198). This processor made possible constant evaluations as well as monthly and annual assessments.

The handbook for tumor clinic secretaries that Miss Macdonald developed in 1956 at MD Anderson was an outgrowth of one used to train workers at the Connecticut State Health Department. That handbook was eventually sent to every hospital in Texas. At the request of the American College of Surgeons (ACoS), the handbook was also sent to every general hospital in the United States and Canada. The handbook was designed to enable workers without any other source of instruction to build a hospital cancer registry and follow-up service that would fulfill the requirements of the ACoS ([2], p. 315).

Miss Macdonald stepped down as head of the department in 1974. When Vincent Guinee, M.D., who had been an epidemiologist for the City of New York Health Department, became the department head in 1976, the database contained information on more than 112,000 patients. Under Dr. Guinee, the department, which changed its name to Patient Studies, continued to collect a well-defined and consistent data set on each patient and to assist researchers within the institution.

In 1979, the 66th Legislature enacted the Texas Cancer Control Act (House Bill 853), which created the Cancer Registry Program within the Texas Department of Health, making cancer a reportable disease [3]. Because of this need to have submittable data and to facilitate internal data retrievals, Dr. Guinee had the registry data moved to a mainframe NOMAD database.

Under the guidance of Dr. Guinee and at the direction of Dr. Clark, MD Anderson founded the International Cancer Patient Data Exchange System, which was funded by the International Union Against Cancer (UICC). Under this system, data from the registries at MD Anderson, Roswell Park Cancer Institute, Memorial Sloan-Kettering Cancer Center, and 11 other institutions in 10 other countries were compiled into one massive database. With this large number of patients, collaborative studies of rare cancers were carried out.

Dr. Guinee was head of the Department of Patient Studies until 1994. When he left, the database had grown to include more than 315,000 patients.

Since 1995, the department has been under the Office of the Physician-in-Chief. That year, the mainframe database was converted to 4th Dimension (4D), where it still resides. The customized in-house software makes possible the continuation of consistency in the collection of data over the span of the institution and makes possible inclusion of past histories of cancer and nonmalignant diagnoses that were originally thought to be cancer. The software also allows retension and expansion of query tools that were initially developed on the mainframe. These query tools are essential for the extensive institutional use of the data for research and administrative purposes. As of December 31, 2011, the database contained information on more than 850,000 patients.

Registry Operations

Information is collected for all malignancies over the life of the patient, benign neoplasms seen at MD Anderson, and nonneoplastic conditions that affect the patient's cancer treatment or constitute the only diagnosis for the patient.

The MD Anderson Tumor Registry staff provide annual vital status follow-up of patients who currently have or had malignant disease, including foreign patients and patients not definitively treated at MD Anderson. This comprehensive follow-up structure provides the fundamental outcomes information necessary to conduct research on a broad spectrum of clinical research topics.

Responsibilities of the Coding Section

The Coding Section of the Tumor Registry is responsible for abstracting demographic and disease information for all patients registered at MD Anderson. The following describes the specific activities of the Coding Section.

Identification and Processing of New Patient Information

On the sixth day of each month, the Coding Section manager downloads a file of all medical records assigned to new patients during the previous month. Patients' demographic information captured during registration is also downloaded. The medical record numbers and demographic data are read into the 4D database, the transactional database used by the Tumor Registry. This read-in process includes several edits. Designated coders are responsible for resolving errors in the data and assigning codes for each patient's referral diagnosis. Certain errors are reported back to the Referral Office so the correction can be made to the institution's system. Once demographic information has been processed, it becomes part of the available Tumor Registry data and awaits abstracting of disease information by the coding staff.

New Patient Abstracting

The Coding Section of the Tumor Registry is responsible for abstracting information from the charts (either electronic or paper) of each patient who registers at MD Anderson. Abstracting is done no sooner than 4 months after a patient registers.

This allows adequate time to elapse for the charts to contain definitive staging information and final pathology reports and for the first course of therapy (defined as therapy given during the first 4 months after registration) to be completed at MD Anderson. Completion of coding of data for newly registered patients from any given month usually takes 2 months. Categories of data abstracted include additional demographic information, malignant neoplasm information (including site, histology, stage, treatment before admission to MD Anderson, treatment at MD Anderson, and sites of metastases), benign neoplasm information (including site, histology, treatment before admission to MD Anderson, and treatment at MD Anderson), and pertinent nonneoplastic conditions and follow-up information (including vital status, date of last contact/death, method of follow-up). The staff of 13 abstracters recorded information for approximately 44,000 new patients during 2011.

Once new patient abstracting is completed for a given month, the disease information becomes available for data retrievals by department staff and is also available to hospital staff from Clinic Station and the institution's data warehouse.

Reabstracting After Notification of Death

The Follow-up Section of the Tumor Registry identifies patients who have died (see Responsibilities of the Follow-up Section) and provides that information to the Coding Section. The Follow-up Section is currently verifying approximately 10,000 patient deaths per year. The Coding Section is responsible for recoding the charts of these patients. At this final death coding, any new cancers, treatments, or metastases that occurred since the last coding (usually the coding that was done 4 months after registration) are abstracted, and the vital status and death information are updated in the database.

Second Primaries

Once a month, the Pathology Department provides the Tumor Registry Department with a file of all pathology reports from the previous month. The Coding Section uses this file to identify living patients with primaries that developed after initial coding. The file of more than 8,000 pathology report codes is reduced electronically to about 300 possible new cancers. A review by the abstracting staff of each of these 300 reports results in about 100 new cancers per month being coded and added to the database.

Quality Assurance of Coded Data

Once data have been abstracted from a chart, they are "saved," at which point the computer edit program is run. Any errors detected by the edit program are corrected by the coder. The coder then gives the chart to another coder who accesses the checking screen to verify site, histology, and stage. Through this process, the coders are able to provide visual verification of the site, histology, and stage for 100% of the charts abstracted. In more difficult cases, the manager of the Coding Section contacts physicians to ensure that the most accurate information is abstracted. In addition, feedback from data users is used to enhance data quality.

Responsibilities of the Follow-Up Section

The Follow-up Section is responsible for obtaining the vital status of every MD Anderson patient with a diagnosis of cancer on an annual basis. During 2011, last contact information was updated for almost 140,000 patients in our registry.

The records of patients who have been seen at the institution within the year are updated by computer matches with information from appointment data, resulting in an updated "alive" status. In 2011, the last contact date was updated with the appointment date for more than 85,000 patients. Passive follow-up includes matching patients with a malignant diagnosis and a "vital" status of not known dead with death certificate tapes from the Bureaus of Vital Statistics (BVS) in Texas, New Mexico, and Oklahoma. Monthly death information from the BVS is compared with data for MD Anderson patients with cancer who are not known to be dead. Typically, data for more than 200,000 MD Anderson patients are compared with data for more than 15,000 new BVS-recorded deaths each month.

Active follow-up involves directly contacting the patient. The active follow-up process is separated into follow-up cycles during the given year to break the workload into manageable groups of patients. The active follow-up process includes selecting patients to be monitored in the cycle, creating computer-generated letters to be sent to patients, and making telephone calls to patients who do not reply to letters.

In the past year, more than 70,000 computer-generated letters were sent to more than 40,000 patients. A second letter is sent only if there is no response to the first letter, and a third letter is sent if neither of the first two letters is responded to. A maximum of three letters is sent, and the text of each of the three letters varies from that of the other letters. These letters have a response rate of 70–75%. Of the letter responses, 4 of 10 include a positive comment such as "thanks for your concern," "we appreciate your interest," or "thank you for caring." Patients who do not reply to the correspondence are contacted by telephone. This information is updated into the patient database, and the returned bar-coded letter is now scanned into the patient's chart.

A patient is eligible for a follow-up letter if the following criteria are met:

- Registered on or after January 1, 1962
- Not known to be dead
- Diagnosed with cancer (excluding non-melanotic skin malignancy)

From the above, the following patients are removed:

- Patients contacted within the past 12 months
- Patients with an appointment scheduled within the next 6 months

- Patients registered when younger than 18 years who are currently younger than age 18
- Patients with stop contact flags
- Patients in the Suspected Dead File (Hold File)

The follow-up letters are sent directly to the patient, not to a physician.

Death Processing

The three major sources of death information are (1) the Bureau of Vital Statistics of Texas, (2) follow-up letters and phone calls, and (3) communication from MD Anderson employees. The follow-up staff verify death information of more than 10,000 patients annually. A verified death list, averaging 900 patients, is distributed monthly to more than 40 MD Anderson departments.

Suspected Death File (Hold File)

The Follow-up Section maintains the Suspected Death File, also known as the Hold File. The Hold File is a database that lists all patients about whom death information has been received but not yet coded. The purpose of the Hold File is to avoid contacting patients who are suspected dead and to start the process of verifying their deaths. After the patient death has been verified, it can be coded and updated to the registry.

ACoS Follow-Up Results

In April 2010, the ACoS conducted an accreditation site visit at MD Anderson. The Tumor Registry's annual follow-up rates were calculated for the site visit based on the following ACoS criteria for identifying patients who are eligible for follow-up: (1) the patient has been registered since our reference date of January 1962; (2) the patient has a malignant diagnosis (not including carcinoma in situ of the cervix or basal or squamous cell skin cancer); (3) the patient is a U.S. resident; and (4) the patient is an "analytic" case (i.e., the first course of treatment was received at MD Anderson). Of the patients registered at MD Anderson between January 1962 and August 2009, a total of 148,942 analytic cases were, by ACoS definition, eligible for follow-up. The follow-up rates for this population were 92% of all patients and 97% for patients who were registered within the past 5 years.

Data Utilization Activities

The Tumor Registry database is designed to be used for clinical and epidemiologic research. The database contains demographic information about the patients and a set of variables that are applicable to all cancers. The data allow a researcher to identify a population meeting specific criteria from which the researcher can focus on a specific topic. Because of the large volume of patients accessible from the database, researchers are able to have ample patients for retrospective case control studies, comparative studies within the institution's patient population, and survival studies comparing subsets of study populations.

The data are also used in combination with other data sets here at the institution, particularly data contained in the institution's data warehouse. The Tumor Registry data have been used to enhance financial data and operational data from our patient population that can then be used to analyze operations and projections for decisions on the institution's future operations, create financial models, carry out strategic planning, and determine market shares.

In addition to in-house use, Tumor Registry data are submitted to the Texas Cancer Registry and to the American College of Surgeons' National Cancer Database to fulfill the institution's compliance requirements.

Summary

In many ways, the functionality of the department has not changed much in the past 60-plus years. The mission of the Tumor Registry Department continues to be to collect, analyze, and disseminate high-quality data on each patient registered at MD Anderson. The abstractors continue to collect a well-defined and consistent set of data on each patient who registers at the institution. The follow-up staff continue to update the vital status of our patients. The epidemiologists continue to provide information to our researchers. In other ways, things have changed dramatically. Collection of data has moved from index cards to paper code sheets to electronic entry. Where once paper medical records, some weighing up to 20 pounds, were the only source for patient data, clinical information is now available virtually entirely in electronic form. Furthermore, the ability to link to other data sets within the institution has added tremendously to the value of the registry data.

References

1. Macdonald EJ. Answers.com Web site. http://www.answers.com/topic/eleanor-josephine-macdonald. Accessed 2 Mar 2011.
2. Cumley RW, McCay J, editors. The first twenty years of The University of Texas M. D. Anderson Hospital and Tumor Institute. Houston: The University of Texas M. D. Anderson Hospital and Tumor Institute; 1964.
3. Texas Cancer Data Center. IMPACT of Cancer on Texas [Internet]. 6th ed. Houston, TX: Texas Cancer Information. State Cancer Resources, Texas Department of Health. http://www.texas-cancer.info/impact/txdept.html. Updated March 1998. Accessed 22 Mar 2011.

Chapter 3
Statistical Methods

Geoffrey G. Giacco, Sarah H. Taylor, and Kenneth R. Hess

Introduction

Long-term progress in cancer treatment can be assessed meaningfully with high-quality data from a cancer registry. This monograph examines changes in cancer survival by decade over a 60-year period at a single institution. However, these statistical assessments are subject to several difficulties in interpretation. These potential biases notwithstanding, measurements based on high-quality data that are collected in a standard way over a long period can add to our compendium of knowledge.

Patient Selection Criteria

The patient data used in this monograph came from The University of Texas MD Anderson Cancer Center Tumor Registry. To be included in the analyses, patients had to have registered and presented at MD Anderson between March 1944 and December 2004. Patients were included if they had received definitive treatment at MD Anderson but were excluded if they had received any cancer treatment before coming to this institution. Patients were also excluded if they had had primary tumors at more than one site, except for superficial skin cancers. If a patient had

G.G. Giacco (✉) • S.H. Taylor
Department of Tumor Registry, The University of Texas MD Anderson Cancer Center,
1400 Pressler Street, Unit 1442, Houston, TX 77030, USA
e-mail: ggiacco@mdanderson.org

K.R. Hess
Department of Biostatistics, The University of Texas MD Anderson Cancer Center,
Houston, TX, USA

M.A. Rodriguez et al. (eds.), *60 Years of Survival Outcomes at The University of Texas MD Anderson Cancer Center*, DOI 10.1007/978-1-4614-5197-6_3,

more than one primary cancer of the same site, the patient was included in these analyses only if the first of those cancers had been treated at MD Anderson.

Observed survival was calculated from the date of initial presentation to MD Anderson until the date of last contact or death. Ten-year survival analyses were performed for patients who initially presented between 1944 and 2004. This time span was selected because it would result in at least 10 years of follow-up for patients initially presenting between 1944 and 1999 and allow adequate follow-up for patients presenting between 2000 and 2004.

Time periods were defined in 10-year increments, except for the first period, which covered March 1944 to December 1954. The 10-year increments display changes in survival over the operating span of the institution. Although the break-points may not coincide with dates of changes in treatments that affected survival for specific sites, the narrative within the chapters will address those changes as appropriate.

Extent of Disease and Summary Stage

For all cancer patients registered since 1 March 1944, the MD Anderson Cancer Center Tumor Registry has captured the Surveillance Epidemiology, and End Results (SEER) stage of cancer at the time the patient first presents to MD Anderson. The SEER staging system is consistent across all cancer sites and therefore accommodates epidemiologic activities and comparisons.

The chapters in this monograph for solid tumors refer to localized, regional, and distant stages, which were based on the SEER stages [1]. Patients with *in situ* and unknown stages were included in the overall survival curves but were excluded from the stage-specific curves. In this monograph, only overall survival curves are presented for patients with lymphoma, leukemia, and myeloma.

The SEER program uses a basic staging system with five levels: *in situ* tumors are those that have not yet broken through the adjacent basement membrane. The term *localized* describes tumors, regardless of size, that are confined to the organ of origin. *Regional* tumors are those that have metastasized to the regional lymph nodes or have extended directly from the organ of origin. *Distant* describes a tumor whose metastases have traveled to other parts of the body or extended to a distant site (leukemia and myeloma are considered distant at diagnosis). When information is not sufficient to assign a stage, a cancer is said to be *unstaged* or *unknown* [2].

Follow-Up

The follow-up section of the MD Anderson Cancer Center Tumor Registry has maintained a 92–95% follow-up rate (based on American College of Surgeon Standards) for vital status in analytical patients over the past two decades. Patients who presented in December 2004 have potentially 55 months of follow-up at the time of analysis in August 2009. Most of the analyses were conducted in August 2009.

For further description of the follow-up procedures, see the "History of MD Anderson's Tumor Registry" chapter.

Analyses

Data were analyzed with use of PASW Statistics (formerly SPSS statistics) 17.0 (Chicago, IL). Survival-time distributions were estimated by using the Kaplan–Meier product-limit method [3]. This approach provides valid estimates of survival probabilities, even when patients are lost to follow-up or are still alive at the time of data collection. We used the trend-version of the log-rank test [4] to assess the differences in survival time distributions between groups. This test is sensitive to survival differences that are ordered with respect to the year of initial presentation at MD Anderson.

Potential Biases

Early Detection and Screening

The introduction of successful screening programs typically leads to earlier detection of lower-stage tumors and thus to improved overall survival rates (since patients with lower-stage tumors tend to live longer than those with higher-stage tumors). Therefore, observed improvements in overall survival rates may be the result of successfully implemented screening rather than the result of improvements in treatment.

In rare cases, a new screening program may result in the detection of cancer in the preinvasive phase and subsequent decrease in survival of invasive cancers (since such screening is more likely to detect lower-stage slow-growing tumors, but not the higher-stage faster-growing tumors, resulting in lower survival).

Although early detection due to screening may lead to changes in the overall survival curves, it does not affect the stage-specific survival curves. Thus, it is important to consider stage-specific survival in addition to overall survival when assessing changes in survival over long periods of time.

Changes in Diagnostic Criteria and Procedures

The introduction of new criteria and/or procedures for diagnosing cancer can lead to a phenomenon known as *stage migration*, which occurs because the new approach is more sensitive and leads to some patients being diagnosed at more advanced stages. In particular, as technology has improved, metastatic tumors have become easier to diagnose; thus, in some cases, previously diagnosed local/regional-stage disease is now being diagnosed as distant-stage disease. As a result of this phenomenon, patients with the worst prognoses (i.e., those with occult metastatic disease) have been moved from the local/regional-stage designation to the distant-stage designation. Since these patients tend to have a better prognosis than do patients with frank metastatic disease, this "migration" from the local/regional stage to the distant stage resulted in an apparent improvement in survival among patients with a distant-stage designation. Since patients with occult metastatic disease (previously in the local/regional stage) tend to have a worse prognosis than do those with true local/regional disease, their removal from the local/regional stage designation resulted in an apparent improvement in survival among patients with a local/regional-stage designation. Thus, this instance of stage migration seemed to improve the survival of both local/regional-stage and distant-stage patients.

Although stage migration does not change overall survival rates for a given cancer, it can change stage-specific survival rates. Thus, it is important to consider stage migration as a potential explanation for improvements seen in stage-specific survival over time. It is also important to consider changes in overall survival in addition to changes in stage-specific survival.

Improvements in Supportive Care

Improvements in supportive and palliative care over time can lead to improvements in survival over time, even in the absence of improvements in cancer-directed therapy. Supportive care consists of nursing, respiratory therapy, physical therapy, cognitive therapy, behavioral therapy, cardiotherapy, infection control, and pain management, among others. Some improvements might be institution-wide, whereas others might occur in specific cancer clinics. Such improvements can lead to both improvements in quality of life for patients and improvements in survival and should be considered when interpreting improving trends in survival over time.

Changes in Patients' Prognostic Profile

Because our comparisons span such a long period of time, it is possible that the prognostic mix of patients with a particular cancer has changed over that period. If increasingly lower-risk patients were seen over time, then the overall survival may appear to improve over time, even without any improvements in cancer therapy. Since survival analyses are not adjusted for these changes in prognostic risk, care must be taken when interpreting improvements in survival over time. Improvements in survival may be wholly due to improvements in cancer-directed therapy, or they may be in part due to improvements in patients' risk profile.

Conclusion

This monograph assesses changes in cancer survival over a 60-year period at MD Anderson Cancer Center. For most cancer sites, we provide overall survival curves and stage-specific survival curves. We computed 10-year survival curves grouped by decade. In this chapter, we have described the methods used for identifying the patients for analysis, for collecting follow-up data, and for estimating survival curves. We also pointed out some potential biases that complicate the interpretation of the reported survival curves.

References

1. Shambaugh EM, Weiss MA, Axtell LM, editors. The 1977 summary staging guide for the cancer Surveillance, Epidemiology and End Results reporting program. Bethesda: National Cancer Institute, SEER Program; 1977.
2. Ries LAG, Young JL, Keel GE, Eisner MP, Lin YD, Horner M-J, editors. SEER survival monograph: cancer survival among adults: U.S. SEER Program, 1988–2001, patient and tumor characteristics. Bethesda: National Cancer Institute, SEER Program; 2007. NIH Pub. No. 07–6215.
3. Kaplan E, Meier P. Nonparametric estimation from incomplete observations. J Am Stat Assoc. 1958;53:457–81.
4. Tarone R. Tests for trend in life table analysis. Biometrika. 1975;62:679–82.

Chapter 4
Breast Cancer

Aman U. Buzdar, Thomas A. Buchholz, Sarah H. Taylor, Gabriel N. Hortobagyi, and Kelly K. Hunt

Introduction

The treatment of breast cancer has evolved over the past 60 years. Earlier efforts, focused on achieving optimal control of local disease, ranged from radical mastectomies to lesser surgeries combined with irradiation. Surgery has been and remains an integral part of the overall therapy for this disease. With developments in therapeutic radiation technology at MD Anderson Cancer Center, the concept of breast-preserving surgery combined with irradiation became a reality in selected patients. In patients with locally advanced breast cancer, before the availability of effective systemic therapies, preoperative irradiation followed by surgery was a standard approach at this institution, and in a number of patients treated with this approach, adequate local control and long-term benefits were achieved [1] (Figs. 4.1, 4.2, and 4.3).

A.U. Buzdar (✉) • G.N. Hortobagyi
Department Breast Medical Oncology, The University of Texas MD Anderson Cancer Center, 1515 Holcombe Boulevard, Unit 1435, Houston, TX 77030, USA
e-mail: abuzdar@mdanderson.org

T.A. Buchholz
Department of Radiation Oncology, The University of Texas MD Anderson Cancer Center, Houston, TX, USA

S.H. Taylor
Department of Tumor Registry, The University of Texas MD Anderson Cancer Center, 1400 Pressler Street, Unit 1442, Houston, TX 77030, USA

K.K. Hunt
Department of Surgical Oncology, The University of Texas MD Anderson Cancer Center, Houston, TX, USA

M.A. Rodriguez et al. (eds.), *60 Years of Survival Outcomes at The University of Texas MD Anderson Cancer Center*, DOI 10.1007/978-1-4614-5197-6_4,

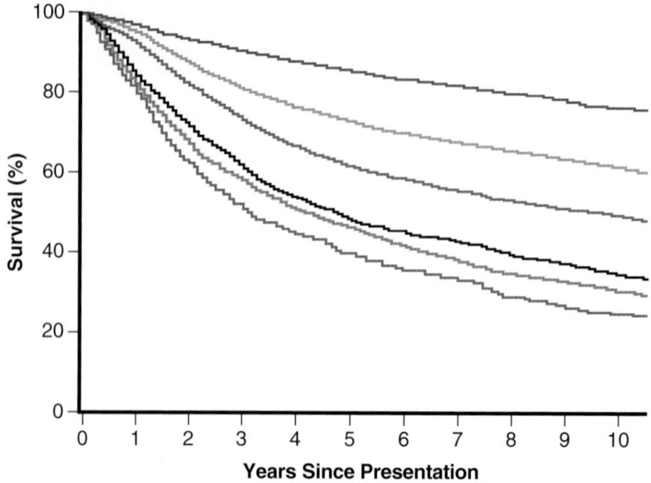

Initial Presentation Year	% Survival 5 Years	10 Years
1944-54	40.0	25.1
1955-64	46.4	30.5
1965-74	48.1	34.6
1975-84	61.8	49.3
1985-94	72.9	61.6
1995-04	85.8	76.5

Fig. 4.1 Overall survival rates for women with breast cancer (1944–2004) ($P<0.0001$, log-rank test for trend).

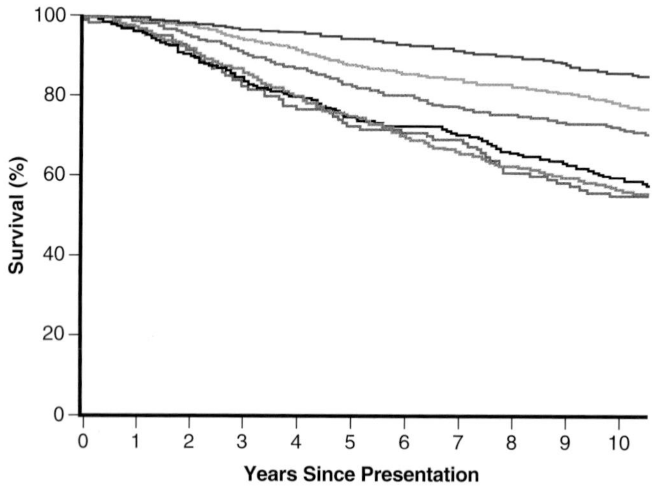

Initial Presentation Year	% Survival 5 Years	10 Years
1944-54	72.5	55.0
1955-64	75.1	56.0
1965-74	74.4	59.3
1975-84	82.7	72.0
1985-94	88.3	78.5
1995-04	94.5	86.1

Fig. 4.2 Survival rates for women with local (SEER stage) breast cancer (1944–2004) ($P<0.0001$, log-rank test for trend).

Historical Perspective

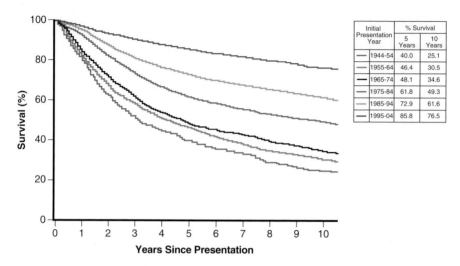

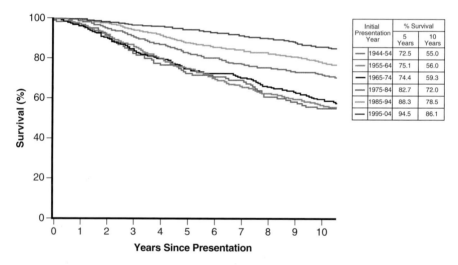

The increased availability of systemic therapies with significant antitumor activity in patients with metastatic breast cancer and the subsequent incorporation of some of these therapies in the combined-modality approach of locally advanced breast cancer have resulted in better local control of the disease and have improved survival rates

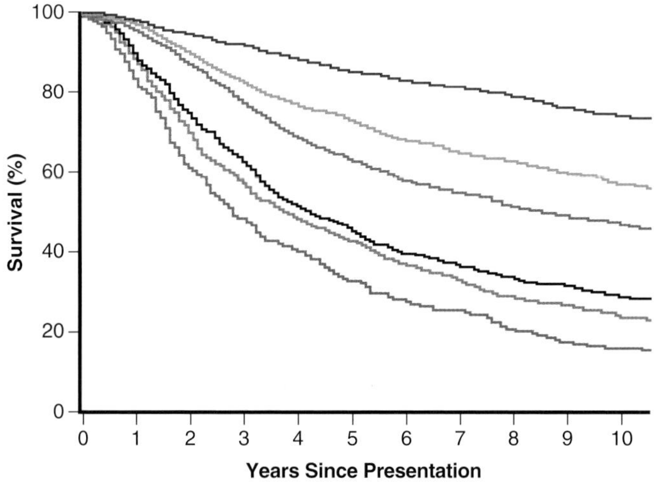

	Initial Presentation Year	% Survival 5 Years	10 Years
	1944-54	33.0	16.2
	1955-64	42.8	23.9
	1965-74	44.7	28.8
	1975-84	62.6	46.9
	1985-94	72.4	57.4
	1995-04	85.5	74.1

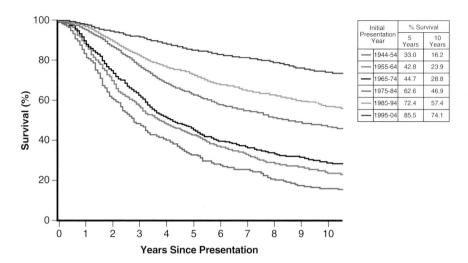

Fig. 4.3 Survival rates for women with regional (SEER stage) breast cancer (1944–2004) ($P<0.0001$, log-rank test for trend).

in this subset of patients [2–6]. At MD Anderson Cancer Center, new therapeutic advances are incorporated into the clinical care of patients early on, and this approach has resulted in improved survival rates in patients within each stage of disease, as illustrated in this chapter. Early in the history of our institution, a combined-modality approach for cancer treatment, and more specifically for breast cancer, was implemented and remains the cornerstone for management of this disease. In this chapter, the progressive improvements in survival rates in female breast cancer at MD Anderson are discussed.

The MD Anderson Cancer Center Experience

Patients and Methods

Between 1944 and 2004, a total of 56,864 patients with breast cancer were seen at MD Anderson Cancer Center. Of these patients, 15,327 had received no prior therapy. The population that was included in further analyses (12,809 patients) consisted of those with no history of other invasive cancers except superficial skin cancer who received their definitive therapy for breast cancer at MD Anderson (Table 4.1).

The extent of disease on initial presentation was determined according to the Surveillance, Epidemiology, and End Results (SEER) staging system (Table 4.2).

Table 4.1 Distribution by SEER stage of women with breast cancer treated at MD Anderson, 1944–2004

	SEER stage at presentation					
	In situ	Local	Regional	Distant	Unstaged	Total
Decade	[No. (%) of patients]					
1944–1954	1 (0.2)	120 (29.3)	191 (46.6)	92 (22.4)	6 (1.5)	410 (100.0)
1955–1964	9 (0.6)	462 (31.9)	656 (45.3)	306 (21.1)	16 (1.1)	1,449 (100.0)
1965–1974	35 (2.5)	440 (31.7)	566 (40.8)	321 (23.1)	25 (1.8)	1,387 (100.0)
1975–1984	55 (2.8)	701 (35.4)	828 (41.8)	367 (18.5)	32 (1.6)	1,983 (100.0)
1985–1994	182 (6.2)	1,036 (35.4)	1,268 (43.3)	364 (12.4)	77 (2.6)	2,927 (100.0)
1995–2004	585 (12.6)	1,898 (40.8)	1,569 (33.7)	455 (9.8)	146 (3.1)	4,653 (100.0)
Total	*867 (6.8)*	*4,657 (36.4)*	*5,078 (39.6)*	*1,905 (14.9)*	*302 (2.4)*	*12,809 (100.0)*

SEER Surveillance, Epidemiology, and End Results program

Results

Overall survival of patients, regardless of the stage of disease, is illustrated in Fig. 4.1. This figure illustrates a steady improvement in survival duration among breast cancer patients treated at this institute during the past six decades. The management of breast cancer evolved over these decades and is briefly discussed below.

Survival Outcomes and Localized Disease

Adjuvant Therapies

Chemotherapies. Anthracycline-based adjuvant chemotherapies have been evaluated at MD Anderson Cancer Center since the mid-1970s. Data from the initial studies demonstrated a significant reduction in the risk of recurrence in breast cancer patients after local therapy [7–10]. This reduced risk of recurrence was independent of stage of disease, nodal status, and age of the patient. In the initial studies, chemotherapy was continued for 2 years [9]. In subsequent clinical trials, a shorter duration of chemotherapy resulted in similar benefit. Inclusion of alternate non-cross-resistant therapies with methotrexate and vinblastine after FAC adjuvant therapy further reduced the risk of recurrence. After taxanes became available, the addition of paclitaxel in adjuvant therapy achieved a further reduction in the risk of recurrence.

Endocrine therapies. After anastrozole was shown to have a better therapeutic index than that of either progestin or tamoxifen therapy in hormone receptor-positive metastatic breast cancer in postmenopausal women, the role of anastrozole was evaluated in a large multinational trial. In the Arimidex, Tamoxifen, Alone or in Combination (ATAC) study, the safety and efficacy of anastrozole alone, of tamoxifen alone, and of combined anastrozole and tamoxifen were compared. On the basis of the initial data

Table 4.2 Initial presentation according to SEER staging system

In Situ (including noninfiltrating intraductal or lobular)

Localized

Primary tumor involving:

Breast tissue only (may be described clinically as fixation of tumor within breast, but not to skin, skin dimpling, tethering, or retraction)

Nipple and/or areola (may be described clinically as nipple and/or areola attachment, thickening, induration, retraction, or involvement, Paget's disease of nipple [including ulceration of nipple] with or without underlying invasive cancer)

Clinical observation such as adherence, attachment, fixation, induration, thickening of skin do not alter classification

Regional

Direct extension

Primary tumor of any size with:

Invasion of subcutaneous tissue, skin infiltration of primary breast, skin edema, peau d'orange, "pigskin," en curraise, lenticular nodules, inflammation of skin, erythema, ulceration of skin of breast, satellite nodules in skin of primary breast

Pectoral fascia or pectoral muscle involvement (may be described clinically as underlying tissue fixation or attachment)

Invasion of (or fixation to) chest wall, ribs, intercostal or serratus anterior muscles

Regional lymph nodes

Low axillary (adjacent to tail of breast)

Mid axillary: central, inter-pectoral, Rotter's node

High axillary: subclavicular, axillary vein nodes, apical

Axillary, NOS

Internal mammary (parasternal)

Nodules in axillary fat

Distant

Direct extension or metastasis

Skin over sternum, upper abdomen, axilla or opposite breast

Satellite nodule(s) in adjacent skin

Breast, contralateral

Adrenal gland

Ovary

Other distant involvement: bone, brain, liver, lung

Distant lymph nodes

Infraclavicular

Supraclavicular (transverse cervical)

Cervical, NOS

Axillary and/or internal mammary, contralateral

Other distant nodes

from this 33-month trial, anastrozole-alone adjuvant therapy was associated with lower risk of recurrence than was tamoxifen-alone therapy; the combination of anastrozole and tamoxifen, however, did not demonstrate an advantage in efficacy or safety and was discontinued [11]. The initial study results changed our approach to endocrine adjuvant therapy, and anastrozole was accepted as the preferred initial endocrine therapy for postmenopausal women with hormone receptor-positive disease at our institution [12]. Subsequently, follow-up data from this trial and from other aromatase inhibitor trials have confirmed the superiority of aromatase inhibitors over tamoxifen.

Biologic Therapies

In patients with metastatic HER-2-positive breast cancer, inclusion of trastuzumab with chemotherapy resulted in higher response rates compared with chemotherapy alone, longer disease control, and improved survival [13]. In the late 1990s, the role of trastuzumab was evaluated at our institution in a randomized trial of patients with localized breast cancer and HER-2-positive disease [14]. In this clinical trial, patients were treated with either paclitaxel for 12 weeks followed by four cycles of 5-fluorouracil, epirubicin, and cyclophosphamide (FEC) chemotherapy alone for 24 weeks or with the same chemotherapy with concurrent trastuzumab therapy. Initial data from this study illustrated that patients treated with combined chemotherapy and trastuzumab had significantly higher pathologic complete remission rates than did those treated with chemotherapy alone. The control arm of this study was stopped, and an additional cohort of patients treated with combined chemotherapy and trastuzumab experienced similarly high pathologic complete remission rates [15]. Currently, combined chemotherapy and trastuzumab is considered standard therapy for patients with HER-2-positive breast cancer.

Survival Outcomes and Locoregional Disease

Local Therapies

With the development of systemic therapies that were effective in palliating disease in patients with metastatic breast cancer [16], anthracycline-based therapies were quickly incorporated into the preoperative setting in patients with locally advanced breast cancer [1]. In earlier trials, three cycles of preoperative chemotherapy resulted in significant reduction in tumor volume in a large proportion of patients, resulting in adequate local control with surgery and radiation therapy. Additional chemotherapy was delivered postoperatively to reduce the risk of recurrence. In another group of selected patients with locally advanced breast cancer who previously would have needed to initially undergo mastectomy to achieve local control, the use of preoperative systemic therapies allowed for breast preservation [17]. The preoperative systemic therapy approach has further evolved over the decades and is now used in patients with operable breast cancer who may not be candidates for breast preservation at initial presentation.

Inflammatory Carcinoma of the Breast

A combined-modality approach using chemotherapy, mastectomy, and radiation has been used since the early 1970s for patients with inflammatory carcinoma of the breast [4, 5]. Of these patients treated with combined systemic therapy, surgery, and radiation therapy, 25–30% remain free of disease [18]. With the established efficacy of taxanes in metastatic disease in the late 1980s, paclitaxel was incorporated into the treatment of patients with inflammatory carcinoma of the breast, and a further reduction in the risk of recurrence in this subset of patients was observed [19]. Inflammatory carcinoma of the breast remains a challenge today, but ≥30% of patients with this disease can be expected to remain disease-free when treated with currently available therapies.

Breast Preservation in Early-Stage Breast Cancer

Breast preservation for patients with early-stage breast cancer was explored by clinicians at MD Anderson Cancer Center as early as the 1970s. Simple excision of the tumor was performed with or without positive margins in patients with favorable types of breast cancer, followed by radiation therapy to the whole breast. Since this initial approach demonstrated excellent local and regional control rates, the technique was compared with both radical mastectomy and modified radical mastectomy, and the results showed similar survival rates and local control rates. With the publication of multicenter randomized trials comparing breast preservation to more radical surgery, breast-conserving surgery became an accepted alternative to mastectomy for patients with unifocal early-stage breast cancer (stages 0, I, and II) [20–22].

Treatment advances in surgery, irradiation, pathologic analyses, diagnostic imaging, and systemic treatments have reduced the risk of local recurrence for patients with stage I disease to approximately 0.5% per year [23–25]. On the basis of our 27-year institutional experience with treating 1,355 patients with breast-conserving therapy for invasive disease, the 5-year rate of in-breast recurrence was significantly lower in patients treated between 1994 and 1996 than in the subgroup treated before 1994 (1.3% versus 5.7%; $P=0.0001$) [26].

A well-recognized role of preoperative chemotherapy is the ability to improve surgical options for patients by reducing tumor size and increasing the chances for breast conservation [17]. The success of this approach depends on the involvement of a multidisciplinary team. Investigators at MD Anderson described the feasibility of breast preservation after chemotherapy in the 1980s and subsequently incorporated this approach into the treatment of patients with locally advanced and large operable breast cancers in the 1980s and 1990s. The 5-year rates of ipsilateral breast tumor recurrence-free survival and locoregional recurrence-free survival were 95% and 91%, respectively. Factors that correlated with ipsilateral breast tumor recurrence and locoregional recurrence were clinical N2 or N3 disease, pathologic residual tumor size of >2 cm, a multifocal pattern of residual disease, and lymphovascular space invasion. A prognostic scoring index based on these factors has also been published to assist clinicians in counseling their patients about the use of breast-conserving therapy after chemotherapy [27].

Imaging of the breast with mammography and of the breast and regional nodal basins with ultrasonography allows for the most accurate assessment of the locoregional disease burden at presentation. Performing a biopsy of any suspicious lesions facilitates appropriate staging and disease management. Once the extent of disease is defined, the potential treatment options can be outlined. Response to therapy should be assessed at defined intervals during treatment. Placement of metallic markers to facilitate subsequent localization of the tumor under ultrasonographic or mammographic guidance and to facilitate radiographic examination of the specimen has become standard. At the conclusion of preoperative chemotherapy, patients undergo breast imaging again so that their options for local treatment can be determined. The preferred residual tumor size after preoperative chemotherapy is <4 cm, but the size of the tumor in relation to the size of the breast is a major consideration. Patients who have extensive microcalcifications on mammography, multicentric disease on physical examination or mammography, or persistent skin edema on physical examination are not considered to be candidates for breast-conserving therapy.

Regional Nodal Treatment

The status of the axillary nodes has been one of the most important prognostic factors in breast cancer. Findings from axillary lymph node dissection (ALND) are important in defining the stage of breast cancer and have been used to guide decisions about systemic therapy and radiation therapy. The use of ALND has been standard practice for management of the axilla in patients with both early-stage and advanced breast cancers for several decades. Sentinel lymph node (SLN) biopsy, introduced in the 1990s, allowed for the selective use of ALND in patients with positive lymph nodes. The *sentinel lymph node* is defined as the first node to receive lymphatic drainage from a specific area of the breast and is the node most likely to contain metastases if the tumor has indeed metastasized to the regional nodes. Thus, when properly identified, the SLN should indicate whether metastases are present in a lymph node basin. Feasibility studies confirmed the proof of concept, and numerous subsequent studies have shown that the SLN biopsy technique is accurate. With this approach, patients with a positive SLN undergo completion ALND, but patients with negative SLNs can be spared completion ALND and its associated morbidity. Furthermore, the use of SLN surgery can identify the most important nodes to the pathologist and may increase the chance that metastases, if present, will be detected. With ALND, detailed analysis of all removed lymph nodes is not feasible. In contrast, the SLN technique directs attention to a smaller number of nodes, allowing more careful analysis of the lymph node most likely to contain metastases. SLN surgery was incorporated as the standard of care at our institution in early 2000 for patients presenting with clinically negative lymph nodes.

As the use of SLN dissection (SLND) gained acceptance in early-stage breast cancer and was shown to reduce the need for ALND in node-negative patients, our surgeons were among the first to use this procedure after chemotherapy [28].

It has been our practice to perform SLND after chemotherapy in patients who present with clinically negative lymph nodes. We have reported that SLN identification rates and false-negative rates are similar in patients who undergo surgery first and in those who undergo neoadjuvant chemotherapy followed by surgery [29]. Overall, there were fewer positive SLNs in the neoadjuvant chemotherapy group, confirming previous reports that chemotherapy eradicates disease in the regional nodal basins. After adjusting for clinical stage, there were no differences in locoregional recurrence, disease-free survival, or overall survival rates between the groups. SLN surgery is equally accurate performed before or after chemotherapy for axillary staging. Chemotherapy eradicates disease in the breast and regional lymph nodes, and the use of SLN surgery after chemotherapy results in fewer positive SLNs and decreases unnecessary axillary dissections. SLND after chemotherapy has become standard practice at our institution for patients undergoing chemotherapy who present with clinically node-negative disease, but it has not yet been proven to be accurate in women with node-positive disease at presentation, a group who should continue to undergo ALND after chemotherapy.

Survival Outcomes and Distant Disease

Chemotherapies

In the 1950s and 1960s, the only available chemotherapy drugs were methotrexate, melphalan, 5-fluorouracil, vincristine, thiotepa, and mitomycin C. These drugs, when used as single agents, had very modest antitumor activity in breast cancer. In the late 1960s, initial data in metastatic breast cancer research suggested that a combination of chemotherapeutic agents (specifically, cyclophosphamide, methotrexate, and 5-fluorouracil [CMF]) used in a metastatic setting could achieve higher response rates. In the early 1970s, doxorubicin (an anthracycline drug) was evaluated in phase I/II studies at our institution and was shown to have significant antitumor activity as a single agent in a number of cancers, including breast cancer.

Subsequently, doxorubicin was evaluated in a combination of 5-fluorouracil, doxorubicin (Adriamycin), and cyclophosphamide (FAC) in metastatic breast cancer, which resulted in objective responses in 60–70% of patients [30]. Use of this combination in patients with metastatic disease illustrated for the first time that a small fraction of patients with metastatic disease (2–3%) can remain in remission for an extended length of time without continued therapy; this finding resulted in the first published documentation showing that a subset of patients with metastatic disease could be rendered free of disease by systemic therapy [31]. In subsequent randomized studies, the FAC combination was established as superior to CMF, with higher response rates, longer control of disease, and a more favorable impact on survival duration [32, 33].

FAC combinations became a standard of care for patients with metastatic disease. The routine use of this combination at MD Anderson Cancer Center in patients

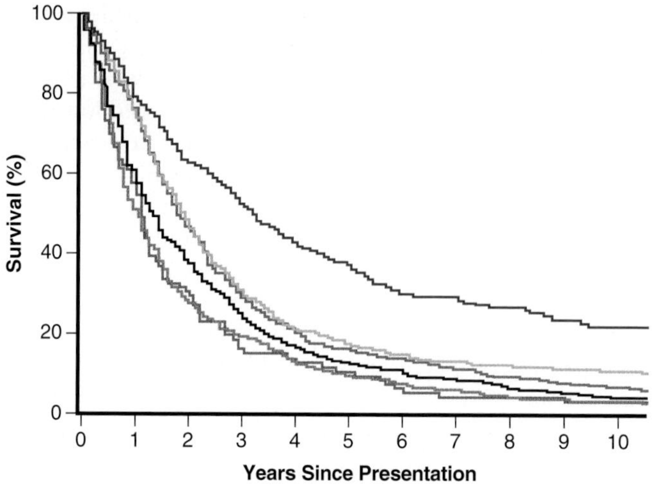

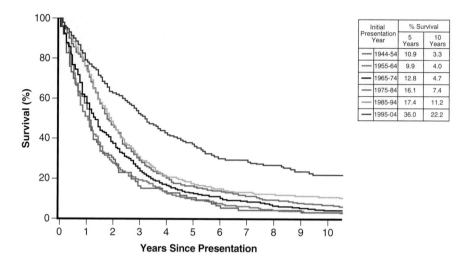

Initial Presentation Year	% Survival 5 Years	% Survival 10 Years
1944-54	10.9	3.3
1955-64	9.9	4.0
1965-74	12.8	4.7
1975-84	16.1	7.4
1985-94	17.4	11.2
1995-04	36.0	22.2

Fig. 4.4 Survival rates for women with distant (SEER stage) breast cancer (1944–2004) ($P<0.0001$, log-rank test for trend).

with metastatic disease resulted in improved survival compared with the survival experience of patients treated here two decades earlier, in the era before combination chemotherapy [34, 35] (Fig. 4.4). A survival advantage of several months, compared with our experience of earlier decades, was evident in most subsets of patients with metastatic disease [34].

Further studies involving patients with isolated metastatic disease after local control (surgery with or without irradiation) of recurrent disease who received the FAC combination resulted in disease-free survival rates of 25–30% after 5 years in contrast to the earlier experience involving patients with disease-free survival rates of <10% [36, 37]. These gains in patients with metastatic disease have been modest, but with the availability of each additional new therapeutic option, survival rates have steadily improved over the decades [37].

Even with the use of anthracycline-containing combination chemotherapy and in spite of the significant palliation achieved in a large number of patients with metastatic disease and the small gains in survival, most patients develop recurrent disease, indicating a need for new drugs; new drugs were also needed for patients with anthracycline-resistant disease. A methotrexate and vinblastine combination developed at our institution in the early 1980s had modest antitumor activity in patients with anthracycline-resistant metastatic disease [38].

Subsequently, in randomized studies involving both patients with locally advanced disease and those with high-risk operable breast cancer, the use of a methotrexate and vinblastine combination after anthracycline-containing chemotherapy resulted in a further reduction in the risk of recurrence and provided the potential for additional modification in the natural history of breast cancer [4, 5, 7, 8]. The reports describing this systemic combination of chemotherapy regimens with alternate non-cross-resistant therapies that affected the biology of this disease were the first to be published.

To enhance the therapeutic index of doxorubicin and vinca alkaloids, various schedules of administration were evaluated in the late 1970s and early 1980s [39, 40]. It was established that doxorubicin's cardiac toxicity could be reduced by infusional therapy [39]; this therapy was therefore incorporated into the standard of care. Infusion therapy was also found to enhance the efficacy of vinblastine, and it remained an effective therapeutic option for patients with anthracycline-resistant disease [38].

Taxanes, such as paclitaxel and docetaxel, were a new class of agents that showed significant antitumor activity in patients with previously treated breast cancer [41, 42]. Both drugs were evaluated at our institution, and their significant antitumor activity was established in patients previously treated with anthracycline-containing combinations. Subsequent studies with these two agents illustrated schedule-dependent efficacy for both drugs [43, 44]. Paclitaxel was most effective (had higher response rates and a better therapeutic index) when administered once a week and has been a standard of care at MD Anderson for the past two decades [43]; docetaxel was most effective when given once every 3 weeks [44]. The drug capecitabine was also evaluated at MD Anderson and showed significant antitumor activity in patients previously treated with anthracyclines and taxanes [45].

Endocrine Therapies

Endocrine therapy in metastatic breast cancer has evolved over the past 100 years. The oldest form of endocrine therapy is ovarian ablation, which results in palliation of metastatic disease. Although patients achieved clinical benefit from ovarian ablation, a significant fraction could achieve additional benefit with sequential ablative therapies, which included either bilateral adrenalectomies or ablation of the pituitary gland (hypophysectomy). Secondary ablative procedures were associated with significant morbidity and a life-long need for replacement therapies. However, with the availability of pharmacological agents, ablative endocrine therapies were replaced with ovarian suppression achieved with luteinizing hormone-releasing hormone agonists, which have similar biological antitumor activity. With the availability of other pharmacological endocrine therapies, including estrogens, progestins, and androgens, patients with metastatic disease could be offered sequential hormonal therapies. Tamoxifen was the first available antiestrogen with efficacy comparable to that of estrogen therapy but had a better safety profile than that of estrogen; tamoxifen therefore replaced the pharmacological doses of estrogens used in treating metastatic breast cancer [46].

Aminoglutethimide with concurrent steroid replacement therapy initially replaced second-line ablative surgical endocrine therapies in metastatic breast cancer [47, 48]. However, aminoglutethimide, a nonselective inhibitor of aromatase, was associated with significant adverse effects. With the availability of selective aromatase inhibitors (anastrozole, letrozole, and exemestane), which were more effective agents, aminoglutethimide as second-line hormonal therapy was replaced [49].

Randomized studies illustrated that selective aromatase inhibitors were superior to progestin (megestrol acetate) and subsequently to tamoxifen; selective aromatase inhibitors therefore became the preferred initial therapy for postmenopausal women with metastatic breast cancer [49, 50]. In earlier decades, endocrine therapies were offered to women with indolent disease. With the discovery of hormone receptors, however, endocrine therapies are now offered to women with hormone receptor-positive disease; in those with hormone receptor-negative disease, endocrine therapies have had negligible benefit [51, 52].

Another new hormonal agent, fulvestrant, an estrogen receptor down-regulator, is now available to treat postmenopausal women with hormone receptor-positive disease who were previously treated with antiestrogens and/or aromatase inhibitors [53]. With the increasing number of available endocrine agents, their sequential use can result in the control of metastatic disease for an extended length of time in a significant number of patients (Fig. 4.4).

Other Supportive Agents

Bisphosphonates have been evaluated in metastatic breast cancer, and initial multi-institutional trials were performed at MD Anderson [54, 55]. The data from these trials have significantly changed the biology of metastatic breast cancer. These drugs have reduced the risk of pathologic fractures of bones, reduced the need for surgeries for bone-related events, and improved the quality of life of patients with metastatic breast cancer. Their role in early-stage breast cancer is now being evaluated in multi-institutional trials.

Current Management Approaches

In the current era, most patients with newly diagnosed breast cancer are candidates for breast-conserving therapy. Preoperative systemic chemotherapy has traditionally been administered in cases of inoperable or locally advanced disease to facilitate locoregional treatment with surgery and radiation. The success of this approach, in addition to the known benefits of adjuvant chemotherapy, has led to its increased use for the treatment of patients with operable breast cancer.

Radiation treatment is important to all patients undergoing breast-conserving surgery and to selected patients treated with mastectomy. Radiation treatment complements surgery as a method for treating the primary cancer and the lymph nodes, and many patients achieve the best locoregional treatment outcome when both modalities are used. Over the six decades that radiation has been used for treatment of breast cancer at MD Anderson, a number of advances in this treatment have occurred. Currently, three-dimensional treatment planning is used with all types of treatment, which allows each treatment plan to be customized to an individual patient's anatomy. Areas at risk of containing disease can be contoured and their inclusion within the treatment volume ensured. In addition, unnecessary radiation doses to important normal structures such as the heart and lung can be minimized or completely eliminated. For patients with tumors in the left breast located directly over the heart, techniques are now available that displace the heart from the left breast by limiting treatments to periods of deep inspiration, during which the diaphragm naturally pulls the heart away from the left breast. These advances have resulted in radiation treatments that are much safer and more effective.

Currently, paclitaxel and FAC chemotherapy are used sequentially as one standard of care in adjuvant chemotherapy for patients with early-stage breast cancer.

The initial data from the ATAC study changed our approach to endocrine adjuvant therapy, and anastrozole became the preferred initial endocrine therapy for postmenopausal women with hormone receptor-positive disease at our institution instead of tamoxifen.

Patients with localized breast cancer who have HER-2-positive disease are treated with preoperative systemic therapy with weekly paclitaxel (12 weeks) and concurrent trastuzumab, followed by FEC chemotherapy (4 cycles) and concurrent trastuzumab. A large study of the American College of Surgeons Oncology Group (ACOSOG) is ongoing to further define the safety and efficacy of this FEC–trastuzumab combination [56].

In summary, over the past six decades, continued improvements in surgical strategy, radiotherapy, endocrine therapy, and chemotherapy (many developed within our institution) have gradually enhanced the safety and tolerance of combined-modality therapy. Furthermore, such advances have led to gradual improvements in overall survival, local control rate, and disease-free survival. As our understanding of the molecular abnormalities that drive breast cancer development, progression, and metastases improves, this information is being used increasingly to develop molecularly targeted agents and to select optimal therapy for individual patients on the basis of their tumor and host characteristics. This focus on the development of personalized medicine in breast cancer is expected to lead to more effective and better-tolerated treatments, while reducing or eliminating undertreatment and overtreatment.

References

1. Rodger A, Montague ED, Fletcher G. Preoperative or postoperative irradiation as adjunctive treatment with radical mastectomy in breast cancer. Cancer. 1983;51:1388–92.
2. Hortobagyi GN, Ames FC, Buzdar AU, et al. Management of stage III primary breast cancer with primary chemotherapy, surgery, and radiation therapy. Cancer. 1988;62:2507–16.
3. Hortobagyi GN, Blumenschein GR, Spanos W, et al. Multimodal treatment of locoregionally advanced breast cancer. Cancer. 1983;51:763–8.
4. Koh EH, Buzdar AU, Ames FC, et al. Inflammatory carcinoma of the breast: results of a combined-modality approach—M.D. Anderson Cancer Center experience. Cancer Chemother Pharmacol. 1990;27:94–100.

5. Buzdar AU, Montague ED, Barker JL, Hortobagyi GN, Blumenschein GR. Management of inflammatory carcinoma of breast with combined modality approach—an update. Cancer. 1981;47:2537–42.
6. Thomas E, Holmes FA, Smith TL, et al. The use of alternate, non-cross-resistant adjuvant chemotherapy on the basis of pathologic response to a neoadjuvant doxorubicin-based regimen in women with operable breast cancer: long-term results from a prospective randomized trial. J Clin Oncol. 2004;22:2294–302.
7. Buzdar AU, Hortobagyi GN, Smith TL, et al. Adjuvant therapy of breast cancer with or without additional treatment with alternate drugs. Cancer. 1988;62:2098–104.
8. Assikis V, Buzdar A, Yang Y, et al. A phase III trial of sequential adjuvant chemotherapy for operable breast carcinoma—final analysis with 10-year follow-up. Cancer. 2003;97:2716–23.
9. Buzdar AU, Blumenschein GR, Gutterman JU, et al. Postoperative adjuvant chemotherapy with fluorouracil, doxorubicin, cyclophosphamide, and BCG vaccine. A follow-up report. JAMA. 1979;242:1509–13.
10. Buzdar AU, Singletary SE, Theriault RL, et al. Prospective evaluation of paclitaxel versus combination chemotherapy with fluorouracil, doxorubicin, and cyclophosphamide as neoadjuvant therapy in patients with operable breast cancer. J Clin Oncol. 1999;17:3412–7.
11. The ATAC Trialists' Group. Anastrozole alone or in combination with tamoxifen versus tamoxifen alone for adjuvant treatment of postmenopausal women with early breast cancer: first results of the ATAC randomised trial. Lancet. 2002;359:2131–9.
12. Morandi P, Rouzier R, Altundag K, Buzdar AU, Theriault RL, Hortobagyi G. The role of aromatase inhibitors in the adjuvant treatment of breast carcinoma: the M. D. Anderson Cancer Center evidence-based approach. Cancer. 2004;101:1482–9.
13. Slamon DJ, Leyland-Jones B, Shak S, et al. Use of chemotherapy plus a monoclonal antibody against HER2 for metastatic breast cancer that overexpresses HER2. N Engl J Med. 2001;344:783–92.
14. Buzdar AU, Ibrahim NK, Francis D, et al. Significantly higher pathologic complete remission rate after neoadjuvant therapy with trastuzumab, paclitaxel, and epirubicin chemotherapy: results of a randomized trial in human epidermal growth factor receptor 2-positive operable breast cancer. J Clin Oncol. 2005;23:3676–85.
15. Buzdar AU, Valero V, Ibrahim NK, et al. Neoadjuvant therapy with paclitaxel followed by 5-fluorouracil, epirubicin, and cyclophosphamide chemotherapy and concurrent trastuzumab in human epidermal growth factor receptor 2-positive operable breast cancer: an update of the initial randomized study population and data of additional patients treated with the same regimen. Clin Cancer Res. 2007;13:228–33.
16. Gutterman JU, Cardenas JO, Blumenschein GR, et al. Chemoimmunotherapy of advanced breast cancer: prolongation of remission and survival with BCG. Br Med J. 1976;2:1222–5.
17. Vlastos G, Mirza NQ, Lenert JT, et al. The feasibility of minimally invasive surgery for stage IIA, IIB, and IIIA breast carcinoma patients after tumor downstaging with induction chemotherapy. Cancer. 2000;88:1417–24.
18. Ueno NT, Buzdar AU, Singletary SE, et al. Combined-modality treatment of inflammatory breast carcinoma: twenty years of experience at M. D. Anderson Cancer Center. Cancer Chemother Pharmacol. 1997;40:321–9.
19. Cristofanilli M, Gonzalez-Angulo AM, Buzdar AU, Kau SW, Frye DK, Hortobagyi GN. Paclitaxel improves the prognosis in estrogen receptor negative inflammatory breast cancer: the M. D. Anderson Cancer Center experience. Clin Breast Cancer. 2004;4:415–9.
20. Buchholz TA, Hunt KK, Amosson CM, et al. Sequencing of chemotherapy and radiation in lymph node-negative breast cancer. Cancer J. 1999;5:159–64.
21. Mirza NQ, Vlastos G, Meric F, et al. Ductal carcinoma-in-situ: long-term results of breast-conserving therapy. Ann Surg Oncol. 2000;7:656–64.
22. Buchholz TA, Tucker SL, Erwin J, et al. Impact of systemic treatment on local control for patients with lymph node-negative breast cancer treated with breast-conservation therapy. J Clin Oncol. 2001;19:2240–6.

23. Mirza NQ, Vlastos G, Meric F, et al. Predictors of locoregional recurrence among patients with early-stage breast cancer treated with breast-conserving therapy. Ann Surg Oncol. 2002;9: 256–65.
24. Meric F, Buchholz TA, Mirza NQ, et al. Long-term complications associated with breast-conservation surgery and radiotherapy. Ann Surg Oncol. 2002;9:543–9.
25. Meric F, Mirza NQ, Vlastos G, et al. Positive surgical margins and ipsilateral breast tumor recurrence predict disease-specific survival after breast-conserving therapy. Cancer. 2003;97:926–33.
26. Cabioglu N, Hunt KK, Buchholz TA, et al. Improving local control with breast-conserving therapy: a 27-year single-institution experience. Cancer. 2005;104:20–9.
27. Chen AM, Meric-Bernstam F, Hunt KK, et al. Breast conservation after neoadjuvant chemotherapy. Cancer. 2005;103:689–95.
28. Breslin TM, Cohen L, Sahin A, et al. Sentinel lymph node biopsy is accurate after neoadjuvant chemotherapy for breast cancer. J Clin Oncol. 2000;18:3480–6.
29. Hunt KK, Yi M, Mittendorf EA, et al. Sentinel lymph node surgery after neoadjuvant chemotherapy is accurate and reduces the need for axillary dissection in breast cancer patients. Ann Surg. 2009;250(4):558–66.
30. Hortobagyi GN, Gutterman JU, Blumenschein GR, et al. Combined chemoimmunotherapy for advanced breast cancer: a comparison of BCG and levamisole. Cancer. 1979;43:1112–22.
31. Greenberg PA, Hortobagyi GN, Smith TL, Ziegler LD, Frye DK, Buzdar AU. Long-term follow-up of patients with complete remission following combination chemotherapy for metastatic breast cancer. J Clin Oncol. 1996;14:2197–205.
32. Levine MN, Bramwell VH, Pritchard KI, et al. Randomized trial of intensive cyclophosphamide, epirubicin, and fluorouracil chemotherapy compared with cyclophosphamide, methotrexate, and fluorouracil in premenopausal women with node-positive breast cancer. National Cancer Institute of Canada Clinical Trials Group.[see comment]. J Clin Oncol. 1998;16:2651–8.
33. Bull JM, Tormey DC, Li SH, et al. A randomized comparative trial of adriamycin versus methotrexate in combination drug therapy. Cancer. 1978;41:1649–57.
34. Ross MB, Buzdar AU, Smith TL, et al. Improved survival of patients with metastatic breast cancer receiving combination chemotherapy. Cancer. 1985;55:341–6.
35. Giordano SH, Buzdar AU, Smith TL, Kau SW, Yang Y, Hortobagyi GN. Is breast cancer survival improving? Cancer. 2004;100:44–52.
36. Buzdar AU, Blumenschein GR, Smith TL, et al. Adjuvant chemoimmunotherapy following regional therapy for isolated recurrences of breast cancer (stage IV NED). J Surg Oncol. 1979;12:27–40.
37. Rivera E, Holmes FA, Buzdar AU, et al. Fluorouracil, doxorubicin, and cyclophosphamide followed by tamoxifen as adjuvant treatment for patients with stage IV breast cancer with no evidence of disease. Breast J. 2002;8:2–9.
38. Hortobagyi GN, Yap HY, Blumenschein GR, et al. Phase II evaluation of vinblastine, methotrexate, and calcium leukovorin rescue in patients with refractory metastatic breast cancer. Cancer. 1983;51:769–72.
39. Legha SS, Benjamin RS, Mackay B, et al. Reduction of doxorubicin cardiotoxicity by prolonged continuous intravenous infusion. Ann Intern Med. 1982;96:133–9.
40. Yau JC, Yap YY, Buzdar AU, Hortobagyi GN, Bodey GP, Blumenschein GR. A comparative randomized trial of vinca alkaloids in patients with metastatic breast carcinoma. Cancer. 1985;55:337–40.
41. Holmes FA, Walters RS, Theriault RL, et al. Phase II trial of Taxol, an active drug in the treatment of metastatic breast cancer. J Natl Cancer Inst. 1991;83:1797–805.
42. Valero V, Holmes FA, Walters RS, et al. Phase II trial of docetaxel: a new, highly effective antineoplastic agent in the management of patients with anthracycline-resistant metastatic breast cancer [see comments]. J Clin Oncol. 1995;13:2886–94.
43. Green MC, Buzdar AU, Smith T, et al. Weekly paclitaxel followed by FAC as primary systemic chemotherapy of operable breast cancer improves pathologic complete remission rates

when compared to every 3-week (q3wk) paclitaxel therapy followed by FAC—final results of a prospective phase III randomized trial [abstract 135]. Proc Annu Meet Am Soc Clin Oncol. 2002;21:35a.
44. Rivera E, Mejia JA, Arun BK, et al. Phase 3 study comparing the use of docetaxel on an every-3-week versus weekly schedule in the treatment of metastatic breast cancer. Cancer. 2008;112: 1455–61.
45. Blum JL, Jones SE, Buzdar AU, et al. Multicenter phase II study of capecitabine in paclitaxel-refractory metastatic breast cancer. J Clin Oncol. 1999;17:485–93.
46. Ingle JN, Ahmann DL, Green SJ, et al. Randomized clinical trial of diethylstilbestrol versus tamoxifen in postmenopausal women with advanced breast cancer. N Engl J Med. 1981;304:16–21.
47. Wells Jr SA, Worgul TJ, Samojlik E, et al. Comparison of surgical adrenalectomy to medical adrenalectomy in patients with metastatic carcinoma of the breast. Cancer Res. 1982;42: 3454s–7.
48. Buzdar AU, Powell KC, Legha SS, Blumenschein GR. Treatment of advanced breast cancer with aminoglutethimide after therapy with tamoxifen. Cancer. 1982;50:1708–12.
49. Buzdar AU, Jones SE, Vogel CL, Wolter J, Plourde P, Webster A. A phase III trial comparing anastrozole (1 and 10 milligrams), a potent and selective aromatase inhibitor, with megestrol acetate in postmenopausal women with advanced breast carcinoma. Arimidex Study Group. Cancer. 1997;79:730–9.
50. Nabholtz JM, Buzdar A, Pollak M, et al. Anastrozole is superior to tamoxifen as first-line therapy for advanced breast cancer in postmenopausal women: results of a North American multicenter randomized trial. Arimidex Study Group. J Clin Oncol. 2000;18:3758–67.
51. Samaan NA, Buzdar AU, Aldinger KA, et al. Estrogen receptor: a prognostic factor in breast cancer. Cancer. 1981;47:554–60.
52. Jensen EV. Estrogen receptors in hormone-dependent breast cancers. Cancer Res. 1975;35: 3362–4.
53. Osborne CK, Pippen J, Jones SE, et al. Double-blind, randomized trial comparing the efficacy and tolerability of fulvestrant versus anastrozole in postmenopausal women with advanced breast cancer progressing on prior endocrine therapy: results of a North American trial.[comment]. J Clin Oncol. 2002;20:3386–95.
54. Hortobagyi GN, Theriault RL, Porter L, et al. Efficacy of pamidronate in reducing skeletal complications in patients with breast cancer and lytic bone metastases. Protocol 19 Aredia Breast Cancer Study Group [see comments]. N Engl J Med. 1996;335:1785–91.
55. Theriault RL, Lipton A, Hortobagyi GN, et al. Pamidronate reduces skeletal morbidity in women with advanced breast cancer and lytic bone lesions: a randomized, placebo-controlled trial. Protocol 18 Aredia Breast Cancer Study Group. J Clin Oncol. 1999;17:846–54.
56. Buzdar AU, Ballman KV, Meric-Bernstam F, et al. Initial safety data of a randomized phase III trial comparing a preoperative regimen of FEC-75 alone followed by paclitaxel plus trastuzumab with a regimen of paclitaxel plus trastuzumab followed by FEC-75 plus trastuzumab in patients with HER2 positive operable breast cancer (ACOSOG Z1041) [abstract]. American Society of Clinical Oncology Breast Cancer Symposium 2009.

Chapter 5
Prostate Cancer

Deborah A. Kuban, Karen E. Hoffman, Paul Corn, and Curtis Pettaway

Introduction

Prostate cancer is one of the most common malignancies in American men, second only to non-melanoma skin cancer. In 2009, an estimated 192,280 new cases of prostate cancer were diagnosed in the United States, and about 27,360 men died of this disease [1]. The median age at diagnosis is 68 years, and the risk of developing the disease increases in men with advancing age, in those with an affected first-degree relative, and in African American men. The behavior of prostate cancer can vary from a microscopic, well-differentiated cancer with a slow clinical course to an aggressive, poorly differentiated cancer with the potential to invade and spread. Men with prostate cancer can be broadly staged as having localized disease (confined to the prostate), regional disease (i.e., spread to periprostatic fat, seminal vesicles, or pelvic lymph nodes), or distant disease (which metastasizes most commonly to distant lymph nodes and bone).

Current American Joint Committee on Cancer staging definitions for the extent of disease are outlined in Table 5.1. Since the introduction of serum prostate-specific antigen (PSA) testing in the 1990s, most cases of prostate cancer have been diagnosed while the disease is confined to the prostate. "Localized" (i.e., nonmetastatic) prostate cancer is further categorized into "low-risk," "intermediate-risk," and "high-risk"

D.A. Kuban (✉) • K.E. Hoffman
Department of Radiation Oncology, The University of Texas MD Anderson Cancer Center,
1515 Holcombe Boulevard, Unit 1202, Houston, TX 77030, USA
e-mail: dakuban@mdanderson.org

P. Corn
Department of GU Medical Oncology, The University of Texas MD Anderson Cancer Center,
Houston, TX, USA

C. Pettaway
Department of Urology, The University of Texas MD Anderson Cancer Center,
Houston, TX, USA

M.A. Rodriguez et al. (eds.), *60 Years of Survival Outcomes at The University of Texas MD Anderson Cancer Center*, DOI 10.1007/978-1-4614-5197-6_5,

Table 5.1 Prostate cancer staging by 2009 American Joint Committee on Cancer staging system

Primary tumor (T)	
Clinical	
Tx	Primary tumor cannot be assessed
T0	No evidence of primary tumor
T1	Clinically inapparent tumor neither palpable nor visible by imaging
T1a	Tumor incidental histologic finding in 5% or less of tissue resected
T1b	Tumor incidental histologic finding in more than 5% of tissue resected
T1c	Tissue identified by needle biopsy (e.g., because of elevated PSA)
T2	Tumor confined within the prostate
T2a	Tumor involves one-half of one lobe or less
T2b	Tumor involves more than one-half of one lobe but not both lobes
T2c	Tumor involves both lobes
T3	Tumor extends through the prostatic capsule
T3a	Extracapsular extension (unilateral or bilateral)
T3b	Tumor invades the seminal vesicle(s)
T4	Tumor is fixed or invades adjacent structures other than seminal vesicles such as external sphincter, rectum, bladder, levator muscles and/or pelvic wall
Pathologic (pT)	
pT2	Organ confined
pT2a	Unilateral, involving one-half of one side or less
pT2b	Unilateral, involving more than one-half of side but not both sides
pT2c	Bilateral disease
pT3	Extraprostatic extension
pT3a	Extraprostatic extension
pT3b	Seminal vesicle invasion
pT4	Invasion of rectum, levator muscles, and/or pelvic wall
Regional lymph nodes (N)	
Clinical	
Nx	Regional lymph nodes were not assessed
N0	No regional lymph node metastasis
N1	Metastases in regional lymph node(s)
Pathologic (pN)	
pNx	Regional lymph node not sampled
pN0	No positive regional lymph nodes
pN1	Metastases in regional lymph node(s)
Distant metastasis (M)	
M0	No distant metastasis
M1	Distant metastasis
M1a	Non-regional lymph node(s)
M1b	Bone
M1c	Other site(s) with or without bone disease

PSA prostate-specific antigen

Table 5.2 National Comprehensive Cancer Network categorization of recurrence risk (v.1.2010)

Category	Tumor characteristics
Very low risk	T1a; Gleason score ≤6; PSA <10 ng/mL; fewer than 3 biopsy cores positive, ≤50% cancer in each core; and PSA density <0.15 ng/mL/g
Low	T1-T2a, Gleason score 2–6, and PSA <10 ng/mL
Intermediate	T2b-T2c, Gleason score 7, or PSA 10–20 ng/mL
High	T3a, Gleason score 8–10, or PSA >20 ng/mL
Very high	T3b-T4
Metastatic	Any T, N1, M0; or any T, any N, M1

PSA prostate-specific antigen

groups on the basis of the extent of local disease, Gleason score, and PSA level. These groups, which reflect the potential (or actual) spread beyond the prostate and the likelihood of recurrence after treatment, are commonly used to guide pretreatment evaluations and treatment recommendations. The current National Comprehensive Cancer Network risk categories are listed in Table 5.2.

In this chapter, we present six decades of the MD Anderson Cancer Center prostate cancer experience.

Historical Perspective

Diagnosing and staging of prostate cancer have evolved over the past six decades. Historically, prostate cancer was diagnosed when men developed obstructive or irritative urinary symptoms, palpable soft tissue metastases, or symptomatic bony metastases (i.e., back or hip pain). The introduction of PSA testing in the 1990s, however, dramatically changed the stage at which prostate cancer was diagnosed [2], in most cases shifting from an advanced metastatic stage at diagnosis to an asymptomatic, localized, and highly curable stage.

Radiologic advances over the past six decades have led to improved methods of identifying men with only local disease or with disease that has spread only to local lymph node basins. In the 1940s and 1950s, plain radiographs were available for diagnostic purposes. Plain radiographs can visualize bone changes but cannot visualize pelvic lymph node involvement. Lymphangiograms were introduced in the 1960s and used throughout the 1990s to image pelvic lymph nodes [3]. Computed tomographic scans were developed in the 1970s, adopted in the 1980s, and continue to be used to evaluate pelvic lymph nodes. Bone scans, introduced in the 1970s, are still used to evaluate men for bone metastases. In addition, endorectal magnetic resonance imaging is used in selected cases to visualize tissue planes and to define the local extent of disease. These imaging advances have improved the accuracy of identifying disease extent at presentation and have no doubt led to stage migration.

Along with advances in scanning technologies, surgical techniques have been refined as well. The anatomic radical prostatectomy technique, described in the early 1980s [4], improved urinary continence and sexual function after surgical resection based on enhanced visualization and precise dissection in a relatively bloodless field. Radical prostatectomy subsequently became a more common treatment for prostate cancer, and a nerve-sparing radical prostatectomy technique was introduced at MD Anderson Cancer Center in the 1990s. The administration of novel therapeutic strategies, such as targeted molecular systemic agents, before radical prostatectomy among patients with high-risk prostate cancer was established in the late 1990s as a mechanism with which to rapidly evaluate both tissue and molecular effects of new potential agents affecting prostate cancer [5]. Recently, less invasive robotic prostatectomy techniques have been adopted that provide enhanced magnification for even greater precision.

The introduction of urologic oncology fellowships provided an opportunity for physicians to refine their surgical technique and enhance their oncologic knowledge base before practicing independently [6]. The first urologic oncology fellowship at MD Anderson Cancer Center was in the early 1970s, and we continue to train four urologic oncology fellows annually.

Radiotherapeutic techniques have also evolved over the past several decades. The introduction of three-dimensional computed tomography-based planning in the 1990s improved targeting in radiotherapy. The development of intensity-modulated radiation therapy improved dose delivery in the 2000s and permitted the escalation of radiation dose [7]. These dose-escalated treatments led to improved treatment outcome in localized prostate cancer, as shown in a randomized trial at MD Anderson Cancer Center [8]. In addition, the integration of hormone therapy with radiotherapy for men with localized and locally advanced prostate cancer led to improved prostate cancer survival rates [9, 10]. Currently, altered radiation fractionation to improve prostate cancer outcome is being investigated at MD Anderson.

Androgen ablative therapy was introduced in the 1940s and remains the primary systemic therapy for men with metastatic or locally advanced prostate cancer [11]. The methods of delivering androgen ablative therapy have changed over time and include maximum androgen blockade and intermittent androgen ablation. Systemic treatment options for men with castrate-resistant prostate cancer are limited; however, improved survival rates after administration of docetaxel were established in 2004 [12]. Clinical trials at MD Anderson are investigating cytotoxic agents, targeted agents, and immunotherapy to improve outcome for men with castrate-resistant prostate cancer.

Currently, in a large portion of men diagnosed with prostate cancer, the disease is still localized to the prostate. There are several treatment options for these men that offer similar efficacy but have different side effect profiles. Therefore, increased attention is being focused on the long-term sequelae of treatment and the impact of treatment on quality of life during treatment selection and treatment evaluation [13]. Ongoing clinical trials at MD Anderson are evaluating the effects of prostate cancer diagnosis and treatments on quality of life. In addition, active surveillance (frequent monitoring with no immediate cancer-directed treatment) is being studied at MD Anderson in men with early disease who may not require intervention and can therefore be spared the adverse effects of treatment and in those with comorbidities that render prostate cancer therapy unnecessary.

The MD Anderson Cancer Center Experience

In total, 28,891 men presented to MD Anderson with a diagnosis of prostate cancer from March 1944 through December 2004. Of this group, 13,711 had no prior treatment for their cancer. Excluding men treated elsewhere and those diagnosed with other primary cancers (except superficial skin cancers), 6,675 men received definitive primary treatment for prostate cancer at MD Anderson and made up the cohort for analysis. Survival was calculated from the date of initial presentation to MD Anderson.

The number of patients presenting by decade is shown in Table 5.3. This number increased considerably over time, from 59 in 1944–1954 to 3,979 in 1995–2004, reflecting both the growth of MD Anderson and the national increase in prostate cancer diagnoses. Diagnoses increased nationally because of improved cancer detection, population growth, longer life expectancies, and the aging population. Of note, the number of prostate cancer patients tripled between 1975–1984 ($n=529$) and 1985–1994 ($n=1,631$), when serum PSA testing became more widespread. Awareness of the potential benefits of early detection with use of PSA testing led to its adoption in early detection programs in the late 1980s at MD Anderson Cancer Center. The widespread use of PSA testing in the 1990s is also reflected in the larger proportion of men with localized disease in later decades; this proportion had remained stable at about 30% through 1984 but increased to 73% in the 1995–2004 period. The proportion of men with localized disease is smaller than that seen nationally, however, because MD Anderson is a referral center that draws men with more advanced cancer.

Over the 60-year period, survival rates after prostate cancer diagnosis have improved significantly at MD Anderson ($P<0.0001$). As illustrated in Fig. 5.1, 5-year survival rates increased from 18.6% to 92.5%, and 10-year survival rates increased from 8.5% to 82.5%. Lengthened survival was the result of both the larger proportion of men being diagnosed with localized disease, when cure is more likely, and the improvements in prostate cancer treatment at MD Anderson, particularly for men with localized and regional disease. Stage migration was a consequence of implementing improved imaging at MD Anderson that could better distinguish men with localized

Table 5.3 Prostate cancer stage distribution by decade

	SEER stage at presentation				
	Local	Regional	Distant	Unstaged	Total
Decade	[No. (%) of men diagnosed]				
1944–1954	18 (30.5)	2 (3.4)	34 (57.6)	5 (8.5)	59 (100.0)
1955–1964	74 (33.9)	26 (11.9)	104 (47.7)	14 (6.4)	218 (100.0)
1965–1974	73 (28.2)	60 (23.2)	119 (45.9)	7 (2.7)	259 (100.0)
1975–1984	174 (32.9)	203 (38.4)	147 (27.8)	5 (0.9)	529 (100.0)
1985–1994	760 (46.6)	642 (39.4)	171 (10.5)	58 (3.6)	1,631 (100.0)
1995–2004	2,914 (73.2)	770 (19.4)	172 (4.3)	123 (3.1)	3,979 (100.0)
Total	*4,013 (60.1)*	*1,703 (25.5)*	*747 (11.2)*	*212 (3.2)*	*6,675 (100.0)*

SEER Surveillance, Epidemiology, and End Results program

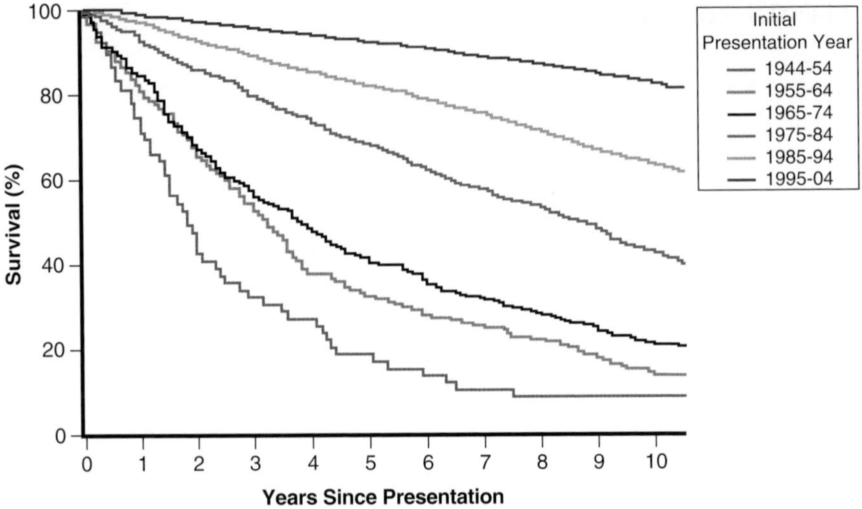

Fig. 5.1 Overall survival rates for patients with prostate cancer (1944–2004) ($P<0.0001$, log-rank test for trend).

disease and regional disease while identifying men with earlier metastatic disease. This contributed to increased survival rates among all groups over time. In addition, improvements in overall health contributed to men living longer over time.

In men with localized disease at diagnosis, 5-year survival rates increased from 38.9% to 96.0%, and 10-year survival increased from 22.2% to 87.3% (Fig. 5.2; $P<0.0001$). Significant improvements were also seen in men with regional disease (Fig. 5.3; $P<0.0001$) and in men with distant disease at diagnosis (Fig. 5.4; $P<0.0001$). In men with distant disease at diagnosis, 5-year survival rates increased from 11.8% to 38.8%, and 10-year rates increased from 2.9% to 16.9%. Androgen deprivation therapy was the mainstay of systemic treatment throughout this period. The benefit of docetaxel for castrate-resistant prostate cancer was not established until 2004; therefore, improvements from docetaxel are not reflected in this analysis.

The significant improvements in prostate-cancer survival over the past six decades reflect the development and implementation of advances in imaging, surgery, radiotherapy, and medical oncology at MD Anderson. In addition, the adoption of routine PSA testing and subsequent earlier diagnosis of prostate cancer have contributed to improved prostate cancer survival.

Current Management Approach

Our current approach to the management of prostate cancer is stratified by using "risk group" criteria and anticipated life expectancy. After initial diagnosis by PSA and prostate biopsy, pelvic imaging and a bone scan are obtained for selected men at

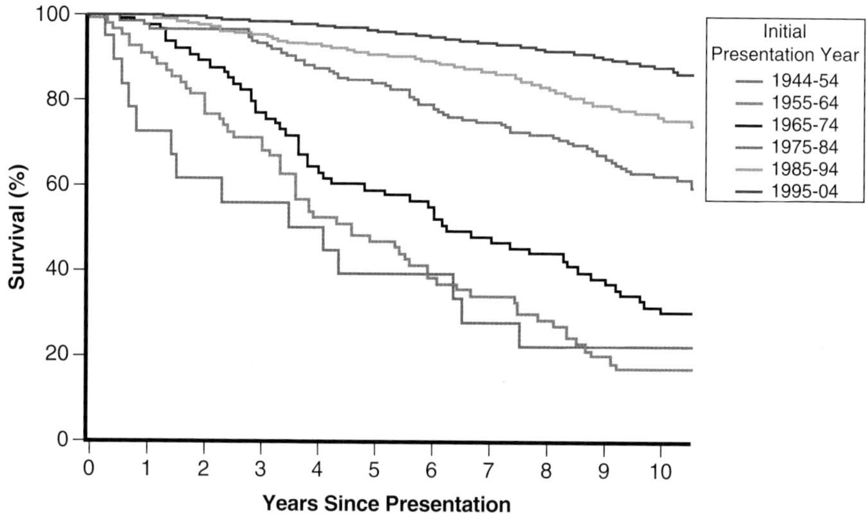

Fig. 5.2 Survival rates for patients with local (SEER stage) prostate cancer (1944–2004) ($P < 0.0001$, log-rank test for trend).

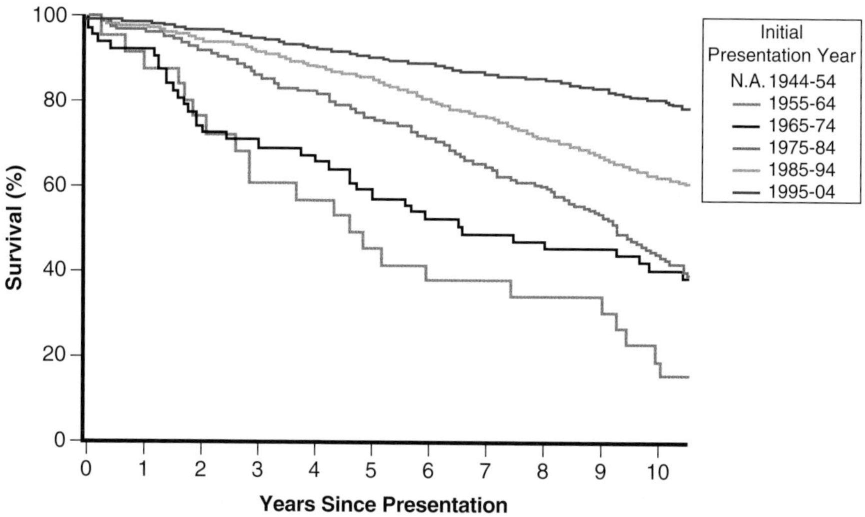

Fig. 5.3 Survival rates for patients with regional (SEER stage) prostate cancer (1944–2004) ($P < 0.0001$, log-rank test for trend). Because of the very small number of individuals with regional prostate cancer seen from 1944 to 1954, data from this period were excluded. N.A., not applicable.

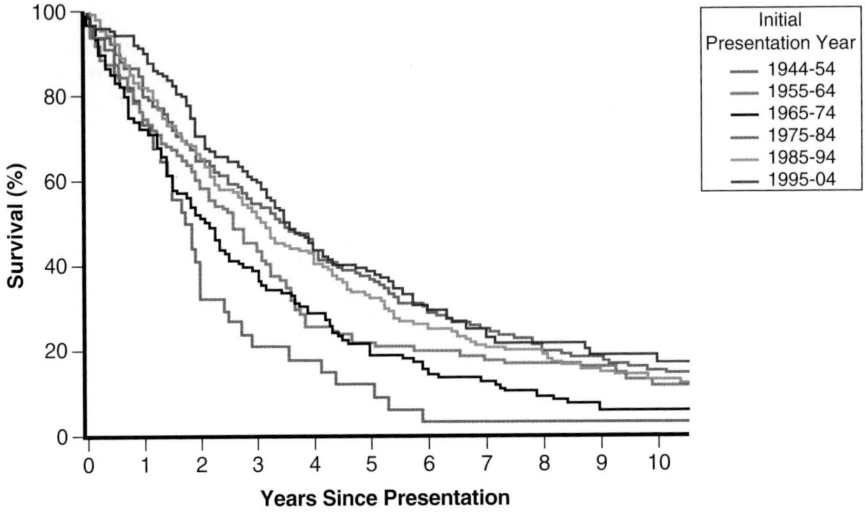

Fig. 5.4 Survival rates for patients with distant (SEER stage) prostate cancer (1944–2004) ($P<0.0001$, log-rank test for trend).

increased risk of disease spread beyond the prostate. Men with localized prostate cancer are offered treatment options on the basis of their overall health, prostate size, pubic bone geometry, and urinary function; these patients can often select from several suitable treatment choices, which include active surveillance, external beam radiotherapy, radical prostatectomy, brachytherapy, and cryotherapy.

Men with low-risk disease or those with a short life expectancy may forgo treatment and instead be monitored for progression of symptoms. For men with high-risk disease and for some men with intermediate-risk disease, androgen deprivation therapy is administered along with external beam radiotherapy. Men with nodal involvement are treated with androgen ablation, and locoregional radiation therapy is administered to some men. Men with metastatic disease are treated with systemic therapy. When appropriate, patients are offered enrollment in clinical trials.

To help patients assimilate all of the complex data associated with their disease process, treatment options, and quality-of-life effects, the Multidisciplinary Prostate Cancer Clinic was established at MD Anderson in 2004. In this setting, patients with localized prostate cancer are seen simultaneously by a urologist and radiation oncologist with a medical oncology consultation as appropriate. Patient visits are facilitated by an advanced practice nurse who helps patients navigate through the treatment selection process [14].

In the future, driven by new knowledge gained through the MD Anderson Cancer Center Prostate Cancer Specialized Program of Research Excellence (SPORE) Program, we anticipate that molecular classifications of prostate cancer will be used to define prognosis and guide management. This move toward personalized medicine should reduce the number of cases of overtreatment and undertreatment in men with prostate cancer.

Among those requiring treatment strategies to reduce the morbidity of local therapies, maintaining quality of life is paramount. Ongoing investigations at MD Anderson will help elucidate the appropriate length of androgen deprivation therapy, the optimal fractionation of radiotherapy, and the optimal time for administration of radiotherapy after prostatectomy. In addition, ongoing laboratory and clinical studies of cytotoxic, targeted, and immunotherapeutic agents will lead to the development of more effective systemic therapies for men with castrate-resistant prostate cancer, the type that presents the greatest threat to life.

Acknowledgements The authors would like to thank and acknowledge Dr. Vikas Kundra and Dr. David Swanson for their contributions regarding the history and advancement of the fields of radiology and urology, respectively.

References

1. Estimated New Cancer Cases and Deaths by Sex, US, 2009. Cancer Facts & Figures 2009. Vol. 2010: American Cancer Society.
2. Catalona WJ, Smith DS, Ratliff TL, Basler JW. Detection of organ-confined prostate cancer is increased through prostate-specific antigen-based screening. JAMA. 1993;270(8):948–54.
3. Darget R. The detection of lymph node invasions in tumors of the bladder and prostate [in French]. J Urol Nephrol (Paris). 1964;70:423–4.
4. Walsh PC, Donker PJ. Impotence following radical prostatectomy: insight into etiology and prevention. J Urol. 1982;128(3):492–7.
5. Pettaway CA, Pisters LL, Troncoso P, et al. Neoadjuvant chemotherapy and hormonal therapy followed by radical prostatectomy: feasibility and preliminary results. J Clin Oncol. 2000;18(5):1050–7.
6. Rosser CJ, Kamat AM, Pendleton J, et al. Impact of fellowship training on pathologic outcomes and complication rates of radical prostatectomy. Cancer. 2006;107(1):54–9.
7. Zelefsky MJ, Fuks Z, Hunt M, et al. High dose radiation delivered by intensity modulated conformal radiotherapy improves the outcome of localized prostate cancer. J Urol. 2001;166(3):876–81.
8. Kuban DA, Tucker SL, Dong L, et al. Long-term results of the MD Anderson randomized dose-escalation trial for prostate cancer. Int J Radiat Oncol Biol Phys. 2008;70(1):67–74.
9. D'Amico AV, Chen MH, Renshaw AA, Loffredo M, Kantoff PW. Androgen suppression and radiation vs radiation alone for prostate cancer: a randomized trial. JAMA. 2008;299(3):289–95.
10. Bolla M, Gonzalez D, Warde P, et al. Improved survival in patients with locally advanced prostate cancer treated with radiotherapy and goserelin. N Engl J Med. 1997;337(5):295–300.
11. Huggins C. Effect of orchiectomy and irradiation on cancer of the prostate. Ann Surg. 1942;115(6):1192–200.
12. Tannock IF, de Wit R, Berry WR, et al. Docetaxel plus prednisone or mitoxantrone plus prednisone for advanced prostate cancer. N Engl J Med. 2004;351(15):1502–12.
13. Sanda MG, Dunn RL, Michalski J, et al. Quality of life and satisfaction with outcome among prostate-cancer survivors. N Engl J Med. 2008;358(12):1250–61.
14. Madsen LT, Craig C, Kuban D. A multidisciplinary prostate cancer clinic for newly diagnosed patients: developing the role of the advanced practice nurse. Clin J Oncol Nurs. 2009;13(3):305–9.

Chapter 6
Non–Small Cell Lung Cancer

Ritsuko Komaki, Anne S. Tsao, and Reza J. Mehran

Introduction

In 2010, approximately 222,520 new cases of lung or bronchial cancer were expected to be diagnosed in the USA, and 157,300 patients are expected to die of this disease [1]. Lung cancer is the leading cause of cancer-related death in both men and women, and non–small cell lung cancer (NSCLC) accounts for about 80% of these cases. Lung cancer is most often asymptomatic in its early stages; consequently, the disease is usually diagnosed at an advanced stage, when it is much more difficult to treat. One or more genes are believed to be responsible for an inherited increase in risk of developing lung cancer in the general population. Smoking remains one of the main environmental factors associated with the development of lung cancer [2]. Although the development of lung cancer seems to be the result of several sequential molecular abnormalities in individuals at high risk of developing the disease, the genetic mechanisms by which an individual develops lung cancer remain largely unknown. These steps involve abnormalities in the expression of angiogenic factors (e.g., vascular endothelial growth factor, or VEGF and epithelial growth factor receptors, or EGFRs) [3]. The heterogeneity of lung cancer and the diversity of its

R. Komaki (✉)
Department of Radiation Oncology, The University of Texas MD Anderson Cancer Center, 1515 Holcombe Boulevard, Houston, TX 77030, USA
e-mail: rkomaki@mdanderson.org

A.S. Tsao
Department of Thoracic Head and Neck Oncology, The University of Texas MD Anderson Cancer Center, Houston, TX, USA

R.J. Mehran
Department of Thoracic and Cardiovascular Surgery, The University of Texas MD Anderson Cancer Center, Houston, TX, USA

M.A. Rodriguez et al. (eds.), *60 Years of Survival Outcomes at The University of Texas MD Anderson Cancer Center*, DOI 10.1007/978-1-4614-5197-6_6,

morphologic appearance and molecular properties make the application of molecular targeted therapies used in other cancers more complex, but such therapies are certainly a goal for the future.

The MD Anderson Cancer Center Experience

The MD Anderson data set is derived from 36,687 patients who presented to the institution on or before 31 December 2004. Of this group, 23,306 patients had had no prior treatment for their malignancy. After the exclusion of patients with multiple primary cancers and those treated elsewhere, 12,044 patients received definitive primary treatment for NSCLC at MD Anderson. The numbers of patients presenting by decade and disease stage at presentation are summarized in Table 6.1. Almost two-thirds of these patients had advanced locoregional or distant disease, consistent with the institution's focus on treating difficult cases.

Figure 6.1 illustrates overall survival curves for the 12,044 patients. Although the group was heterogeneous in terms of several risk factors for survival such as age, race, socioeconomic status, and stage and histology of the disease, survival rates increased nearly 20-fold in the past 50 years; however, these rates remain poor at about 20% at 5 years.

Figures 6.2, 6.3, and 6.4 show survival rates according to the disease stage at presentation. The most dramatic improvement over time has been in the management of resectable lung cancer. Patients with stage I disease can expect survival rates of 60% or more at 5 years; this rate, however, decreases to 25% for those with mediastinal nodal disease and remains poor for those with distant metastatic disease. Improvements seen in locoregional control of the disease are a reflection of MD Anderson's significant advances in surgery and radiation therapy, which we will discuss in the following sections. Although survival rates have improved over the past 60 years, survival with distant metastatic disease, which is treated mainly with systemic therapy, still lags behind, and more effective treatments for disease at this stage are desperately needed.

Table 6.1 Numbers and percentages of patients presenting to MD Anderson (1944–2004) by decade and disease stage

	SEER stage at presentation				
	Local	Regional	Distant	Unstaged	Total
Decade	[No. (%) of patients]				
1944–1954	5 (6.1)	19 (23.2)	47 (57.3)	11 (13.4)	82 (100.0)
1955–1964	101 (12.1)	161 (19.3)	514 (61.6)	59 (7.1)	835 (100.0)
1965–1974	303 (21.0)	228 (15.8)	823 (57.1)	87 (6.0)	1,441 (100.0)
1975–1984	469 (20.0)	661 (28.2)	1,149 (49.0)	64 (2.7)	2,343 (100.0)
1985–1994	423 (13.2)	1,000 (31.2)	1,611 (50.2)	174 (5.4)	3,208 (100.0)
1995–2004	625 (15.1)	1,154 (27.9)	2,189 (52.9)	167 (4.0)	4,135 (100.0)
Total	*1,926 (16.0)*	*3,223 (26.8)*	*6,333 (52.6)*	*562 (4.7)*	*12,044 (100.0)*

SEER Surveillance, Epidemiology, and End Results program

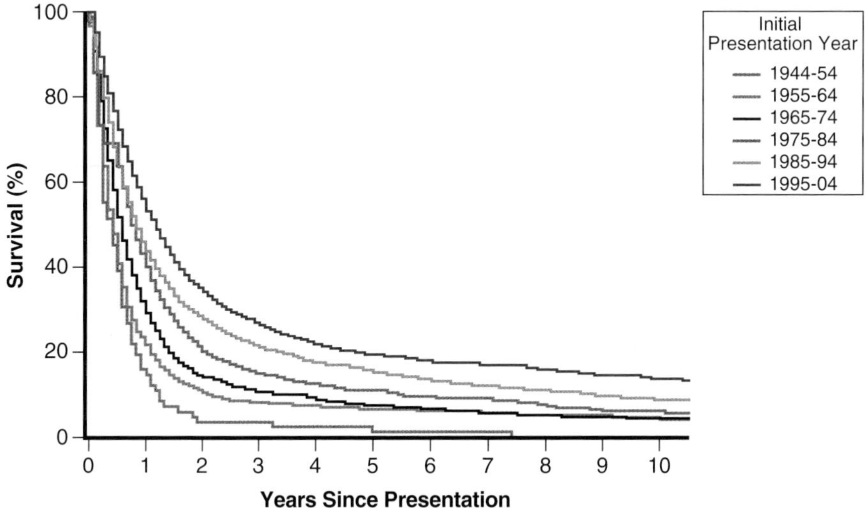

Fig. 6.1 Overall survival rates for 12,044 patients with non–small cell lung cancer at any stage presenting to MD Anderson Cancer Center (1944–2004) according to year of presentation ($P<0.0001$, log-rank test for trend).

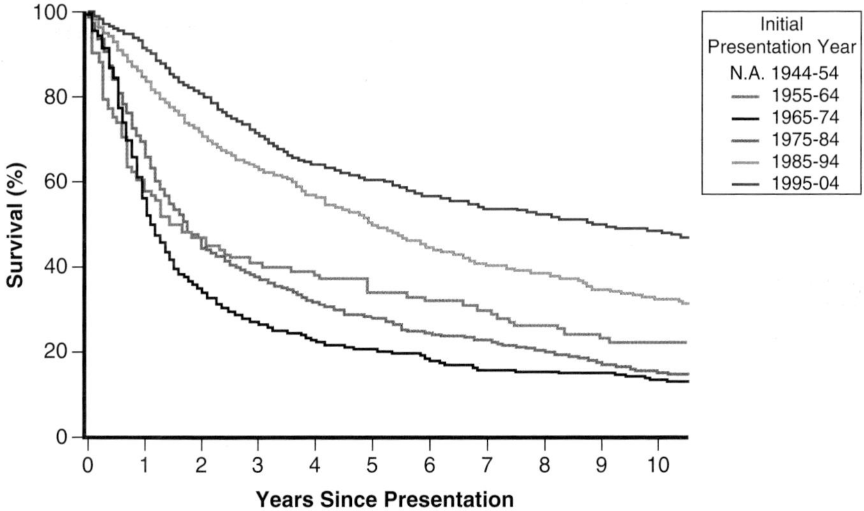

Fig. 6.2 Overall survival rates for 1,926 patients with local (SEER stage) non–small cell lung cancer (confined to primary site) presenting to MD Anderson Cancer Center (1944–2004) according to year of presentation ($P<0.0001$, log-rank test for trend). Because of the very small number of individuals with local non–small cell lung cancer seen from 1944 to 1954, data from this period were excluded. *N.A.* not applicable.

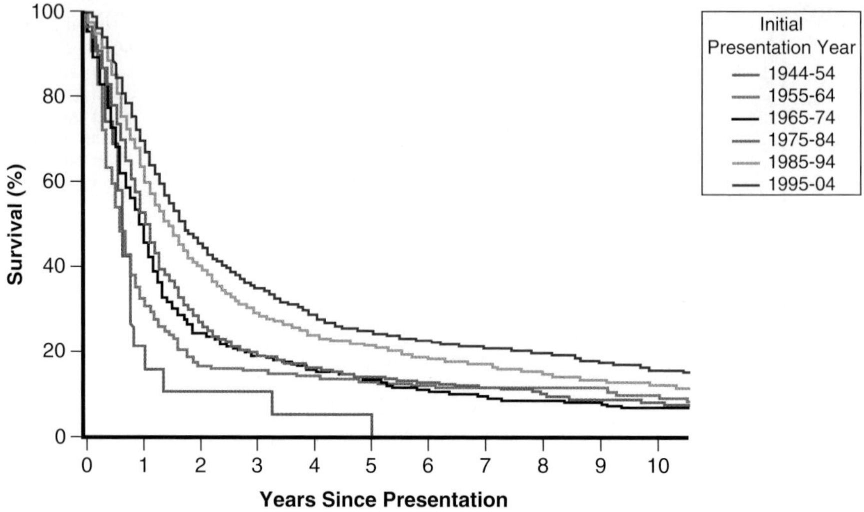

Fig. 6.3 Overall survival rates for 3,223 patients with regional (SEER stage) non–small cell lung cancer (spread to regional lymph nodes) presenting at MD Anderson Cancer Center (1944–2004) according to year of presentation ($P<0.0001$, log-rank test for trend).

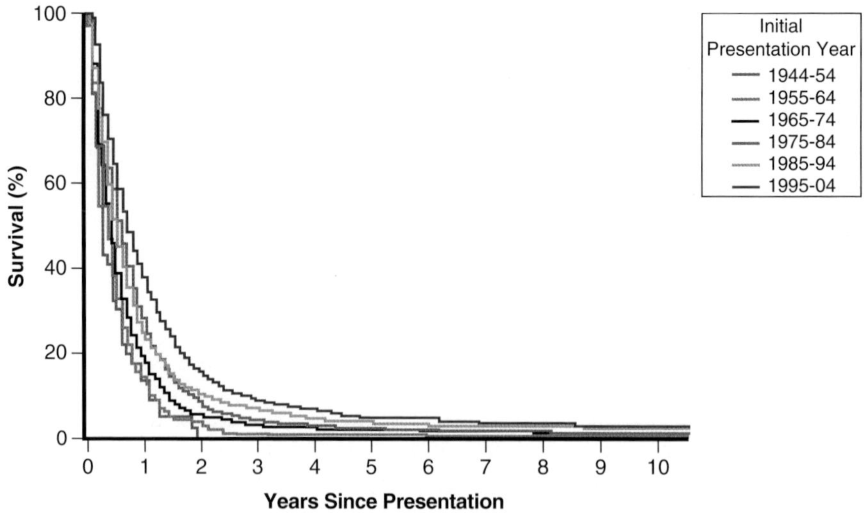

Fig. 6.4 Overall survival rates for 6,333 patients with distant (SEER stage) non–small cell lung cancer (metastasized to distant sites) presenting to MD Anderson Cancer Center (1944–2004) according to year of presentation ($P<0.0001$, log-rank test for trend).

Historical Perspective

Localized Disease

For patients with early-stage lung cancer who are able to undergo surgery, surgery has always offered the best hope of cure. Two great accomplishments during the past three decades—the extension of indications for surgery and improvements in postoperative care—have led to very low rates of morbidity and mortality even after extensive resections. Patients without evidence of mediastinal disease can sustain curative resection of disease extending into the spine, great vessels of the heart, and the carina. Patients with T3–T4 tumors with N0 or N1 disease do significantly better after radical resection than do patients with more extensive nodal disease [4].

Patients who cannot undergo surgery for NSCLC because of coexisting medical problems such as severe chronic obstructive pulmonary disease, cardiac disease, or severe diabetes can sometimes be cured by radiation therapy with or without chemotherapy.

Locally Advanced Disease

Survival rates after complete resection have been disappointing in patients with locally advanced disease. Five-year survival rates decrease from 67% for patients with T1N0 disease to 23% for patients with N2 disease [5]. Attempts to improve these rates have included many investigations of a variety of adjuvant therapies, including chemotherapy and thoracic irradiation. *Induction chemotherapy* has been extensively evaluated, and results from phase II and III trials have been promising [6]. *Adjuvant chemotherapy* with platin-based agents has been validated for patients younger than 75 years who have good performance status, no surgical complications, and stage II or higher disease [7]. *Chemotherapy in combination with radiation therapy* has been used with some success for locally advanced but unresectable lung cancer or in combination with surgery for more advanced (N2) disease [8]. The optimal timing of radiation therapy before or after surgery, however, remains to be determined.

The past several years have also seen substantial advancements in the techniques for delivering radiation therapy. *Three-dimensional conformal radiation therapy* has led to better local control and possibly to better survival rates than traditional two-dimensional radiation therapy has for patients with medically inoperable stage I NSCLC [9]. *Stereotactic body radiation therapy* [SBRT, also known as stereotactic ablative radiation therapy (SABR)] has been used successfully to treat early-stage lung cancer located far enough from the hilum or the mediastinum to allow the delivery of increased radiation doses [10]. The superior distribution of Bragg peaks characteristic of *proton beam therapy* has been shown in treatment-planning studies to reduce the radiation dose to normal tissues adjacent to the target relative to X-ray (photon) therapy. This advantage may make proton beam therapy a better choice for treating central pulmonary lesions close to the heart or the esophagus [11].

Longstanding obstacles to the successful treatment of lung cancer have included the inability of previous imaging modalities to accurately visualize direct tumor extension, regional nodal involvement, and the presence of distant metastasis. Even in patients with localized disease, the inability to control that disease leads to ongoing seeding of cancer cells to distant organs, eventually causing treatment failure and death from lung cancer. Control or eradication of locoregional disease with radiation therapy is difficult for three reasons: (a) geographic "misses" arising from the inadequacies of imaging for both disease staging and radiation therapy planning; (b) the need to account for tumor motion associated with respiration; and (c) the inability to deliver adequate (tumoricidal) radiation doses because of the risk of significant toxicity. However, recent developments in *image-guided radiation therapy* are showing promise for overcoming these difficulties. The use of integrated *positron emission tomography with computed tomography* (PET/CT) can improve targeting accuracy in 25–50% of cases, and *four-dimensional CT scanning* can help individualize radiation therapy based on tumor motion. *Intensity-modulated radiation therapy* (IMRT) and proton beam therapy may allow radiation doses to be escalated without increasing toxicity. SBRT can produce local control rates in excess of 90% by delivering focused, hypofractionated, high biological-equivalent doses of radiation. These approaches, until very recently, were considered experimental; however, they are fast becoming standard treatments for lung cancer at major cancer centers.

Current Management Approach

Imaging Studies to Define Disease Stage

The current management of NSCLC depends on the disease stage at presentation. Every effort must be made to accurately and thoroughly establish the disease stage by using high-quality imaging and invasive staging of the mediastinum with endobronchial ultrasonography, endoesophageal ultrasonography, or mediastinoscopy. PET results should be interpreted with caution, and biopsies of PET-positive lymph nodes should be obtained to rule out false-positive scans, which can occur in up to 20% of cases. Staging of disease outside the chest is reserved for patients who are symptomatic or at high risk of metastatic disease. Magnetic resonance imaging (MRI) of the brain, bone scanning, or PET should be used in those instances.

Multidisciplinary Planning

MD Anderson has championed the model of specialized multidisciplinary care in the management of cancer. Any patient with regional or distant disease must have the benefit of being reviewed by a multidisciplinary team consisting of a pathologist, radiologist, thoracic medical oncologist, radiation oncologist, and surgeon. The decision as to the type of treatment must be based on current practices, which change frequently as new science is introduced. The multidisciplinary approach is also a venue that allows patients to consider new experimental treatments. The treatment guidelines presently used at MD Anderson follow those of the National Comprehensive Cancer Network (NCCN) [12].

Systemic Chemotherapy

The management of NSCLC with systemic therapy depends on the disease stage and the presence of comorbid conditions. For patients with early-stage or locoregionally advanced disease for whom therapy is given with definitive (curative) intent, systemic chemotherapy is now used as a component of adjuvant, neoadjuvant, and concurrent treatment. For patients with metastatic disease for whom therapy is given with palliative intent, significant progress has been made from the addition of targeted agents to chemotherapy and personalized medicine. Advances have also been made in the development of maintenance therapy given after frontline chemotherapy.

Early-Stage or Locally Advanced Disease

Adjuvant Chemotherapy

For patients with surgically resectable disease and good performance status, the following treatment algorithm [13–15] is used with regard to adjuvant chemotherapy:

Stage IA: adjuvant chemotherapy not recommended
Stage IB tumor <3 cm: adjuvant chemotherapy not recommended
Stage IB tumor >3 cm: adjuvant chemotherapy can be considered
Stage II: adjuvant chemotherapy recommended
Stage III: adjuvant chemotherapy recommended

Adjuvant chemotherapy has proven survival benefits for patients with stage II or III disease [13, 14], but its usefulness in stage I disease remains controversial, with no survival benefit evident for stage IA but some evidence of benefit for stage IB when tumors are larger than 3 cm [14, 15]. The choice of chemotherapy is at the oncologist's discretion, but four cycles of a platin-based doublet therapy is usually recommended.

Neoadjuvant Chemotherapy

For patients with potentially resectable disease, neoadjuvant chemotherapy can be considered if it has a good chance of downstaging the disease to the point of allowing surgical resection [16]. The choice of chemotherapy is again at the oncologist's discretion but usually involves a platin-based doublet.

Concurrent Chemotherapy and Radiation

For patients with unresectable disease who are still considered candidates for definitive treatment, concurrent chemotherapy with radiation is the treatment of choice. Several regimens can be used, the choice of which depends on comorbid conditions, tumor histology, and tumor location. Some commonly used regimens are cisplatin with etoposide, weekly cisplatin with a taxane, and cisplatin with pemetrexed. Patients considered for concurrent chemotherapy with radiation may already have received neoadjuvant chemotherapy at systemic doses before the concurrent chemoradiation. On the basis of findings of a Hoosier Oncology Group study [17], consolidation chemotherapy after concurrent chemotherapy with radiation is no longer recommended for patients with stage III disease.

Late-Stage (Metastatic) Disease

The goal of systemic therapy for patients with metastatic disease is palliation, and for most patients the median survival time is 6–9 months. However, the discovery of two genetic alterations associated with lung cancer has changed the standard of care for metastatic disease. The first such alteration, the presence of particular mutations in EGFR [18], may confer sensitivity to EGFR tyrosine kinase inhibitors (TKIs) such as erlotinib and gefitinib, which can produce better response rates and progression-free survival than chemotherapy can [19]. Patients with these mutations should receive an EGFR TKI as early as possible during therapy. The second such alteration is the presence of the fusion protein EML4-ALK, which may confer sensitivity to the ALK inhibitor crizotinib [20]. Findings from the Iressa Pan-Asian Study (IPASS) trial [19] indicate that gefitinib as frontline therapy for patients with lung adenocarcinoma and a minimal smoking history produced better response and progression-free survival rates for patients with EGFR mutations, but carboplatin and paclitaxel were more effective for patients with wild-type (unmutated) EGFR. These findings have led to the recommendation that chemo-naïve patients be screened for the presence of EGFR mutations before beginning frontline therapy. Although intense searches for other biomarkers in NSCLC are under way, only EGFR mutations and EML4-ALK are predictive of clinical benefit at this time.

For patients who have neither EGFR mutations nor the EML4-ALK translocation, several options exist for frontline therapy [21]. However, the addition of targeted agents has improved survival outcomes. The only targeted monoclonal antibody currently approved by the U.S. Food and Drug Administration (FDA) for use as frontline therapy with chemotherapy is *bevacizumab*, a VEGF inhibitor. Bevacizumab is given during four to six cycles of chemotherapy and then continued as monotherapy maintenance until the development of intolerable adverse effects or progression of disease. Bevacizumab is contraindicated for patients with squamous cell lung carcinoma because of a high risk of fatal pulmonary hemoptysis [22]. For patients with nonsquamous cell carcinoma and no EGFR mutations, the NCCN guidelines recommend a platin-based doublet combined with bevacizumab as first-line therapy.

Maintenance Therapy: Switch Vs. Continuation

The NCCN guidelines now recognize two types of maintenance therapy for metastatic NSCLC—switch maintenance and continuation maintenance. In switch maintenance, a doublet or triplet chemotherapy regimen is given as frontline chemotherapy; those patients whose disease responds or stabilizes are then switched to a different class of drug after four cycles of therapy. In continuation maintenance, at least one of the agents used in the original frontline regimen is continued after the frontline therapy is completed; an example is giving bevacizumab with chemotherapy for four to six cycles and then continuing the bevacizumab as monotherapy maintenance.

In July 2009, the FDA approved maintenance therapy with pemetrexed after four cycles of a nonpemetrexed-containing platin-doublet regimen for nonsquamous NSCLC [23]. Currently, the decision as to whether to give maintenance therapy is at the discretion of the treating physician; such a decision should be made only after weighing the quality of life and personal needs of the patient.

Salvage Therapy

Three agents have been approved by the FDA as second-line salvage therapy for metastatic NSCLC: erlotinib and docetaxel for patients with NSCLC of any histology and pemetrexed for patients with nonsquamous cell disease. Erlotinib has also been approved as third-line therapy. Other agents commonly used for salvage therapy include vinorelbine and gemcitabine. We recommend that patients with recurrent metastatic disease consider enrolling in clinical trials of novel therapeutic agents.

Radiation/Proton Beam Therapy

Radiation therapy for NSCLC has advanced considerably with the development of image-guided techniques for that therapy, particularly PET/CT-based treatment planning, four-dimensional CT to account for tumor motion, and "on-board" imaging during the radiation therapy itself. Collectively, these advances are expected to improve the accuracy of tumor targeting and minimize treatment-related adverse effects. The combination of image-guided techniques with radiation dose escalation/acceleration has the potential to significantly improve clinical outcome for many patients with lung cancer. For example, image-guided SBRT has been shown to improve local control and survival in patients with early-stage NSCLC [24–27], and IMRT is better tolerated in terms of its toxicity profile [28, 29] than is three-dimensional conformal radiation therapy.

Early-Stage (I–II) Disease

Surgical resection (lobectomy with mediastinal lymph node dissection or sampling) is considered the standard of care for early-stage NSCLC, with 5-year overall survival rates of 65–70% for stage I (T1-2N0M0) disease and 35–50% for stage II (T1-2N1M0, T3N0M0) disease. Adjuvant platin-based chemotherapy can prolong overall survival in patients with stage II disease [13, 15, 30]. Adjuvant radiation therapy has been shown to suppress local recurrence but to date has not been shown to extend survival. Moreover, adjuvant radiation therapy is indicated only for patients with close or positive surgical margins or disease in several hilar lymph nodes (see the "Radiation After Surgery" section).

Definitive Radiation Therapy

Definitive radiation therapy, either with X-rays (photons) or with proton beams, is used for patients who refuse or are unable to undergo surgery because of coexisting medical conditions such as poor pulmonary function, recent myocardial infarction, or a tendency toward bleeding.

Locoregionally Advanced (Stages IIIA–IIIB) Disease

Concurrent chemotherapy with radiation therapy has become the standard of care for patients with good performance status and inoperable stage IIIA (T3N1M0, T1-3N2M0) or IIIB (TXN3M0, T4NXM0) NSCLC. Several trials of two-dimensional radiation therapy, including RTOG 94-10 [31–33], have shown that concurrent chemotherapy and radiation therapy provide better locoregional control and overall survival than does sequential treatment consisting of chemotherapy followed by radiation therapy. However, those advantages come at the cost of considerably higher toxicity, especially to the esophagus (rates of grade ≥3 esophageal toxicity exceed 50% for twice-daily radiation with concurrent chemotherapy, are 30% for once-daily radiation with concurrent chemotherapy, and are 10% for chemotherapy followed sequentially by radiation therapy). The use of three-dimensional conformal (as opposed to two-dimensional) radiation therapy has been associated with less toxicity and can allow the radiation dose to be escalated from 60 Gy (as in RTOG 94-10) to 74 Gy [34–36]. However, the experience from RTOG 0617, a randomized prospective phase III trial testing dose escalation in the context of concurrent radiation with chemotherapy [37], demonstrates that doses of 74 Gy should be attempted only with the use of image-guided adaptive radiation therapy with four-dimensional CT-based treatment simulation and planning and strict compliance with dose–volume constraints to avoid severe toxicity.

Another approach to allowing dose escalation while simultaneously avoiding toxicity is the addition of molecular targeted agents to concurrent radiation and chemotherapy. In the phase II trial RTOG 0324, the addition of cetuximab, a monoclonal antibody to EGFR and a radiosensitizer [38], to chemoradiation therapy improved median survival time and 2-year overall survival rates without increasing esophageal toxicity [39]. These promising results led to the inclusion of cetuximab in two arms of the RTOG 0617 study. Mature results from this study and others of molecular targeted agents in the treatment of lung cancer are eagerly awaited.

The use of IMRT may further reduce toxicity to the lung and esophagus by reducing the percentage of lung volume exposed to 20 Gy (V_{20}), the V_{10}, and the total mean lung dose (MLD) and by sparing more of the esophagus and heart [40, 41]. Regarding dose escalation, even though radiation doses of about 60 Gy have been considered standard for stage III NSCLC for decades, this dose has been associated with 40–50% locoregional failure rates. Several studies have shown potential benefits in local control and survival from the use of image-guided, three-dimensional conformal radiation therapy or IMRT to escalate radiation doses [34–36, 42].

Radiation with Chemotherapy

Theoretically, full-dose induction chemotherapy is believed to improve clinical outcome by eliminating or suppressing distant metastasis, whereas radiation therapy given concurrently with a radiosensitizing chemotherapeutic agent may further improve clinical outcome by enhancing locoregional control. The recently completed phase II randomized LAMP study [43] compared three treatment strategies: induction chemotherapy followed by radiation, concurrent chemotherapy with radiation followed by adjuvant chemotherapy, and induction chemotherapy followed by concurrent chemotherapy with radiation. Preliminary findings indicate that receipt of concurrent weekly paclitaxel, carboplatin, and thoracic radiation followed by consolidation chemotherapy was associated with the best outcome, although this schedule was associated with greater toxicity.

For patients who have already undergone induction chemotherapy, we usually use concurrent chemotherapy with radiation. If the patients cannot tolerate concurrent therapy, we give two or three cycles of induction chemotherapy followed by radiation therapy alone. If the patient cannot tolerate any chemotherapy, radiation therapy alone can be considered.

For patients with pathologically proven stage III N2 NSCLC, induction chemotherapy followed by surgery has resulted in better overall survival rates than has surgical resection alone [16, 44]. Induction chemoradiation followed by surgery has also yielded better disease-free survival rates than has definitive chemoradiation, although overall survival rates were no different between these two treatment groups [8]. Notably, that same study showed that patients who required pneumonectomy after induction chemoradiation had considerably higher mortality rates than did those who required lobectomy, suggesting that patients who require pneumonectomy should be treated with definitive chemoradiotherapy rather than surgery.

Radiation After Surgery

Postoperative radiation therapy is indicated for close or positive surgical margins or resected N2 (mediastinal) disease. If the resection margins are negative but the mediastinal nodes are positive, two to four cycles of adjuvant chemotherapy should be given, followed by radiation therapy. If the resection margins are positive, postoperative radiation should be given first, followed by chemotherapy.

The role of postoperative radiation therapy for resected N1 disease remains controversial. Because such patients may live for long periods after surgery, the chronic toxicity associated with postoperative radiation should be considered. For patients with positive or close surgical margins but no N1 or N2 involvement, the target volume should be limited to the site of the positive margin and the dose should be 60–66 Gy. Patients with gross positive margins (subtotal resection) should receive definitive chemoradiation. For patients with surgically resected N2 disease, the target volume should be limited to the positive lymph node station, plus or minus the ipsilateral hilar and subcarinal lymph nodes depending on the location of the primary tumor and whether a full lymph node dissection was done. The radiation dose should be limited to about 50 Gy, delivered in standard fractions.

The indications for postoperative therapy are the same for patients treated with induction chemotherapy followed by surgery. Postoperative radiation therapy can improve local control and may extend disease-free survival [45] and overall survival [46] for patients with pathologic N2 disease. Adjuvant chemotherapy can improve survival duration in patients with stage IB-III NSCLC and should be considered standard therapy [13, 15, 30].

Intensity-Modulated Radiation Therapy

IMRT for lung cancer has yet to be widely adopted outside the academic medical community for several reasons, including its technologic complexity, concerns that this technique may result in exposure of large volumes of normal lung tissue to low yet damaging radiation doses relative to radiation delivered by other means, and the need to account for respiration-related tumor movement in both treatment planning and delivery. Our own work has shown that IMRT can provide higher target doses with better conformity and greater normal tissue sparing than three-dimensional conformal radiation therapy can for patients with early-stage or locally advanced NSCLC [37, 38].

IMRT for lung cancer has the potential to reduce toxicity in normal tissues and to allow escalation of the radiation dose to high-risk regions [42]. Our recommendations for using IMRT for lung cancer are as follows.

Patient Selection

IMRT is probably the most beneficial for cases involving tumors in the superior sulcus or close to the esophagus, heart, or spinal cord or cases involving positive lymph nodes. Small, early-stage, mobile tumors may not be good candidates for IMRT unless motion-mitigation techniques are used (see below). The highly conformal dose distribution and high-dose gradients associated with IMRT also mandate reliable means of patient immobilization.

Tumor Motion Considerations

Organ motion during treatment must be considered and addressed individually. We recommend that four-dimensional CT be used for treatment planning; at a minimum, tumor motion should be assessed fluoroscopically. If the tumor moves <10 mm during respiration, the patient can be treated with free-breathing IMRT by using the internal target volume (ITV) approach with an adequate margin. However, if considerable tumor motion is anticipated, the patient should be treated with breath-hold, respiratory-gated therapy, or other means of tumor tracking if such techniques can be used to "freeze" the tumor at reproducible positions.

Tissue Heterogeneity Considerations

Because tissue heterogeneity affects some beamlets more than others, resulting in substantial differences in dose distribution, heterogeneity should be corrected for all IMRT lung cancer treatment plans.

Treatment Plan Evaluation and Quality Assurance

IMRT can cause "cold spots" or "hot spots" in unexpected locations that may not be reflected in dose–volume distribution estimates. Therefore, the isodose distribution should be inspected on every image slice. To reduce the potential for delivering low-dose (<10 Gy) radiation to normal lung issue, we recommend that fewer beams (i.e., 5–7) be used to reduce the beam-delivery time and improve patient comfort. Both IMRT planning and delivery should be done by experienced personnel, meaning that physicians must be aware of the need to balance dose inhomogeneity and lung tissue sparing. Strict quality assurance is also required for both mechanical and dosimetric accuracy. One of the disadvantages of IMRT is the large volumes of tissue exposed to low-dose radiation (e.g., 5 Gy) relative to proton beam therapy. This large volume of lower dose could be harmful to radiosensitive normal tissues such as the alveoli or esophagus or to rapidly dividing normal cells, especially in children.

Proton Beam Therapy

Proton beams, unlike photon or X-ray beams, consist of charged particles that have a well-defined range of penetration into tissue. Tissues that are past this range are not irradiated. Thus, proton beam therapy is ideal for situations in which normal tissue sparing is a priority, as is true for lung cancer given the proximity of critical thoracic structures such as the esophagus, heart, and spinal cord.

Recently published results of prospective phase II studies of proton therapy indicate that this technique has promise in the treatment of NSCLC. One such study, involving patients with early-stage yet inoperable disease, indicated that proton beam therapy to a dose of 74 Gy(RBE) at 2 Gy(RBE)/fraction given concurrently with weekly carboplatin–paclitaxel chemotherapy followed by full-dose adjuvant chemotherapy led to encouraging overall survival and progression-free survival rates and relatively mild toxicity relative to those experienced after photon-based treatment with this type of chemotherapy [47]. That study and another [48] suggested that adaptive replanning (that is, repeated imaging during the course of the radiation therapy, with corresponding adjustments to the radiation treatment plan) can further reduce normal tissue doses and prevent target misses, particularly for patients with large tumors that shrink substantially during therapy.

Other evidence that proton beam therapy may be less toxic to normal tissues than photon-based therapies comes from a comparison of severe pneumonitis, esophagitis, and bone marrow toxicity rates among patients with locally advanced NSCLC treated by proton beam therapy with those among patients treated previously with three-dimensional conformal radiation therapy or IMRT, all with concurrent chemotherapy. The results suggested that proton beam therapy with concurrent chemotherapy led to less bone marrow toxicity, less treatment-related pneumonitis, and less esophageal toxicity than did three-dimensional conformal radiation or IMRT with concurrent chemotherapy [49]. Whether this lesser toxicity would allow further radiation dose escalation or use of more aggressive systemic regimens with proton beam therapy needs to be tested prospectively in a randomized trial. One such trial currently under way is comparing proton beam therapy with IMRT, both with concurrent carboplatin-and-paclitaxel chemotherapy, for locally advanced lung cancer. This trial, funded by the U.S. National Cancer Institute and conducted jointly by MD Anderson Cancer Center and Massachusetts General Hospital, is the first direct comparison of these two techniques in terms of local tumor control and the incidence of severe pneumonitis.

Normal Tissue Toxicity

As noted previously, normal tissue toxicity becomes increasingly important when chemotherapy is given with radiation. Rates of pneumonitis, a potentially lethal late side effect of radiation, have been declining with the use of increasingly more conformal radiation techniques, being highest after two-dimensional radiation therapy and becoming progressively lower after three-dimensional conformal radiation therapy, IMRT, and proton beam therapy [42]. Another approach to minimizing the incidence of severe pneumonitis is by finding ways to identify patients at relatively higher or lower risk of this side effect and tailoring the radiation fields and delivery accordingly. This susceptibility may have a genetic component, as revealed in epidemiologic studies of associations between single nucleotide polymorphisms (SNPs) in certain genes and the incidence of radiation-induced pneumonitis [50–54].

The Future

Much of the improvement in outcomes achieved for patients with NSCLC during the past two decades has resulted from tobacco cessation and early detection through the use of low-dose spiral CT for individuals considered at high risk of developing lung cancer [55]. The importance of eliminating smoking cannot be overemphasized, particularly for young people. As for early detection, if NSCLC is detected early enough, it can be cured by surgery or, if patients are unable or unwilling to undergo surgery, by SBRT. Outcomes for patients with locally advanced or metastatic NSCLC can be improved only through a better understanding of the biological basis of the disease. Such an understanding should lead to the development of "smarter" (more individualized) therapy and more effective chemotherapeutic or molecular targeted agents for use alone or in combination with local treatments such as surgery, SBRT, IMRT, or proton beam therapy. The search for molecular abnormalities in tumors and for agents that target those abnormalities ultimately requires the development of validated predictive biomarkers from prospectively collected tissue samples. A novel strategy for systematically addressing this need, and a major focus of the MD Anderson lung cancer group, is the BATTLE (Biomarker-integrated Approaches of Targeted Therapy for Lung Cancer Elimination) program. This multidisciplinary effort, sponsored by the U.S. Department of Defense, comprises four separate clinical trials, the goal of which is to identify those patients who are most likely to benefit from promising targeted investigational agents. As for other approaches, local therapies involving surgery will become even less invasive, allowing increasing numbers of patients to benefit from surgery, particularly those with borderline pulmonary reserve. Several techniques for planning and delivering radiation therapy that are being investigated for future use include means of explicitly incorporating motion and setup uncertainty into the calculation of radiation doses and means of tracking the motion of a moving target during the delivery of radiation. Future developments in proton beam therapy such as discrete spot scanning and intensity-modulated proton therapy must await resolution of tumor motion issues when these advanced techniques are to be used. Radiation therapy may become, in the near future, as effective as surgical options for many patients. The recent ASCO/NCCN guidelines for screening high-risk patients with chest CT for early detection of NSCLC will hopefully also lead to earlier disease stages at diagnosis, hence higher probability of cure.

Acknowledgments We thank the Thoracic Radiation Oncologists, Thoracic & Head/Neck Medical Oncologists, Thoracic Cardiovascular Surgeons, Pulmonary Medicine Specialists, Thoracic Pathologists and Medical Physicists involved in the care of patients with lung cancer at MD Anderson Cancer Center. We also thank Christine F. Wogan for her efforts in developing this report.

References

1. Jemal A, Siegel R, Xu J, Ward E. Cancer statistics 2010. CA Cancer J Clin. 2010;60:277–300.
2. Kamholz SL. Pulmonary and cardiovascular consequences of smoking. Med Clin North Am. 2004;88:1415–30.
3. Wistuba II, Behrens C, Milchgrub S, et al. Sequential molecular abnormalities are involved in the multistage development of squamous cell carcinoma. Oncogene. 1999;18:643–50.
4. Van Schil PE. Surgery: therapeutic indications. Cancer Radiother. 2007;11(1–2):47–52.
5. Mountain CF. Revisions in the international system for staging lung cancer. Chest. 1997;111:1710–7.
6. Burdett S, Stewart L, Rydzewska L. A systematic review and meta-analysis of the literature: chemotherapy and surgery vs surgery alone in non small cell lung cancer. J Thorac Oncol. 2006;1:611–21.
7. Pignon JP, Tribodet H, Scagliotti GV, et al. Lung adjuvant cisplatin evaluation (LACE): a pooled analysis of five randomized clinical trials including 4,584 patients. J Clin Oncol. 2006;24 Suppl 18:7008.
8. Albain K, Swann R, Rusch V, et al. Radiotherapy plus chemotherapy with or without surgical resection for stage III non-small-cell lung cancer: a phase III randomised controlled trial. Lancet. 2009;374:379–86.
9. Fang C, Komaki R, Allen P, et al. Comparison of outcomes for patients with medically inoperable stage I non-small-cell lung cancer treated with two-dimensional vs. three-dimensional radiotherapy. Int J Radiat Oncol Biol Phys. 2006;66(1):108–16.
10. Grills IS, Mangona VS, Welsh R, et al. Outcomes after stereotactic lung radiotherapy or wedge resection for stage I non-small-cell lung cancer. J Clin Oncol. 2010;28(6):928–35.
11. Zhang X, Li Y, Pan X, et al. Intensity-modulated proton therapy reduces the dose to normal tissue compared with intensity-modulated radiation therapy or passive scattering proton therapy and enables individualized radical radiotherapy for extensive stage IIIB non-small-cell lung cancer: a virtual clinical study. Int J Radiat Oncol Biol Phys. 2010;77(2):357–66.
12. National Comprehensive Care Network. Non-small cell lung cancer. NCCN Practice Guidelines in Oncology v2; 2010. http://www.nccn.org/professionals/physician_gls/PDF/nscl.pdf.
13. Arriagada R, Bergman B, Dunant A, et al. Cisplatin-based adjuvant chemotherapy in patients with completely resected non-small-cell lung cancer. N Engl J Med. 2004;350(4):351–60.
14. Winton T, Livingston R, Johnson D, et al. Vinorelbine plus cisplatin vs. observation in resected non-small-cell lung cancer. N Engl J Med. 2005;352(25):2589–97.
15. Strauss GM, Herndon 2nd JE, Maddaus MA, et al. Adjuvant paclitaxel plus carboplatin compared with observation in stage IB non-small-cell lung cancer: CALGB 9633 with the Cancer and Leukemia Group B, Radiation Therapy Oncology Group, and North Central Cancer Treatment Group Study Groups. J Clin Oncol. 2008;26(31):5043–51.
16. Roth J, Fossella F, Komaki R, et al. A randomized trial comparing perioperative chemotherapy and surgery with surgery alone in resectable stage IIIA non-small-cell lung cancer. J Natl Cancer Inst. 1994;86:673–80.
17. Hanna N, Neubauer M, Yiannoutsos C, et al. Phase III study of cisplatin, etoposide, and concurrent chest radiation with or without consolidation docetaxel in patients with inoperable stage III non-small-cell lung cancer: the Hoosier Oncology Group and U.S. Oncology. J Clin Oncol. 2008;26(35):5755–60.
18. Lynch TJ, Bell DW, Sordella R, et al. Activating mutations in the epidermal growth factor receptor underlying responsiveness of non-small-cell lung cancer to gefitinib. N Engl J Med. 2004;350:2129–39.
19. Mok TS, Wu Y-L, Thongprasert S, et al. Gefitinib or carboplatin-paclitaxel in pulmonary adenocarcinoma. N Engl J Med. 2009;361:947–57.
20. Koivunen JP, Mermel C, Zejnullahu K, et al. EML4-ALK fusion gene and efficacy of an ALK kinase inhibitor in lung cancer. Clin Cancer Res. 2008;14(13):4275–83.

21. Schiller JH, Harrington D, Belani CP, et al. Comparison of four chemotherapy regimens for advanced non-small-cell lung cancer. N Engl J Med. 2002;346:92–8.
22. Johnson DH, Fehrenbacher L, Novotny WF, et al. Randomized phase II trial comparing bevacizumab plus carboplatin and paclitaxel with carboplatin and paclitaxel alone in previously untreated locally advanced or metastatic non-small-cell lung cancer. J Clin Oncol. 2004;22:2184–91.
23. Ciuleanu T, Brodowicz T, Zielinski C, et al. Maintenance pemetrexed plus best supportive care versus placebo plus best supportive care for non-small-cell lung cancer: a randomised, double-blind, phase 3 study. Lancet. 2009;374:1432–40.
24. Xia T, Li H, Sun Q, et al. Promising clinical outcome of stereotactic body radiation therapy for patients with inoperable stage I/II non-small-cell lung cancer. Int J Radiat Oncol Biol Phys. 2006;66:117–25.
25. Onishi H, Araki T, Shirato H, et al. Stereotactic hypofractionated high-dose irradiation for stage I non-small cell lung carcinoma clinical outcome in 245 subjects in a Japanese multi-institutional study. Cancer. 2004;101(7):1623–31.
26. Nagata Y, Takayama K, Matsuo Y, et al. Clinical outcomes of a phase I/II study of 48 Gy of stereotactic body radiotherapy in 4 fractions for primary lung cancer using a stereotactic body frame. Int J Radiat Oncol Biol Phys. 2005;63(5):1427–31.
27. Chang JY, Balter PA, Dong L, et al. Stereotactic body radiation therapy in centrally and superiorly located stage I or isolated recurrent non-small-cell lung cancer. Int J Radiat Oncol Biol Phys. 2008;72(4):967–71.
28. Yom SS, Liao Z, Liu HH, et al. Initial evaluation of treatment-related pneumonitis in advanced-stage non-small-cell lung cancer patients treated with concurrent chemotherapy and intensity-modulated radiotherapy. Int J Radiat Oncol Biol Phys. 2007;68(1):94–102.
29. Chang J, Liu H, Komaki R. Intensity modulated radiation therapy and proton radiotherapy for non-small-cell lung cancer. Curr Oncol Rep. 2005;7:255–9.
30. Douillard JY, Rosell R, De Lena M, et al. Adjuvant vinorelbine plus cisplatin versus observation in patients with completely resected stage IB-IIIA non-small-cell lung cancer (Adjuvant Navelbine International Trialist Association [ANITA]): a randomised controlled trial. Lancet Oncol. 2006;7(9):719–27.
31. Curran Jr WJ, Paulus R, Langer CJ, et al. Sequenial vs. concurrent chemoradiation for stage III non-small cell lung cancer: randomized phase III trial RTOG 9410. J Natl Cancer Inst. 2011;103(19):1452–60.
32. Furuse K, Fukuoka M, Kawahara M, et al. Phase III study of concurrent versus sequential thoracic radiotherapy in combination with mitomycin, vindesine, and cisplatin in unresectable stage III non-small-cell lung cancer. J Clin Oncol. 1999;17(9):2692–9.
33. Fournel P, Robinet G, Thomas P, et al. Randomized phase III trial of sequential chemoradiotherapy compared with concurrent chemoradiotherapy in locally advanced non-small-cell lung cancer: Groupe Lyon-Saint-Etienne d'Oncologie Thoracique-Groupe Francais de Pneumo-Cancerologie NPC 95–01 Study. J Clin Oncol. 2005;23(25):5910–7.
34. Socinski M, Rosenman J, Halle J, et al. Dose-escalating conformal thoracic radiation therapy with induction and concurrent carboplatin/paclitaxel in unresectable stage IIIA/B non-small-cell lung carcinoma. Cancer. 2001;92(5):1213–23.
35. Schild S, McGinnis W, Graham D, et al. Results of a phase I trial of concurrent chemotherapy and escalating doses of radiation for unresectable non-small-cell lung cancer. Int J Radiat Oncol Biol Phys. 2006;65(4):1106–11.
36. Bradley JD, Moughan J, Graham MV, et al. A phase I/II radiation dose escalation study with concurrent chemotherapy for patients with inoperable stages I to III non-small-cell lung cancer: phase I results of RTOG 0117. Int J Radiat Oncol Biol Phys. 2010;77(2):367–72.
37. Bradley J, Paulus R, Komaki R, et al. A randomized phase III comparison of standard-dose (60 Gy) versus high-dose (74 Gy) conformal chemoradiotherapy +/− cetuximab for stage IIIa/IIIb non-small cell lung cancer: preliminary findings on radiation dose in RTOG 0617 (late-breaking abstract 2). Presented at the 53rd Annual Meeting of the American Society of Radiation Oncology, 2–6 October 2011, Miami.

38. Milas L, Mason K, Hunter N, et al. In vivo enhancement of tumor radioresponse by C225 antiepidermal growth factor receptor antibody. Clin Cancer Res. 2000;6:701–8.
39. Blumenschein GR, Paulus R, Curran WJ, et al. Phase II study of cetuximab in combination with chemoradiation in patients with stage IIIA/B non-small-cell lung cancer: RTOG: 0324. J Clin Oncol. 2011;29(17):2312–8.
40. Murshed H, Liu H, Liao Z, et al. Dose and volume reduction for normal lung using intensity-modulated radiotherapy for advanced-stage non-small-cell lung cancer. Int J Radiat Oncol Biol Phys. 2004;58(4):1258–67.
41. Liu H, Wang X, Dong L, et al. Feasibility of sparing lung and other thoracic structures with intensity-modulated radiotherapy for non-small-cell lung cancer. Int J Radiat Oncol Biol Phys. 2004;58(4):1268–79.
42. Liao ZX, Komaki RR, Thames HD, et al. Influence of technologic advances on outcomes in patients with unresectable, locally advanced non-small-cell lung cancer receiving concomitant chemoradiotherapy. Int J Radiat Oncol Biol Phys. 2010;76(3):775–81.
43. Belani C, Choy H, Bonomi P, et al. Combined chemoradiotherapy regimens of paclitaxel and carboplatin for locally advanced non-small-cell lung cancer: a randomized phase II locally advanced multi-modality protocol. J Clin Oncol. 2005;23(25):5883–91.
44. Rosell R, Gomez-Codina J, Camps C, et al. A randomized trial comparing preoperative chemotherapy plus surgery with surgery alone in patients with non-small-cell lung cancer. N Engl J Med. 1994;330(3):153–8.
45. Lung Cancer Study Group. Effects of postoperative mediastinal radiation on completely resected stage II and stage III epidermoid cancer of the lung. N Engl J Med. 1986;315: 1377–81.
46. Douillard JY, Rosell R, De Lena M, et al. Impact of postoperative radiation therapy on survival in patients with complete resection and stage I, II, or IIIA non-small-cell lung cancer treated with adjuvant chemotherapy: the Adjuvant Navelbine International Trialist Association (ANITA) Randomized Trial. Int J Radiat Oncol Biol Phys. 2008;72(3):695–701.
47. Chang JY, Komaki R, Wen HY, et al. Toxicity and patterns of failure of adaptive/ablative proton therapy for early-stage, medically inoperable non-small cell lung cancer. Int J Radiat Oncol Biol Phys. 2011;80(5):1350–7.
48. Koay EJ, Lege D, Mohan R, et al. Adaptive/nonadaptive proton radiation planning and outcomes in a phase II trial for locally advanced non-small cell lung cancer. Int J Radiat Oncol Biol Phys. 2012 Apr 27 [Epub ahead of print].
49. Sejpal S, Komaki R, Tsao A, et al. Early findings on the toxicity of proton beam therapy with concurent chemotherapy for nonsmall cell lung cancer. Cancer. 2011;117(13):3004–13.
50. Yuan X, Liao Z, Liu Z, et al. Single nucleotide polymorphism at rs1982073:T869C of the TGFbeta 1 gene is associated with the risk of radiation pneumonitis in patients with non-small-cell lung cancer treated with definitive radiotherapy. J Clin Oncol. 2009;27(20):3370–8.
51. Yin M, Liao Z, Liu Z, et al. Genetic variants of the nonhomologous end joining gene LIG4 and severe radiation pneumonitis in nonsmall cell lung cancer patients treated with definitive radiotherapy. Cancer. 2012;118(2):528–35.
52. Yin M, Liao Z, Huang YJ, et al. Polymorphisms of homologous recombination genes and clinical outcomes of non-small cell lung cancer patients treated with definitive radiotherapy. PLoS One. 2011;6(5):e20055.
53. Yin M, Liao Z, Liu Z, et al. Functional polymorphisms of base excision repair genes XRCC1 and APEX1 predict risk of radiation pneumonitis in patients with non-small cell lung cancer treated with definitive radiation therapy. Int J Radiat Oncol Biol Phys. 2011;81(3):e67–73.
54. Hildebrandt MA, Komaki R, Liao Z, et al. Genetic variants in inflammation-related genes are associated with radiation-induced toxicity following treatment for non-small cell lung cancer. PLoS One. 2010;5(8):e12402.
55. National Lung Screening Trial Research Team. Reduced lung-cancer mortality with low-dose computed tomographic screening. N Engl J Med. 2011;365(5):395–409.

Chapter 7
Small Cell Lung Cancer

Frank V. Fossella

Introduction

Small cell lung cancer (SCLC) accounts for about 13% of all lung cancer cases, with about 29,000 new cases diagnosed annually in the USA [1]. The incidence of SCLC is declining, due in part to decreased smoking rates, increased use of filtered cigarettes, and changes in pathologic criteria for classifying SCLC [2].

SCLC occurs almost exclusively in smokers. In contrast to non–small cell lung cancer, SCLC generally has a more rapid doubling time, a higher growth fraction, and a greater propensity for early nodal and distant metastases. Although this neoplasm is very sensitive to first-line chemotherapy and radiotherapy (XRT), most patients experience relapse after initial treatment and ultimately die of their recurrent disease.

Staging of SCLC

Except in rare cases of very early stage SCLC with a very small primary lesion and no nodal disease, the TNM staging system is not used in staging this cancer. Instead, this disease is staged as either "limited" or "extensive." *Limited-stage disease* is confined to one hemithorax and can be encompassed within a tolerable radiation port; this includes patients with mediastinal and ipsilateral supraclavicular involvement but excludes patients with pleural/pericardial effusion, contralateral hilar adenopathy, and contralateral supraclavicular adenopathy. *Extensive-stage disease*

F.V. Fossella (✉)
Department of Thoracic/Head and Neck Medical Oncology, The University of Texas MD Anderson Cancer Center, 1515 Holcombe Boulevard, Unit 432, Houston, TX 77030, USA
e-mail: ffossell@mdanderson.org

M.A. Rodriguez et al. (eds.), *60 Years of Survival Outcomes at The University of Texas MD Anderson Cancer Center*, DOI 10.1007/978-1-4614-5197-6_7,

Table 7.1 Small cell lung cancer population at MD Anderson Cancer Center[a]

Population group	No. of patients
Patients with small cell lung cancer initially presenting to MD Anderson Cancer Center on or before 12/31/2004	5,286
No previous treatment	3,408
Definitive MD Anderson treatment	2,536
No other primaries except superficial skin cancers	2,164

[a]Survival calculated from initial presentation to MD Anderson

Table 7.2 Numbers and percentages of patients presenting to MD Anderson (1944–2004) by decade and disease stage

	SEER stage at presentation			
	Limited	Extensive	Unstaged	Total
Decade	[No. (%) of patients]			
1944–1954	1 (100.0)	0 (0)	0 (0)	1 (100.0)
1955–1964	11 (20.4)	42 (77.8)	1 (1.9)	54 (100.0)
1965–1974	84 (23.0)	267 (73.2)	14 (3.8)	365 (100.0)
1975–1984	220 (35.0)	397 (63.1)	12 (1.9)	629 (100.0)
1985–1994	198 (31.9)	378 (61.0)	44 (7.1)	620 (100.0)
1995–2004	133 (26.9)	318 (64.2)	44 (8.9)	495 (100.0)
Total	*647 (29.9)*	*1,402 (64.8)*	*115 (5.3)*	*2,164 (100.0)*

SEER Surveillance, Epidemiology, and End Results program

extends beyond the ipsilateral hemithorax and includes patients with malignant pleural or pericardial effusions [3].

About 30–40% of patients with SCLC present with limited-stage disease. These patients receive multimodality treatment, with curative intent. The remaining 60–70% of SCLC patients have extensive-stage disease at diagnosis. They receive chemotherapy and/or XRT alone, with a goal of symptom palliation and/or prolongation of survival.

Tables 7.1 and 7.2 show the incidence and staging of SCLC at MD Anderson Cancer Center between 1944 and 2004.

Clinical Presentation of SCLC

SCLC usually arises in the proximal airways and spreads submucosally, resulting in airway obstruction. Early nodal spread is common, and the presenting X-rays often show the proximal primary tumor with associated bulky hilar and mediastinal adenopathy. Typical presenting symptoms include dyspnea and/or cough. Due to the submucosal growth pattern of this tumor, hemoptysis is less likely than with other types of lung cancer. Due to the large size of the primary tumor and regional nodes, patients with right-sided tumors may present with superior vena cava obstruction. The 60–70% of patients with distant metastases at diagnosis may present with symptoms referable to their sites of metastases, including pain from skeletal metastasis, headache or neurologic symptoms from brain metastasis, and/or anorexia, weight loss, or jaundice from hepatic metastasis.

Some patients with SCLC present with paraneoplastic syndromes. The paraneoplastic syndromes associated with SCLC are either endocrine syndromes (mediated by peptides produced by the tumor) or neurologic syndromes (autoimmune-related). Although the endocrine syndromes usually improve with effective treatment of the underlying cancer, the neurologic syndromes may persist despite effective anticancer treatment.

The most common endocrine syndrome—syndrome of inappropriate antidiuretic hormone (SIADH)—occurs in 10–15% of SCLC patients. It is due to ectopic ADH production by tumor cells and results in hyponatremia [4]. Cushing syndrome, which occurs in 3–7% of patients, is due to ectopic adrenocorticotropic hormone and results in hypokalemic alkalosis and hyperglycemia [5]. Patients with Cushing syndrome due to SCLC tend to have a worse prognosis, in part due to increased incidence of opportunistic infections [6].

A neurologic paraneoplastic syndrome associated with SCLC includes Eaton–Lambert myasthenic syndrome, which occurs in 3% of patients. It is caused by calcium channel autoantibodies and results in proximal muscle weakness. Unlike some of the other neurologic syndromes, Eaton–Lambert syndrome often improves with anticancer therapy. Other neurologic paraneoplastic syndromes associated with SCLC include cerebellar degeneration, encephalomyelitis, limbic encephalitis, autonomic or sensory neuropathy, retinopathy, and myotonia/Isaacs syndrome. These are mediated by a variety of autoantibodies, including anti-Hu, anti-CV2/CRMP5, and anti-Zic4. Although some of these neurologic syndromes may improve or stabilize with anticancer treatment, others may not improve despite adequate treatment of the underlying cancer [7].

Natural History and Prognosis of SCLC

SCLC has a very aggressive clinical course: the median survival duration for untreated patients is only 2–4 months [8]. Fortunately, SCLC is very responsive to chemotherapy, with response rates to first-line combination chemotherapy ranging from 60% to 80%. The median survival duration with chemotherapy is 18–30 months for limited-stage disease and 8–12 months for extensive-stage SCLC [7]. However, despite the excellent responses seen with first-line therapy, most patients will experience relapse and ultimately die of their disease within 2 years. The cure rate for SCLC is 10–15% for patients with limited-stage disease and only 1–2% for those with extensive-stage disease. Adverse prognostic factors for SCLC include poor performance status, extensive stage, and elevated lactic dehydrogenase level [5].

Figure 7.1 shows the overall survival rates for all patients with SCLC who were treated at MD Anderson Cancer Center between 1944 and 2004.

a

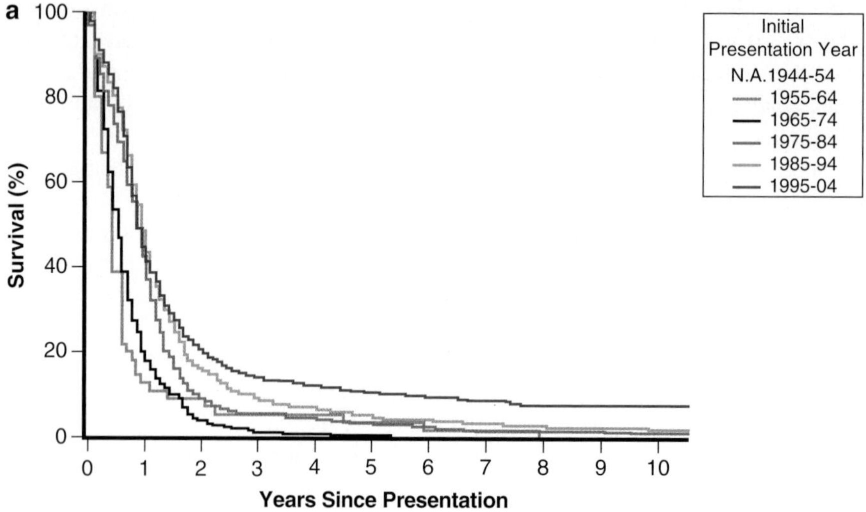

b

	Percent Survival	
Year	60 mo	120 mo
1944-54	0.0	0.0
1955-64	3.7	0.0
1965-74	0.8	0.5
1975-84	3.7	1.6
1985-94	5.3	2.5
1995-04	11.0	7.9

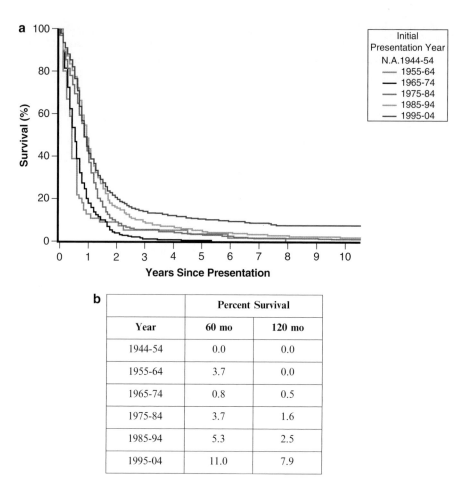

Fig. 7.1 (**a**) Overall survival rates for patients with small cell lung cancer (1944–2004) ($P<0.0001$, log-rank test for trend). Because of the very small number of individuals with small cell lung cancer seen from 1944 to 1954, data from this period were excluded. *N.A.* not applicable. (**b**) Kaplan–Meier survival table.

Principles of Chemotherapy for SCLC

Because SCLC usually presents with early systemic spread, neither surgical resection nor XRT alone is rarely appropriate, even for patients with limited-stage disease. SCLC must be treated as a systemic disease, and as such, chemotherapy is the cornerstone of treatment.

Combination chemotherapy regimens for SCLC are clearly superior to single agents in terms of response rates and survival [7]. One of the original effective combination regimens, cyclophosphamide, doxorubicin (Adriamycin), and vincristine (CAV), was supplanted in the 1980s by etoposide and cisplatin (Platinol) (EP) based on data showing it to be at least as effective at CAV but with a more favorable toxicity profile, particularly when given with concurrent thoracic XRT [9]. EP remains the most widely used regimen for treatment of SCLC, with response rates ranging from 60% to 80%.

Alternating or sequential chemotherapy regimens for SCLC were studied in the 1980s. None of these studies, which used varying combinations and sequences of etoposide, cisplatin, cyclophosphamide, doxorubicin, and vincristine, showed any consistent survival advantage [10–14].

The *addition of other cytotoxic agents* to the backbone of EP has generally yielded greater toxicity without consistent improvement in survival [15–18].

Studies that have sought to improve the efficacy of EP by *substituting the etoposide* with an alternative active agent have yielded conflicting results. An initial Japanese trial that replaced etoposide with a combination of irinotecan and cisplatin (Platinol) (IP) showed favorable results [19]; however, these findings were not borne out in two subsequent North American studies [20, 21]. A European study showed improved response rates and survival with irinotecan/carboplatin versus etoposide/carboplatin [22]. However, interpretation of this study was complicated by the fact that patient outcomes in both arms of the trial were not as favorable as expected compared with historical controls. In a another phase III study, the substitution of topotecan for etoposide, in combination with cisplatin, did not improve survival compared with EP [23]. Therefore, etoposide/platinum doublets remain the gold standard for the treatment of SCLC.

Another strategy that has been used to improve chemotherapy efficacy for SCLC has been to *increase dose density or intensity*. Several randomized studies using a dose-dense approach showed only modest benefit. A Japanese trial [24] used a non-platinum-containing regimen, thus limiting the applicability of this study to standard practice. In a British study [25] of 299 patients randomized to receive vincristine, ifosfamide, etoposide, plus carboplatin every 4 weeks versus every 3 weeks, survival was superior with the 3-week regimen (2-year survival of 18% versus 33%). However, the fact that there were no substantial differences in toxicity between the arms suggests that the 3-week cycle was not truly "dose dense." Another study evaluated cyclophosphamide, doxorubicin, and etoposide at 3-week versus 2-week intervals, with granulocyte colony-stimulating factor support in the dose-dense arm; no survival advantage was observed in the dose-dense arm [26].

A small randomized trial comparing ifosfamide, carboplatin, and etoposide every 4 weeks versus a dose-dense regimen schedule given every 2 weeks (with filgrastim and autologous peripheral blood progenitor cell support) showed improvement in survival and time to progression [27]. However, a larger phase III trial did not support these findings since there were no differences in response rate, time to progression, or survival [28]. Two randomized trials comparing high-dose with standard-dose EP for extensive SCLC did not show any survival advantage with the high-dose approach [29, 30].

And, finally, a meta-analysis of 60 studies that assessed the relationship between intended chemotherapy dose intensity of CAV or EP and response or median survival failed to show any correlation with improved outcome [31].

With regard to *prolonged administration of chemotherapy*, a study which compared four cycles of EP versus six cycles of CAV versus six cycles of alternating CAV/EP for patients with extensive-stage SCLC found the regimens to be equivalent with respect to response rate and survival [12]. Two randomized trials comparing observation versus maintenance chemotherapy (oral etoposide [32] or topotecan [33]) after completion of first-line therapy for extensive-stage SCLC did not show any survival advantage for the patients receiving maintenance therapy. The general standard of care for first-line treatment of SCLC is four cycles and six cycles of EP for patients with limited-stage and extensive-stage disease, respectively. There is probably no role for prolonged or maintenance chemotherapy as first-line treatment.

Treatment of Limited-Stage SCLC

As previously discussed, surgical resection is rarely appropriate for patients with limited-stage SCLC. The optimal treatment for limited-stage SCLC requires a combined-modality approach of both chemotherapy and XRT [34]. The chemotherapy regimen of choice is EP, both because of its favorable toxicity profile (particularly when given concurrently with chest XRT) and improved survival. Data do not support the use of dose-dense, dose-intense, or maintenance chemotherapy, or the addition of other cytotoxics.

Sequential, concurrent, and alternating schedules have been evaluated in integrating thoracic XRT with chemotherapy. Data have shown that the use of concurrent chemoradiation is superior to sequential. The early integration of thoracic XRT with systemic chemotherapy is crucial in treating limited-stage SCLC. In a National Cancer Institute of Canada phase III trial of thoracic XRT (40 Gy over 3 weeks) initiated with either cycle 2 or cycle 6 of chemotherapy (alternating CAV/EP), progression-free survival and overall survival were improved in the patients receiving early chemotherapy [35]. In a similar trial of XRT (1.5 Gy twice daily to 54 Gy) given either during weeks 1–4 or during weeks 6–9 of concurrent chemotherapy with etoposide/carboplatin, survival was improved in the early chemotherapy arm [36]. At least four meta-analyses addressing the timing of thoracic XRT have been published. Although not all individual trials have consistently shown a benefit to early thoracic XRT, the weight of evidence suggests a modest survival benefit with early rather than delayed thoracic XRT [7].

The current standard of care for limited-stage SCLC is based on the INT-0096 study [37]. This study compared 45 Gy given either twice daily (1.5 Gy per fraction) over 3 weeks or once daily (1.8 Gy per fraction) over 5 weeks in 417 patients with limited-stage SCLC. Patients received four cycles of EP, the first two cycles of which were given concurrently with thoracic XRT. There was significant improvement in survival in the hyperfractionated (twice daily) XRT arm (median survival, 23 versus 19 months; 5-year survival rates, 26% versus 16%), although at a cost of more grade 3 esophagitis (27% versus 11%). Because of this increase in toxicity, as well as logistical issues encountered in delivering twice-daily XRT in many communities, the use of accelerated hyperfractionated thoracic XRT has not been uniformly adopted. In those settings in which twice-daily thoracic XRT is not believed to be appropriate or feasible, once-daily thoracic XRT should be given to a total dose of at least 60 Gy.

An ongoing phase III trial is being conducted by the Cancer and Leukemia Group B/Radiation Therapy Oncology Group (CALGB/RTOG) to compare standard 45 Gy twice-daily thoracic XRT with two experimental thoracic XRT regimens: 70 Gy (2 Gy once-daily over 7 weeks) or 61.2 Gy (1.8 Gy once-daily for 16 days followed by 1.8 Gy twice-daily concomitant boost for 9 days). In all three treatment arms, the XRT is started with cycle 1 of EP chemotherapy. The study objective is survival, with toxicity and local/distant rates of control as secondary end points. Pending the outcome of this trial, however, 45-Gy twice-daily thoracic XRT, with four cycles of concurrent EP, should be considered the standard of care for limited-stage SCLC when feasible.

As noted above, patients with SCLC rarely present with disease at an early enough stage to warrant surgery. However, surgery is appropriate for the rare patient who presents with stage I disease, provided that their tumor is peripheral and that nodal metastases have been ruled out preoperatively by mediastinoscopy or endobronchial ultrasonography. Definitive surgery should include a lobectomy with mediastinal dissection. Because of the high rate of microscopic metastases, postoperative adjuvant EP chemotherapy should be administered to all patients. Furthermore, if metastases to hilar and/or mediastinal nodes are found at surgery, concurrent thoracic XRT should also be given.

Figure 7.2 shows the overall survival rates for all patients with limited-stage SCLC who were treated at MD Anderson Cancer Center between 1944 and 2004.

Treatment of Extensive-Stage SCLC

Treatment for extensive-stage SCLC consists of systemic chemotherapy alone; XRT is used only for immediate palliation of cancer-related symptoms. Six cycles of EP is the regimen of choice for these patients, with response rates ranging from 60% to 80%. Despite this good response to first-line chemotherapy, however, most patients experience relapse and eventually die of their disease. Median survival duration of patients with extensive-stage SCLC is 8–12 months, and the 5-year survival rate is less than 5%. Unfortunately, improvements in survival in the past two to three decades have been only modest. Some improvements have occurred, however, which have primarily been due to better supportive care measures; others can be attributed to more common use of second- and third-line chemotherapy for patients whose disease progressed after first-line therapy [7].

Figure 7.3 shows the overall survival rates for all patients with extensive-stage SCLC who were treated at MD Anderson Cancer Center between 1944 and 2004.

a

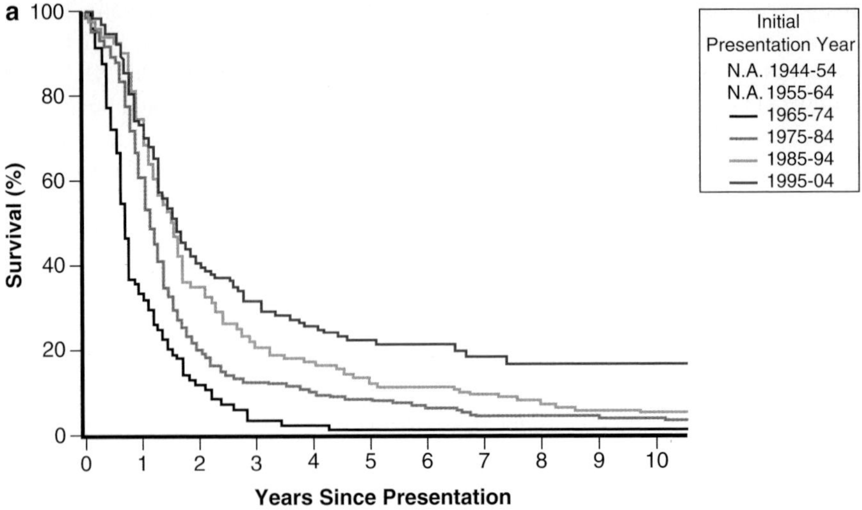

b

	Percent Survival	
Year	60 mo	120 mo
1944-54	0.0	0.0
1955-64	18.2	0.0
1965-74	1.2	1.2
1975-84	8.2	4.1
1985-94	12.6	5.7
1995-04	22.4	16.7

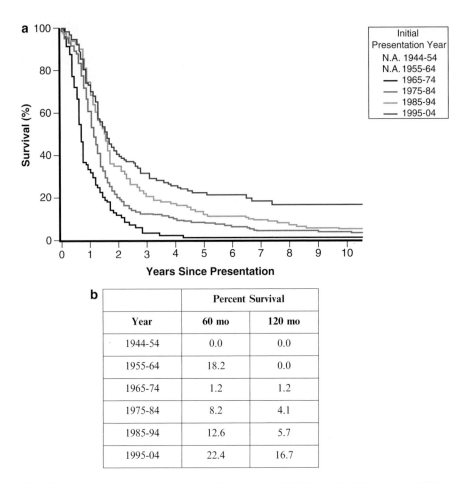

Fig. 7.2 (**a**) Survival rates for patients with limited-stage (SEER) small cell lung cancer (1944–2004) ($P<0.0001$, log-rank test for trend). Because of the very small number of individuals with limited-stage small cell lung cancer seen from 1944 to 1954 and from 1955 to 1964, data from these periods were excluded. *N.A.* not applicable. (**b**) Kaplan–Meier survival table.

Prophylactic Cranial Irradiation

Brain metastasis is a common site of spread in SCLC. Although our treatment of limited-stage disease has improved local control, brain metastasis as a site of relapse in patients treated for limited-stage SCLC is a major challenge, since about 60% of these patients will eventually develop central nervous system recurrence [38].

Between 1977 and 1995, 11 prospective randomized trials evaluated prophylactic cranial irradiation (PCI) in patients with SCLC. Although all but two reported a significant reduction in brain metastasis, none demonstrated a survival advantage. However, a meta-analysis of 987 patients (mostly with limited-stage disease) in complete remission who took part in seven of these trials did show modest but significant improvement in 3-year survival rates, from 15.3% to 20.7%, with the use of PCI [39].

a

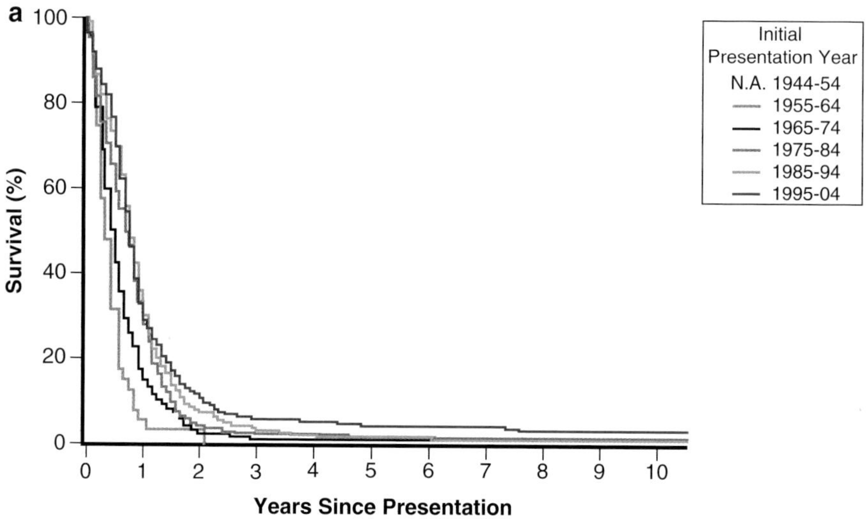

b

	Percent Survival	
Year	60 mo	120 mo
1944-54	NA	NA
1955-64	0.0	0.0
1965-74	0.7	0.4
1975-84	1.3	0.3
1985-94	0.8	0.3
1995-04	3.9	2.6

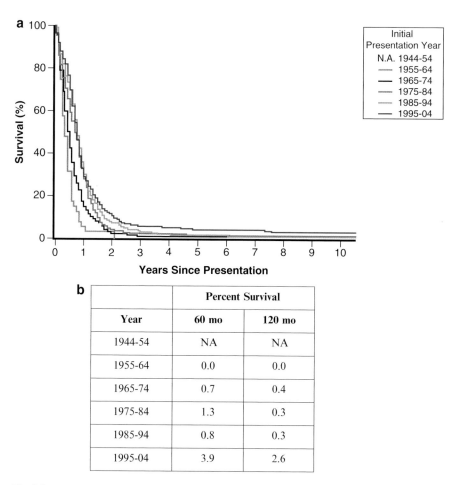

Fig. 7.3 (**a**) Survival rates for patients with extensive-stage (SEER) small cell lung cancer (1944–2004) ($P<0.0001$, log-rank test for trend). Because of the very small number of individuals with extensive-stage small cell lung cancer seen from 1944 to 1954, data from this period were excluded. *N.A.* not applicable. (**b**) Kaplan–Meier survival table.

Until recently, it was unclear whether patients with extensive-stage SCLC would also benefit from PCI. A randomized trial by the European Organisation for Research and Treatment of Cancer (EORTC) Radiation Oncology and Lung Cancer group randomized patients with extensive-stage SCLC who had responded to four to six cycles of chemotherapy to receive PCI or observation. Patients in the PCI group had a lower risk of symptomatic brain metastases (14.6% versus 40.4%) and improvement in 1-year survival rates (27.1% versus 13.3%). The one caveat to this study is that more patients in the PCI arm received second-line chemotherapy than did those in the observation arm, which could account for some of the survival advantage [40].

Thus, on the basis of the meta-analysis and the EORTC study, PCI is recommended for patients with both limited- and extensive-stage SCLC who achieve complete or near-complete remission after first-line therapy.

Despite the survival advantage with PCI, there has been some concern about late treatment-related neurotoxicity in long-term survivors. The EORTC study cited above did not show any neurologic sequelae in the patients who received PCI, at least over the short duration of follow-up reported. Furthermore, four additional randomized trials showed no differences in neurocognitive function in comparing patients who received PCI with those who did not (over follow-up periods as long as 30 months) [7]. However, there may be an increased risk of neurotoxicity from PCI when it is given concurrently with or before chemotherapy, when radiation fractions are greater than 2.5 Gy, and/or when the total radiation dose is more than 30 Gy [41]. Thus, PCI should be administered in 2- to 2.5-Gy daily fractions to a total dose of 25–30 Gy.

Second-Line Chemotherapy for Relapsed Disease After First-Line Therapy

Despite the high response rate to first-line chemotherapy, about 80% of patients with limited-stage SCLC and virtually all patients with extensive-stage SCLC will experience relapse. Generally, the response to second-line therapy, and thus survival from time of relapse, is influenced by the response to first-line chemotherapy and the progression-free interval following completion of first-line therapy [42–46]. Consequently, in considering how to treat patients with relapsed disease, one must classify them as having either "sensitive relapse" (i.e., responsive to first-line therapy, with a progression-free interval of at least 90 days) or "resistant relapse" (i.e., progressive while receiving first-line therapy, or responsive to first-line therapy, but experiencing relapse within 90 days).

Patients with sensitive relapse may respond to the same regimen used in their first-line treatment (usually an etoposide-platinum doublet). This approach is based on four small retrospective series [42–44, 46] that showed that patients with sensitive relapse treated with chemotherapy regimens that included some or all of the drugs used in their initial treatment had high response rates (50–80%). Although this re-induction approach has not been prospectively studied, it is widely accepted that patients with sensitive relapse, especially those with a progression-free interval of 6 months or longer, should be treated again with the regimen to which they responded in the first-line setting.

Other options for second-line treatment, either for patients who do not respond to re-induction or for those with resistant relapse, include CAV or single-agent topotecan or irinotecan. Topotecan is the most extensively studied agent for relapsed SCLC; response rates to topotecan as a second-line agent range from 11% to 31% in sensitive disease and from 2% to 7% in resistant disease; median survival times range from 25 to 36 weeks and from 16 to 21 weeks, respectively [47–53].

Irinotecan, although not studied nearly as extensively as topotecan in patients with recurrent disease, appears to have similar activity [54]. The taxanes have undergone limited study in the second-line treatment of SCLC. Response rates with paclitaxel and docetaxel have ranged from 20% to 29% [55–57]. And finally, palliative radiation is effective and is used commonly in drug-resistant and recurrent SCLC.

References

1. American Cancer Society. Cancer facts and figures 2009. Atlanta: American Cancer Society; 2009.
2. Govindan R, Page N, Morgensztern D, et al. Changing epidemiology of small-cell lung cancer in the United States over the last 30 years: analysis of the surveillance, epidemiologic, and end results database. J Clin Oncol. 2006;24:4539–44.
3. Micke P, Faldun A, Metz T, et al. Staging small cell lung cancer: Veterans Administration Lung Study Group versus International Association for the Study of Lung Cancer – what limits limited disease? Lung Cancer. 2002;37:271–6.
4. List AF, Hainsworth JD, Davis BW, Hande KR, Greco FA, Johnson DH. The syndrome of inappropriate secretion of antidiuretic hormone (SIADH) in small-cell lung cancer. J Clin Oncol. 1986;4:1191–8.
5. Yip D, Harper PG. Predictive and prognostic factors in small cell lung cancer: current status. Lung Cancer. 2000;28:173–85.
6. Shepherd FA, Laskey J, Evans WK, Goss PE, Johansen E, Khamsi F. Cushing's syndrome associated with ectopic corticotropin production and small-cell lung cancer. J Clin Oncol. 1992;10:21–7.
7. Hanrahan EO, Glisson B. Small cell carcinoma of the lung. In: Stewart D, editor. Lung cancer: prevention, management, and emerging therapies. Houston: The University of Texas MD Anderson Cancer Center; 2010. p. 395–434.
8. Green RA, Humphrey E, Close H, Patno ME. Alkylating agents in bronchogenic carcinoma. Am J Med. 1969;46:516–25.
9. Evans WK, Shepherd FA, Feld R, Osoba D, Dang P, Deboer G. VP-16 and cisplatin as first-line therapy for small-cell lung cancer. J Clin Oncol. 1985;3:1471–7.
10. Evans WK, Feld R, Murray N, et al. Superiority of alternating non-cross-resistant chemotherapy in extensive small cell lung cancer. A multicenter, randomized clinical trial by the National Cancer Institute of Cancer. Ann Intern Med. 1987;107:451–8.
11. Fukuoka M, Furuse K, Saijo N, et al. Randomized trial of cyclophosphamide, doxorubicin, and vincristine versus etoposide and cisplatin versus alternation of these two regimens in extensive small-cell lung cancer. J Natl Cancer Inst. 1991;83:855–61.
12. Roth BJ, Johnson DH, Einhorn LH, et al. Randomized study of cyclophosphamide, doxorubicin, and vincristine versus etoposide and cisplatin versus alternation of these two regimens in extensive small-cell lung cancer: a phase II trial of the Southeastern Cancer Study Group. J Clin Oncol. 1992;10:282–91.
13. Feld R, Evans WK, Coy P, et al. Canadian multicenter randomized trial comparing sequential and alternating administration of two non-cross-resistant chemotherapy combinations in patients with limited small-cell carcinoma of the lung. J Clin Oncol. 1987;5:1401–9.
14. Goodman GE, Crowley JJ, Blasko JC, et al. Treatment of limited small-cell lung cancer with etoposide and cisplatin alternating with vincristine, doxorubicin, and cyclophosphamide versus concurrent etoposide, vincristine, doxorubicin, and cyclophosphamide and chest radiotherapy: a Southwest Oncology Group Study. J Clin Oncol. 1990;8:39–47.
15. Hanna N, Ansari R, Fisher W, Shen J, Jung SH, Sandler A. Etoposide, ifosfamide, and cisplatin (VIP) plus concurrent radiotherapy for previously untreated limited small cell lung cancer: a Hoosier Oncology Group (HOG) phase II study. Lung Cancer. 2002;35:293–7.
16. Niell HB, Herndon JE, Miller AA, et al. Randomized phase II intergroup trial of etoposide and cisplatin with or without paclitaxel and granulocyte colony-stimulating factor in patients with extensive-stage small-cell lung cancer: cancer and leukemia group B trial 9732. J Clin Oncol. 2005;23:3752–9.
17. Mavroudis D, Papadakis E, Veslemes M, et al. A multicenter randomized clinical trial comparing paclitaxel-cisplatin-etoposide versus cisplatin-etoposide as first-line treatment in patients with small-cell lung cancer. Ann Oncol. 2001;12:463–70.

18. Reck M, von Pawel J, Macha HN, et al. Randomized phase III trial of paclitaxel, etoposide, and carboplatin versus carboplatin, etoposide, and vincristine in patients with small cell lung cancer. J Natl Cancer Inst. 2003;95:1118–27.
19. Noda K, Nishiwaki Y, Kawahara M, et al. Irinotecan plus cisplatin compared with etoposide plus cisplatin for extensive small-cell lung cancer. N Engl J Med. 2002;346:85–91.
20. Hanna N, Bunn PA, Langer C, et al. Randomized phase III trial comparing cisplatin with etoposide/cisplatin in patients with previously untreated extensive-stage disease small-cell lung cancer. J Clin Oncol. 2006;24:2038–43.
21. Natale RB, Lara PN, Chansky K, et al. S0124: a randomized phase III trial comparing irinotecan/cisplatin with etoposide/cisplatin in patients with previously untreated extensive stage small cell lung cancer [abstract 7512]. J Clin Oncol. 2008;26 Suppl 15:7512.
22. Hermes A, Bergman B, Bremnes R, et al. Irinotecan plus carboplatin versus oral etoposide plus carboplatin in extensive small-cell lung cancer: a randomized phase III trial. J Clin Oncol. 2008;26:4261–7.
23. Eckardt JR, von Pawel J, Papai Z, et al. Open-label, multicenter, randomized, phase III study comparing oral topotecan/cisplatin versus etoposide/cisplatin as treatment for chemotherapy-naïve patients with extensive-disease small-cell lung cancer. J Clin Oncol. 2006;24:2044–51.
24. Fukuoka M, Masuda N, Negoro S, et al. CODE chemotherapy with and without granulocyte colony-stimulating factor in small-cell lung cancer. Br J Cancer. 1997;75:306–9.
25. Steward WP, von Pawel J, Gatzemeier U, et al. Effects of granulocyte-macrophage colony-stimulating factor and dose intensification of V-ICE chemotherapy in small-cell lung cancer: a prospective randomized study of 300 patients. J Clin Oncol. 1998;16:642–50.
26. Thatcher N, Girling DJ, Hopwood P, Sambrook RJ, Qian W, Stephens RJ. Improving survival without reducing quality of life in small-cell lung cancer patients by increasing the dose-intensity of chemotherapy with granulocyte colony-stimulating factor support: results of a British Medical Research Council Multicenter Randomized Trial. J Clin Oncol. 2000;18:395–404.
27. Buchholz E, Manegold C, Pilz L, Thatcher N, Drings P. Standard versus dose-intensified chemotherapy with sequential reinfusion of hematopoietic progenitor cells in small cell lung cancer patients with favorable prognosis. J Thorac Oncol. 2007;2:51–8.
28. Lorigan P, Woll PJ, O'Brien ME, Ashcroft LF, Sampson MR, Thatcher N. Randomized phase III trial of dose-dense chemotherapy supported by whole-blood hematopoietic progenitors in better-prognosis small-cell lung cancer. J Natl Cancer Inst. 2005;97:666–74.
29. Ihde DC, Mulshine JL, Kramer BS, et al. Prospective randomized comparison of high-dose and standard-dose etoposide and cisplatin chemotherapy in patients with extensive-stage small-cell lung cancer. J Clin Oncol. 1994;12:2022–34.
30. Heigener DF, Manegold C, Jäger E, Saal JG, Zuna I, Gatzemeier U. Multicenter randomized open-label phase III study comparing efficacy, safety, and tolerability of conventional carboplatin plus etoposide versus dose-intensified carboplatin plus etoposide plus lenograstim in small-cell lung cancer in extensive disease stage. Am J Clin Oncol. 2009;32:61–4.
31. Klasa RJ, Murray N, Coldman AJ. Dose-intensity meta-analysis of chemotherapy regimens in small-cell carcinoma of the lung. J Clin Oncol. 1991;9:499–508.
32. Hanna NH, Sandler AB, Loehrer PJ, et al. Maintenance daily oral etoposide versus no further therapy following induction chemotherapy with etoposide plus ifosfamide plus cisplatin in extensive small-cell lung cancer: a Hoosier Oncology Group randomized study. Ann Oncol. 2002;13:95–102.
33. Schiller JH, Adak S, Cella D, DeVore RF, Johnson DH. Topotecan versus observation after cisplatin plus etoposide in extensive-stage small cell lung cancer: E7593 – a phase III trial of the Eastern Cooperative Oncology Group. J Clin Oncol. 2001;19:2114–22.
34. Arriagada R, Le Chevalier T, Pignon JP, et al. Initial chemotherapeutic doses and survival in patients with limited small-cell lung cancer. N Engl J Med. 1993;329:1848–52.
35. Murray N, Coy P, Pater JL, et al. Importance of timing for thoracic irradiation in the combined modality treatment of limited-stage small-cell lung cancer. The National Cancer Institute of Canada Clinical Trials Group. J Clin Oncol. 1993;11:336–44.

36. Jeremic B, Shibamoto Y, Acimovic L, Milisavljevic S. Initial versus delayed accelerated hyperfractionated radiation therapy and concurrent chemotherapy in limited small-cell lung cancer: a randomized study. J Clin Oncol. 1997;15:893–900.
37. Turrisi AT, Kim K, Blum R, et al. Twice-daily compared with once-daily thoracic radiotherapy in limited small-cell lung cancer treated concurrently with cisplatin and etoposide. N Engl J Med. 1999;340:265–71.
38. Pöttgen C, Eberhardt W, Stuschke M. Prophylactic cranial irradiation in lung cancer. Curr Treat Options Oncol. 2004;5:43–50.
39. Aupérin A, Arriagada R, Pignon JP, et al. Prophylactic cranial irradiation for patients with small-cell lung cancer in complete remission. Prophylactic Cranial Irradiation Overview Collaborative Group. N Engl J Med. 1999;341:476–84.
40. Slotman B, Faivre-Finn C, Kramer G, et al. Prophylactic cranial irradiation in extensive small-cell lung cancer. N Engl J Med. 2007;357:664–72.
41. Fonseca R, O'Neill BP, Foote RL, Grill JP, Sloan JA, Frytak S. Cerebral toxicity in patients treated for small cell carcinoma of the lung. Mayo Clin Proc. 1999;74:461–5.
42. Postmus PE, Berendsen HH, van Zandwijk N, Splinter TA, Burghouts JT, Bakker W. Retreatment with the induction regimen in small cell lung cancer relapsing after an initial response to short term chemotherapy. Eur J Cancer Clin Oncol. 1987;23:1409–11.
43. Giaccone G, Ferrati P, Donadio M, Testore F, Calciati A. Reinduction chemotherapy in small cell lung cancer. Eur J Cancer Clin Oncol. 1987;23:1697–9.
44. Vincent M, Evans B, Smith I. First-line chemotherapy rechallenge after relapse in small cell lung cancer. Cancer Chemother Pharmacol. 1988;21:45–8.
45. Giaccone G, Donadio M, Bonardi G, Testore F, Calciati A. Teniposide in the treatment of small-cell lung cancer: the influence of prior chemotherapy. J Clin Oncol. 1988;6:1264–70.
46. Batist G, Ihde DC, Zabell A, et al. Small-cell carcinoma of the lung: reinduction therapy after late relapse. Ann Intern Med. 1983;98:472–4.
47. Eckardt JR, von Pawel J, Pujol JL, et al. Phase III study of oral compared with intravenous topotecan as second-line therapy in small-cell lung cancer. J Clin Oncol. 2007;25:2086–92.
48. von Pawel J, Schiller JH, Shepherd FA, et al. Topotecan versus cyclophosphamide, doxorubicin, and vincristine for the treatment of recurrent small-cell lung cancer. J Clin Oncol. 1999;17:658–67.
49. O'Brien ME, Ciuleanu TE, Tsekov H, et al. Phase III trial comparing supportive care alone with supportive care with oral topotecan in patients with relapsed small-cell lung cancer. J Clin Oncol. 2006;24:5441–7.
50. Ardizzoni A, Manegold C, Debruyne C, et al. European Organization for Research and Treatment of Cancer (EORTC) 08957: phase II study of topotecan in combination with cisplatin as second line treatment of refractory and sensitive small cell lung cancer. Clin Cancer Res. 2003;9:143–50.
51. Eckardt J, Gralla R, Palmer MC, et al. Topotecan as second line therapy in patients with small cell lung cancer: a phase II study [abstract 513P]. Ann Oncol. 1996;7:107.
52. Depierre A, von Pawel J, Hans K, et al. Evaluation of topotecan in relapsed small cell lung cancer. A multicentre phase II study [abstract]. Lung Cancer. 1997;18:35.
53. von Pawel J, Gatzemeier U, Pujol JL, et al. Phase II comparator study of oral versus intravenous topotecan in patients with chemosensitive small-cell lung cancer. J Clin Oncol. 1999;19:1743–9.
54. Masuda N, Fukuoka M, Kusunoki Y, et al. CPT-11: a new derivative of camptothecin for the treatment of refractory or relapsed small-cell lung cancer. J Clin Oncol. 1992;10:1225–9.
55. Joos G, Schallier D, Pinson P, et al. Paclitaxel as second line treatment in patients with small cell lung cancer refractory to carboplatin-etoposide: a multicenter phase II study [abstract 7211]. Proc ASCO. 2004. pp. 22.
56. Smit EF, Fokkema E, Biesma B, Groen HJ, Snoek W, Postmus PE. A phase II study of paclitaxel in heavily pretreated patients with small-cell lung cancer. Br J Cancer. 1998;77:347–51.
57. Smyth JF, Smith IE, Sessa C, et al. Activity of docetaxel (Taxotere) in small cell lung cancer. The Early Clinical Trials Group of the EORTC. Eur J Cancer. 1994;30:1058–60.

Chapter 8
Colon Cancer

Cathy Eng, Patrick Lynch, and John Skibber

Introduction

Globally, colorectal cancer is one of the leading causes of cancer morbidity and mortality. In the USA, it is the third leading cause of cancer and the second leading cause of cancer death; colorectal cancer will be diagnosed in approximately 141,210 Americans this year and in 1 of every 20 Americans in their lifetime [1]. More than two-thirds of these cases will originate from the colon vs. the rectum. For the purpose of this chapter, we will focus on the more common colon cancer.

Most patients present with early-stage colon cancer and are treated by surgery with curative intent. However, approximately 25% of patients present with advanced stage IV disease. A minority of these patients (20%) will be considered for surgical resection. Successful eradication of metastatic disease requires multidisciplinary management by a team of pathology, medical, surgical, and radiation oncology professionals. Although several developments in cancer biology, systemic chemotherapy, targeted therapy, surgery, diagnostic imaging, and radiation oncology have evolved over the past two decades, our purpose is not to discuss each individual entity or approach. We propose to describe here the overall impact of these

C. Eng (✉)
Department of Gastrointestinal Medical Oncology, The University of Texas MD Anderson Cancer Center, 1515 Holcombe Boulevard, Houston, TX 77030, USA
e-mail: ceng@mdanderson.org

P. Lynch
Department of Gastroenterology, Hepatology, & Nutrition, The University of Texas MD Anderson Cancer Center, Houston, TX, USA

J. Skibber
Department of Surgical Oncology, The University of Texas MD Anderson Cancer Center, Houston, TX, USA

M.A. Rodriguez et al. (eds.), *60 Years of Survival Outcomes at The University of Texas MD Anderson Cancer Center*, DOI 10.1007/978-1-4614-5197-6_8,

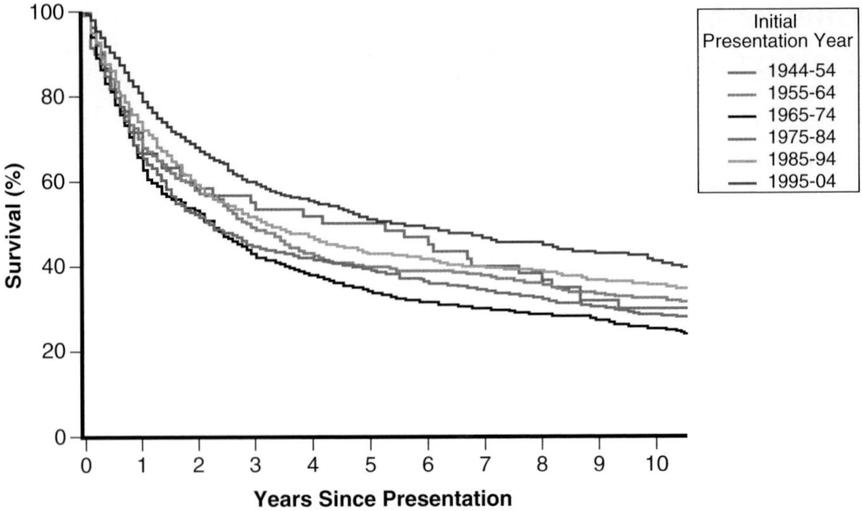

Fig. 8.1 Overall survival rates for patients with colon cancer (1944–2004) ($P<0.0001$, log-rank test for trend).

developments on the outcome of patients with local, regional, or distant (advanced) colon cancer (Figs. 8.1, 8.2, 8.3, and 8.4) who were treated at MD Anderson Cancer Center over six decades.

Historical Perspective

An early diagnosis of colon cancer is imperative for optimal outcome. Patients with stage I disease have an excellent 5-year overall survival (OS) rate of 95% and remain on surveillance after surgical resection. Yet the majority of patients present with locally advanced disease (AJCC stage II or stage III), for which adjuvant chemotherapy is considered in order to reduce the risk of recurrence, the overall survival benefit for these patients is <10%. Patients with stage IV disease are rarely cured with chemotherapy alone and have a 5-year OS rate of 11%. However, advances in chemotherapy have dramatically improved response rates, allowing reduction in tumor burden and consideration of metastatic surgical resection. Hence, for these selected patients, the expected 5-year OS rate increases to 30–60% [2].

Risk Factors

In a minority of patients, colorectal cancer develops because of inherited genetic disorders including familial adenomatous polyposis (FAP) or hereditary nonpolyposis colorectal cancer (HNPCC) syndrome, as well as chronic inflammatory

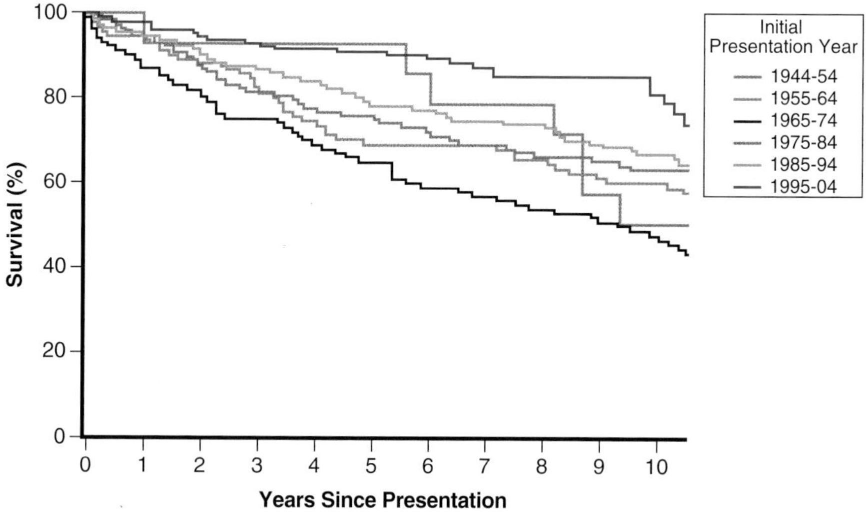

Fig. 8.2 Survival rates for patients with local (SEER stage) colon cancer (1944–2004) ($P<0.0001$, log-rank test for trend).

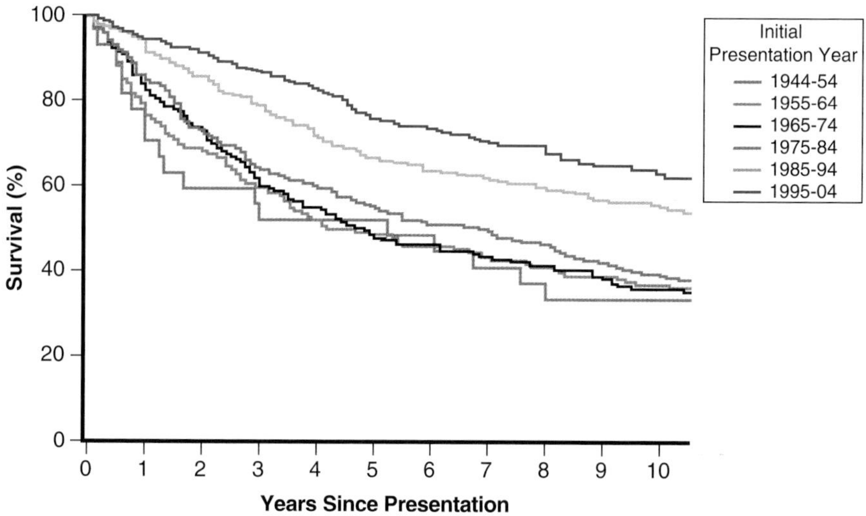

Fig. 8.3 Survival rates for patients with regional (SEER stage) colon cancer (1944–2004) ($P<0.0001$, log-rank test for trend).

bowel diseases such as ulcerative colitis and Crohn's disease. However, in most cases, sporadic colorectal cancer is diagnosed, a multifactorial process attributed to both somatic and germline mutations. Recent literature indicates that a defect in the microsatellite DNA mismatch repair gene may result in a microsatellite instability (MSI) defect, commonly associated with HNPCC and sporadically

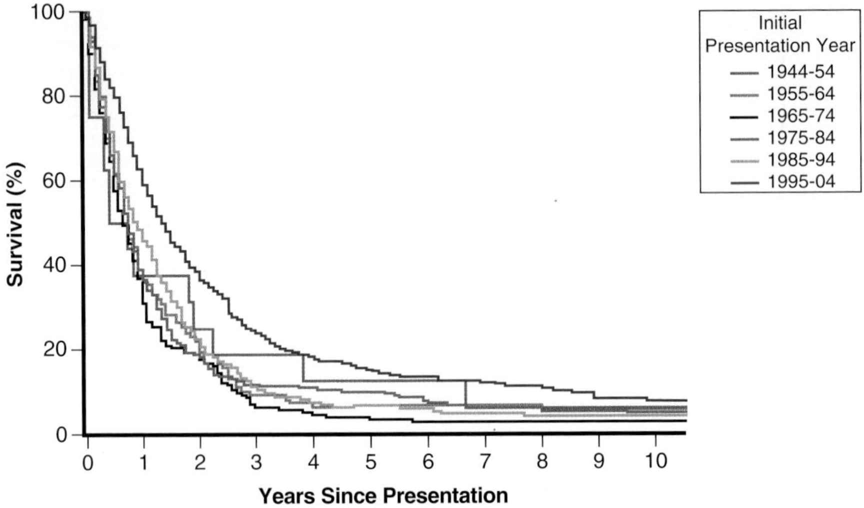

Fig. 8.4 Survival rates for patients with distant (SEER stage) colon cancer (1944–2004) ($P<0.0001$, log-rank test for trend).

due to hypermethylation of the promoter region (associated with MSI-high or MSI-deficient mismatch repair protein).

The main limitation to use MSI testing is the fact that 12–15% of nonfamilial colorectal cancers exhibit somatically acquired MSI, generally seen in older patients with right-sided tumors. Despite this limitation in the use of MSI in predicting HNPCC, there is an important reason to consider the use of routine MSI testing. One characteristic that sporadic MSI shares with HNPCC is that patients with MSI-H tumors have improved prognosis and survival [3]. Oddly, this trend exists regardless of the relative insensitivity of MSI tumors to the agent most commonly used in the adjuvant chemotherapy setting, 5-fluorouracil (5-FU), and its analogs [4]. Retrospective studies have indicated that MSI status may affect the efficacy of 5-FU monotherapy and overall prognosis.

At MD Anderson, we have attempted to be one of the pioneers in addressing some of the limitations in the use of MSI tumor testing. We have recently begun performing MSI testing by immunohistochemical (IHC) analysis for mismatch repair protein expression in all new cases of colorectal cancer surgically resected at MD Anderson. We have not yet initiated MSI testing in patients who undergo surgical resection in outside institutions because of the logistic challenges encountered when requesting unstained slides. However, this will be an initiative in the near future.

Since sporadic MSI exists in 12–15% of all colorectal cancer, but HNPCC exists in only 1–2%, it would be very undesirable to conduct expensive germline mutation testing (>$2,000 just for hMSH2 and hMLH1 tests) in all cases of MSI. Furthermore, to do so would carry a predicted uninformative rate of >90%. Fortunately, assays are now in place that can distinguish sporadic MSI from HNPCC-associated MSI.

Polymerase chain reaction-based methylation assays and BRAF mutation testing also work very well in this regard and are routinely reported as a supplement to pathological testing in which MSI/IHC analysis has shown abnormalities warranting further evaluation [5, 6].

Treatment

Radical surgical resection with curative intent is appropriate for 80–90% of patients with colon carcinoma and is the only treatment required for most tumors limited to the bowel wall. In these cases, adequate surgical resection is the major treatment factor affecting local control and cure [7, 8].

The primary principles of surgical management in colon cancer are as follows:

- Removal of the primary tumor along with proximal, distal, and radial resection margins
- Treatment and drainage of lymphatics
- Restoration of function by anastomosis and avoidance of a permanent colostomy

These principles of surgical management have remained largely constant over the years. Surgical management must also include assessment for the presence of liver metastases. Although this is commonly accomplished by palpation and inspection, intraoperative ultrasonography of the liver has been observed to increase the likelihood of detecting small metastases. The extent of colonic resection is determined by the blood vessels that must be divided to remove the lymphatic drainage of the tumor-bearing portion of the colon with tumor-free margins. This is the primary treatment approach in patients with colon carcinoma. Resection of intermediate and principal nodes requires ligation and division of the main vascular trunks to the affected colon segment. Tumor-free margins are usually accomplished by resection of >5 cm of normal bowel proximal and distal to the tumor [9].

Excellent results have been obtained with wide mesenteric resection and adequate lymphadenectomy. In addition to the therapeutic benefits of this procedure, by prevention of local progression, lymphadenectomy is critical in the staging of colon carcinoma. In colon cancer, recovery of involved lymph nodes is the parameter most often used as an indicator of the need for adjuvant therapy within treatment guidelines applicable in the USA. Mesenteric resection should be extensive enough to harvest at least 12 lymph nodes for examination to allow for accurate staging. The number of examined lymph nodes is a process outcome that involves the patient and tumor characteristics, as well as the quality of the surgery and the pathology examination [10].

Laparoscopic techniques are widely used in the management of benign and malignant colorectal conditions. These techniques can be carried out safely and successfully, especially when conducted by an experienced laparoscopic surgeon. Laparoscopic techniques have been shown to reduce the duration of hospitalization and hasten recovery. The shortened stay associated with laparoscopic colectomy, attributable to early postoperative feeding, has resulted in changes to the treatment of patients with colon cancer who undergo resection techniques. Available data on the extent of lymphadenectomy and resection margins achieved by oncologic laparoscopic resection indicate that this technique is comparable to open colectomy for cancer. Rates of recurrence in port sites after laparoscopic resection have ranged between 1.1% and 3.6%, similar to rates associated with laparotomy wounds in patients treated by open resection. Similarly, there are equivalent results in terms of local recurrence, distant metastases, and survival.

For those patients for whom chemotherapy must be considered, 5-FU has served as the foundation for chemotherapy for almost five decades in both adjuvant and metastatic settings, regardless of stage and purpose of therapy. Given the limited variety of treatment, modifications in intravenous 5-FU administration have been attempted, including bolus, continuous infusion (7 days), and most recently, the De Gramont method of continuous infusion over 46–48 h. The oral fluoropyrimidine capecitabine is an alternative to intravenous 5-FU, with similar toxic effects, and is currently approved in early- and advanced-disease settings. Therapeutic advances outside of 5-FU were not noted until 1998, when the topoisomerase-1 inhibitor irinotecan was the first drug for metastatic colorectal cancer administration as a single agent and in combination with 5-FU [IFL (bolus 5-FU) or FOLFIRI (infusional 5-FU)]. Multiple trials have determined that irinotecan has no role in the adjuvant setting but only in the metastatic setting.

FDA approval of the third-generation platinum analog oxaliplatin in 2004 added to the treatment armamentarium. Unlike irinotecan, it is inactive as a single agent and must be given in combination with either infusional 5-FU (FOLFOX), bolus 5-FU (FLOX), or the oral fluoropyrimidine capecitabine (XELOX). Oxaliplatin has been determined to be efficacious in both early and advanced disease. The most recent treatment advances (since 2006) have focused less on traditional cytotoxic agents and more on biologic "targeted" agents, specifically the monoclonal antibodies against the vascular endothelial growth factor (anti-VEGF) bevacizumab and the epidermal growth factor receptors (anti-EGFRs) cetuximab and panitumumab. These targeted therapies work best in combination with chemotherapy and are suited at this time for the metastatic disease setting [11, 12]. Overall, these therapeutic advances have improved the response, progression-free survival, and overall survival for patients with metastatic disease.

The MD Anderson Cancer Center Experience

The intent of this chapter is to discuss the historical outcome of patients who were treated at MD Anderson for all stages of colorectal cancer. Between 1944 and 2004, a total of 20,880 patients initially presented to MD Anderson with a diagnosis of colon cancer (Table 8.1); the number of patients presenting to our institution increased linearly over this interval. Of these patients, 3,182 had no other cancers and received their first course of treatment at MD Anderson (Table 8.1).

Table 8.1 Colon cancer population

Patient demographics	No. of patients
Patients with cancer of the colon initially presenting to MD Anderson Cancer Center on or before 12/31/2004	20,880
No previous treatment	5,073
Definitive MD Anderson treatment	4,176
No other primaries except superficial skin cancers[a]	3,182

[a]Survival calculated for this subgroup of 3,182 from initial presentation at MD Anderson

Table 8.2 Patients with colon cancer treated at MD Anderson, 1944–2004

	SEER stage at presentation					
	In situ	Local	Regional	Distant	Unstaged	Total
Decade	[No. (%) of patients]					
1944–1954	1 (1.7)	14 (23.3)	27 (45.0)	16 (26.7)	2 (3.3)	60 (100.0)
1955–1964	3 (0.8)	91 (25.6)	144 (40.4)	113 (31.7)	5 (1.4)	356 (100.0)
1965–1974	3 (0.7)	102 (22.7)	162 (36.1)	180 (40.1)	2 (0.4)	449 (100.0)
1975–1984	5 (0.8)	114 (18.9)	216 (35.8)	263 (43.6)	5 (0.8)	603 (100.0)
1985–1994	0 (0)	143 (18.5)	284 (36.7)	332 (42.9)	14 (1.8)	773 (100.0)
1995–2004	3 (0.3)	147 (15.6)	350 (37.2)	418 (44.4)	23 (2.4)	941 (100.0)
Total	*15 (0.5)*	*611 (19.2)*	*1,183 (37.2)*	*1,322 (41.5)*	*51 (1.6)*	*3,182 (100.0)*

SEER Surveillance, Epidemiology, and End Results program

Among these 3,182 patients over this 60-year period, 611 (19.2%) had local disease, 1,183 (37.2%) had regional disease, and 1,322 (41.5%) presented with metastatic disease. There is an evident trend from seeing more patients with locoregional disease (23.3% vs. 15.6%) to seeing those with more distant disease (26.7% vs. 44.4%), which probably reflects the fact that more patients with local disease are receiving treatment in outside institutions, resulting in our seeing the more advanced cases (Table 8.2).

For all stages, the 5-year OS rates appear to have remained fairly stagnant, but clear improvement was seen in 10-year OS (30–41.1%) for all patients. The greatest improvements in 5-year OS were notably in the past two decades for regional disease (51.9–75.6%) and distant disease (12.5–15.2%), likely due to modifications in adjuvant and distant chemotherapy as well as to surgical approaches.

It should be noted again that for the 60-year duration, from 1944 to 2004, innovations in chemotherapy for colon cancer were few. Thus, many significant chemotherapeutic developments of this past decade are not truly visualized in these data.

Conclusions

Over the past six decades, we have seen exponential growth in patients treated for colon cancer at our institution for both early and advanced disease. During this period, we have seen treatment developments expand beyond 5-FU alone to include four other chemotherapy agents. We have also seen great advances in surgical techniques as well as in genetic and molecular testing. We have moved beyond the standard chemotherapeutic cytotoxic agents and are focused on biologic agents that are created as inhibitors of various receptors or ligands involved in colon carcinogenesis. We envision that this methodology will continue to evolve as various molecular markers are validated as predictive for efficacy of therapy. Colon cancer treatment has manifested as one of the most advanced fields in oncology. The landscape continues to change in its treatment, and it is presumed that MD Anderson Cancer Center will continue to evolve with all future methodology.

References

1. American Cancer Society. Cancer facts and figures, 2011. Atlanta: American Cancer Society; 2011.
2. Gleisner AL, Choti MA, Assumpcao L, et al. Colorectal liver metastases: recurrence and survival following hepatic resection, radiofrequency ablation, and combined resection-radiofrequency ablation. Arch Surg. 2008;143:1204–12.
3. Popat S, Hubner R, Houlston RS. Systematic review of microsatellite instability and colorectal cancer prognosis. J Clin Oncol. 2005;23:609–18.
4. Ribic CM, Sargent DJ, Moore MJ, et al. Tumor microsatellite-instability status as a predictor of benefit from fluorouracil-based adjuvant chemotherapy for colon cancer. N Engl J Med. 2003;349:247–57.
5. Deng G, Bell I, Crawley S, et al. BRAF mutation is frequently present in sporadic colorectal cancer with methylated hMLH1, but not in hereditary nonpolyposis colorectal cancer. Clin Cancer Res. 2004;10:191–5.
6. Deng G, Peng E, Gum J, et al. Methylation of hMLH1 promoter correlates with the gene silencing with a region-specific manner in colorectal cancer. Br J Cancer. 2002;86:574–9.
7. Compton CC, Fielding LP, Burgart LJ, et al. Prognostic factors in colorectal cancer. College of American Pathologists Consensus Statement 1999. Arch Pathol Lab Med. 2000;124:979–94.
8. Nelson H, Petrelli N, Carlin A, et al. Guidelines 2000 for colon and rectal cancer surgery. J Natl Cancer Inst. 2001;93:583–96.
9. West NP, Hohenberger W, Weber K, et al. Complete mesocolic excision with central vascular ligation produces an oncologically superior specimen compared with standard surgery for carcinoma of the colon. J Clin Oncol. 2010;28:272–8.
10. Joseph NE, Sigurdson ER, Hanlon AL, et al. Accuracy of determining nodal negativity in colorectal cancer on the basis of the number of nodes retrieved on resection. Ann Surg Oncol. 2003;10:213–8.
11. Alberts SR, Sargent DJ, Smyrk TC, et al. Adjuvant mFOLFOX6 with or without cetuxiumab (Cmab) in KRAS wild-type (WT) patients (pts) with resected stage III colon cancer (CC): results from NCCTG intergroup phase III Trial N0147 [abstract CRA3507]. J Clin Oncol. 2010;28(Suppl):959s.
12. Allegra CJ, Yothers G, O'Connell MJ, et al. Phase III trial assessing bevacizumab in stages II and III carcinoma of the colon: results of NSABP Protocol C-08. J Clin Oncol. 2011;29:11–6.

Chapter 9
Ovarian Cancer

Robert L. Coleman and David M. Gershenson

Introduction

Primary malignancy of the ovary is fortunately a relatively uncommon condition. In 2011, however, more than 20,000 new cases will likely be diagnosed. Ovarian cancer has a poor reputation for survivorship: nearly three-quarters of all diagnosed patients succumb to the disease, distinguishing it as the most lethal gynecologic malignancy. These statistics largely reflect the clinicopathologic course of the most common type of ovarian cancer, epithelial ovarian cancer, which accounts for more than 80% of primary cases. However, ovarian cancer may also arise from the germ cells, ovarian stroma, and other supporting tissues; expected survivorship in such cases is generally more favorable as a result of the early stage at diagnosis and the high degree of chemotherapy and radiotherapy sensitivity, when adjuvant therapy is recommended. Generally, younger women with ovarian cancer have a proliferative but noninvasive element designated as "low malignant potential" or "borderline" epithelial ovarian tumor. Clearly distinguishing the individual risk factors and therapeutic options for these subtypes is important, given their occurrence in women of reproductive potential and unique natural history.

Risk factors for epithelial ovarian carcinoma are well established. Age is the strongest patient-related risk factor. Overall, an estimated 1 in 70 women will develop ovarian cancer in their lifetime, with age-specific incidence peaking at 75–80 years of age. This is especially startling considering the aging population in the United States. The second-strongest risk factor is a family history of ovarian and/or breast cancer. Women who are heterozygous for mutations of either *BRCA1*

R.L. Coleman • D.M. Gershenson (✉)
Department of Gynecologic Oncology and Reproductive Medicine,
The University of Texas MD Anderson Cancer Center,
P.O. Box 301439, Houston, TX 77230-1439, USA
e-mail: dgershen@mdanderson.org

M.A. Rodriguez et al. (eds.), *60 Years of Survival Outcomes at The University of Texas MD Anderson Cancer Center*, DOI 10.1007/978-1-4614-5197-6_9,

or *BRCA2* have an estimated lifetime risk of 16–60%. Other risk factors associated with increased risk include nulliparity, involuntary infertility, early menarche, and late menopause. Interestingly, oral contraceptive use, pregnancy, lactation, and tubal ligation are associated with reduced risk. Collectively, on the basis of these observations, the investigation into the etiology of this disease has been focused on factors governing ovulation in the adnexa.

Although the exact process of malignant transformation is not known and is likely not a solitary event, three interrelated theories have been proposed to explain the epidemiological observations. The first posits that incessant ovulation leads to repetitive wounding of the ovarian surface epithelium and generates cellular proliferation in postovulatory repair. Such events could increase the probability of accumulated genomic abnormalities. In addition, this cyclic reparative process is believed to generate ovarian epithelial inclusion cysts, whose epithelia undergo carcinogenic transformation in an environment of aberrant autocrine and paracrine growth factor stimulation. Genomic profiling of these cells has demonstrated that they differ significantly from surface epithelia, and although not overtly phenotypically malignant, they express many factors associated with the cancer genotype.

A second theory postulates that surges of pituitary gonadotropins at ovulation and persistently high concentrations after menopause stimulate surface epithelial cells, which result in accumulation of genetic changes and carcinogenesis.

The third theory, supported by observations of increased risk associated with endometriosis, pelvic inflammatory disease, mumps, and talc or asbestos exposure, is associated with factors governing the inflammatory response. Changes in the redox potential in the setting of ovulation and surface-epithelium repair might account for accumulation of genetic injury promoting cancer transformation. Since the inflammation-like setting in which ovulation occurs is dependent on cyclooxygenase-2 (COX2), this theory lends support to the exploration of the chemopreventive potential of COX2 inhibitors.

Historical Perspective

When MD Anderson opened its doors in 1944, few diagnostic tools or therapeutic modalities were available for the treatment of ovarian cancer. Primary surgery was rather primitive; the aggressive and ultraradical surgical approaches to the treatment of ovarian cancer had not yet evolved. Rather, surgery included possible removal of the ovarian mass(es) without omentectomy or maximum cytoreductive surgery of all gross diseases. The postoperative therapy available from 1944 to approximately 1954 included various radiotherapeutic techniques: intraperitoneal instillation of radioactive gold or chromic phosphate solutions, open-field whole abdominal radiation techniques, or the moving strip technique of delivering whole abdominal radiation. The intraperitoneal techniques were primarily used to control malignant effusions. With these treatments, 5-year survival rates were approximately 65% for stage I, 40% for stage II, 18% for stage III, and 12% for stage IV.

The period between 1955 and 1964 was dominated by alkylating agent chemotherapy, used at MD Anderson for the management of ovarian cancer. The agents used in this treatment included cyclophosphamide, melphalan, chlorambucil, nitrogen mustard, and thio-TEPA. By 1960, early reports indicated objective responses in a high percentage of patients, some of which were dramatic, although drug deaths were also reported. Based on preliminary results, melphalan (L-sarcolysin) was selected as the alkylating agent worthy of further clinical trials.

By 1960, MD Anderson physicians were treating women with ovarian cancer with surgery, irradiation, and chemotherapy in various sequences. Response rates to chemotherapy were generally higher than 50%, and control of malignant effusions was noted. Treatment guidelines that had evolved by this time included the following: (1) Total abdominal hysterectomy and bilateral salpingo-oophorectomy was used if surgically feasible; the omentum was removed only if gross tumor was present. (2) For stage I disease, surgery was used, followed by abdominal strip irradiation. (3) For stages II and III with no tumor implants larger than 2 cm, surgery was used, followed by abdominal strip irradiation with a pelvic boost. (4) For cases with tumor implants larger than 3 cm and/or ascites, chemotherapy with melphalan was administered postoperatively. For patients who had a good response, abdominal strip irradiation was then administered. In addition, during this era, second-look surgery after a designated number of chemotherapy cycles was routinely performed to assess response. For patients who developed progressive disease on melphalan, 5-fluorouracil was occasionally used as second-line chemotherapy. Overall, however, it was difficult to evaluate whether chemotherapy improved survival.

By the mid-1960s, second-look surgery after chemotherapy had become standard. However, only about 12% of patients receiving chemotherapy were candidates for this procedure; the remainder generally developed progressive disease during chemotherapy. Combination chemotherapy was introduced into clinical practice at MD Anderson at this time in the form of the AcFuCy regimen—actinomycin-D, 5-fluorouracil, and cyclophosphamide. This combination regimen was initially used for patients who experienced disease progression while taking melphalan, and response rates in early trials ranged from 35% to 40%. However, compared with melphalan, more serious toxic effects were noted; of the first 47 patients so treated, 6 experienced serious toxic effects, and 3 died of drug complications.

Throughout the mid- to late-1960s, little progress was made. Furthermore, because the options for treatment were extremely limited, all subtypes of ovarian cancer—epithelial tumors, malignant germ cell tumors, and sex cord-stromal tumors—were treated similarly. As the 1970s approached, the only major advance was seen in a number of patients with disseminated ovarian dysgerminoma who had been treated and cured with surgery followed by postoperative irradiation.

By 1970, a number of advances were on the horizon, the most dramatic being the evolution of treatment for girls and young women with malignant ovarian germ cell tumors [1]. About this time, the combination of vincristine, actinomycin-D, and cyclophosphamide (VAC) was first used for nondysgerminomatous germ cell tumors, resulting in significant improvement in survival rates. For patients with stage I disease, the 5-year survival rates ranged from 85% to 90%, and for those with stage III disease, these 5-year rates were approximately 50%. For patients with sex cord-stromal ovarian tumors, surgery remained the cornerstone of therapy throughout the 1970s. No standard postoperative therapy was established, but for patients with newly diagnosed disseminated disease or those with recurrent disease, common treatments during this era included whole abdominal or pelvic irradiation or combination chemotherapy with either AcFuCy or VAC. By the mid-1970s, single-agent doxorubicin was being investigated as well.

For patients with epithelial ovarian cancers, a number of different strategies and treatments were being studied during the 1970s. In 1970, a randomized clinical trial was initiated for women with stage III epithelial ovarian cancer that compared whole abdominal radiation using the moving strip technique with single-agent melphalan. The results of this trial indicated relatively equivalent outcomes but with different toxicities. Melphalan remained the standard postoperative chemotherapy during most of this period.

Beginning in 1973 and ending in 1980, a series of four contract studies sponsored by the National Cancer Institute were conducted. The initial study, conducted between 1973 and 1974, consisted of a three-arm trial of melphalan vs. 5-fluorouracil vs. hexamethylmelamine. The second trial, conducted between 1974 and 1976, randomized patients to melphalan, hexamethylmelamine, doxorubicin, or the combination of hexamethylmelamine and cyclophosphamide. The third trial, conducted between 1976 and 1978, randomized patients to melphalan, the combination of hexamethylmelamine and cyclophosphamide, cisplatin, or the combination of hexamethylmelamine, doxorubicin, and cyclophosphamide. And the final trial, conducted between 1978 and 1980, randomized patients to either the combination of hexamethylmelamine, doxorubicin, and cyclophosphamide or the combination of melphalan and cisplatin.

The major advance during the 1970s was the introduction of cisplatin, which emerged as the most active drug to date for the treatment of ovarian cancer. The other major advance was the standard use of combination chemotherapy by the end of the 1970s. Starting in the early 1980s, the combination of cisplatin and cyclophosphamide became the standard postoperative regimen, and the standard number of cycles was 12, which was simply extrapolated from the melphalan era.

By the end of the 1970s, primary surgery was becoming more aggressive, according to preliminary reports from Boston. Also during this period, neoadjuvant chemotherapy was beginning to be used selectively for women with extensive metastatic disease, massive malignant effusions, or severe comorbidities.

Also of note in the late 1970s, the combination of vinblastine, bleomycin, and cisplatin (Platinol) (VBP) was introduced for patients with malignant ovarian germ cell tumors, leading to further improvement in sustained remissions approaching 100% for stage I disease and 75% for advanced-stage disease. The VBP combination continued to be used during the early part of the 1980s. For patients with ovarian sex cord-stromal tumors, use of VAC gave way to the new combination of cisplatin, doxorubicin (Adriamycin), and cyclophosphamide (PAC) by the early 1980s.

For postoperative treatment of high-risk early-stage epithelial ovarian cancers and advanced-stage cancers during most of the 1980s, the combination of cisplatin and cyclophosphamide continued to be studied in a series of investigator-initiated trials. By the mid-1980s, the number of cycles was abbreviated to 6. Carboplatin was studied in clinical trials during the 1980s, and by the end of the decade, it was being used primarily as a single agent for patients with recurrent disease.

For patients with malignant ovarian germ cell tumors, by the mid-1980s, etoposide (in the combination chemotherapy regimen bleomycin, etoposide, and cisplatin [Platinol] [BEP]) had replaced vinblastine (in the combination regimen vinblastine, bleomycin, and cisplatin [Platinol] [VBP]) [2]. A major advance during this period was the substitution of postoperative BEP chemotherapy for irradiation in patients with ovarian dysgerminoma. This allowed MD Anderson gynecologic oncologists to much better preserve fertility in young patients. In the 1980s, fertility-sparing surgery had become a treatment standard in these patients. For patients with metastatic sex cord-stromal tumors, a clinical trial focused on BEP was initiated in 1988.

In the 1980s, surgical cytoreduction was becoming progressively more aggressive, with the objective of achieving minimal residual disease. However, by the mid-1980s, second-look surgery was becoming obsolete, primarily because of its lack of clinical benefit.

For patients with epithelial ovarian cancers, primary cytoreductive surgery followed by combination cisplatin and cyclophosphamide chemotherapy continued to be the standard until paclitaxel was introduced into clinical trials in the early 1990s. By the mid-1990s, after the publication of the Gynecologic Oncology Group (GOG) 111 protocol, combined paclitaxel and cisplatin became the new standard [3].

For patients with malignant germ cell tumors or sex cord-stromal tumors, treatment advanced little during this period. With the introduction of paclitaxel, some of the latter patients began to be treated with paclitaxel alone or with combined paclitaxel and cisplatin [4].

By the early 2000s, primary cytoreductive surgery was becoming even more aggressive to achieve minimal residual disease, with diaphragmatic stripping or debulking, a greater frequency of splenectomy, and more common bowel surgery or lymph node debulking. Also during this period, findings from the GOG 158 trial were published, which demonstrated that paclitaxel/carboplatin and paclitaxel/cisplatin were equivalent in terms of efficacy, but a better therapeutic index was reported with the former [5]. As a result, carboplatin replaced cisplatin almost completely as the standard regimen for both epithelial tumors and sex cord-stromal tumors. For epithelial ovarian cancer, this combination remains a standard postoperative therapy.

The MD Anderson Cancer Center Experience

The MD Anderson Tumor Registry data set was derived from 12,411 women who were diagnosed as having ovarian cancer between 1950 and 2004. Of this group, 2,536 women had received no previous treatment for ovarian cancer. After excluding patients who had received treatment elsewhere and those who had multiple

Table 9.1 Women with ovarian cancer treated at MD Anderson, 1944–2004

	SEER stage at presentation					
	In situ	Local	Regional	Distant	Unstaged	Total
Decade	[No. (%) of patients]					
1944–1954	0 (0)	2 (13.3)	3 (20.0)	10 (66.7)	0 (0)	15 (100.0)
1955–1964	0 (0)	10 (5.6)	10 (5.6)	143 (80.8)	14 (7.9)	177 (100.0)
1965–1974	0 (0)	13 (4.3)	19 (6.3)	260 (86.4)	9 (3.0)	301 (100.0)
1975–1984	0 (0)	36 (10.2)	10 (2.8)	304 (86.1)	3 (0.8)	353 (100.0)
1985–1994	2 (0.5)	79 (18.8)	22 (5.2)	301 (71.7)	16 (3.8)	420 (100.0)
1995–2004	0 (0)	82 (14.7)	24 (4.3)	412 (74.0)	39 (7.0)	557 (100.0)
Total	*2 (0.1)*	*222 (12.2)*	*88 (4.8)*	*1,430 (78.4)*	*81 (4.4)*	*1,823 (100.0)*

SEER Surveillance, Epidemiology, and End Results program

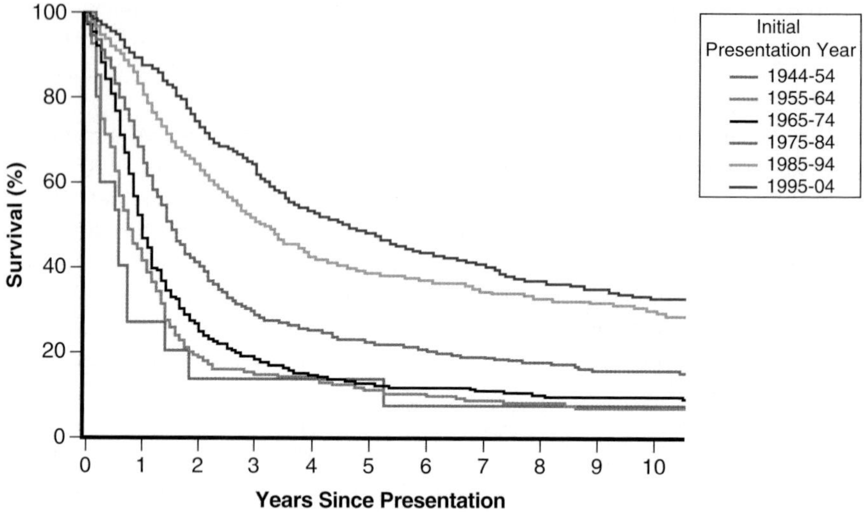

Fig. 9.1 Overall survival rates for patients with ovarian cancer (1944–2004) ($P<0.0001$, log-rank test for trend).

primary cancers, 1,823 patients received definitive primary treatment at MD Anderson Cancer Center. Thus, based on consistent referral patterns over the years, the majority of women who had been referred with a diagnosis of ovarian cancer had received some types of previous treatment.

Table 9.1 shows the number of patients treated with definitive primary therapy by time period and stage of disease. As expected, almost 80% of women had advanced-stage (stage III or IV) disease. The computed survival curves represent the clinical outcomes for women who received definitive primary treatment at MD Anderson Cancer Center. Figure 9.1 reveals the overall survival rates for all stages of disease. As noted, during this 60-year period, there has been incremental improvement in 5-year survival (from 13.3% to 48%) and in 10-year survival (from 6.7% to 32.6%) ($P<0.0001$).

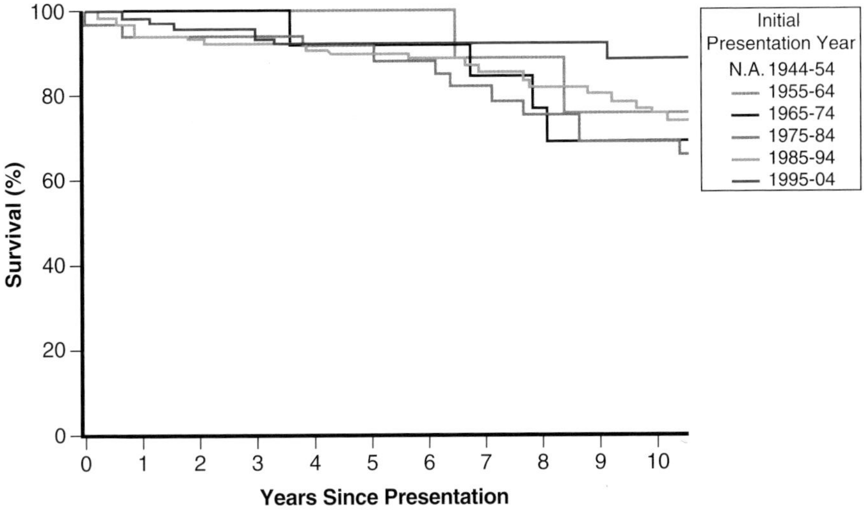

Fig. 9.2 Survival rates for patients with local (SEER stage) ovarian cancer (1944–2004) (P=0.39, log-rank test for trend). Because of the very small number of individuals with local ovarian cancer seen from 1944 to 1954, data from this period were excluded. *N.A.* not applicable.

In the following sections, the change in overall survival over time by stage of disease is discussed. Although the data are presented with use of the typical Tumor Registry methodology—categorizing disease into local, regional, and distant—this is somewhat problematical for ovarian cancer. The primary method of determining stage for ovarian cancer has historically been based on findings at primary surgery, and this system has been relatively consistent during the period under study. However, the rigor with which surgical staging has been practiced has changed dramatically. In the early decades, surgical staging for apparent early disease was less than optimal in many instances. Thus, the data for both local disease (stage I) and regional disease (stage II) patients may be somewhat suspect during the first half of the study period.

Survival in Women with Localized Disease

As noted in Fig. 9.2, there is no clear trend in improvement over the study period. There are several possible explanations for this finding. First, the number of patients with localized (stage I) disease is relatively small. Furthermore, the inclusion of all histotypes and histologic grades complicates analysis. For instance, we know that women with low-risk disease—stage I low-grade endometrioid carcinomas, low-grade serous carcinomas, mucinous carcinomas, malignant ovarian germ cell tumors, and granulosa cell tumors—have an excellent prognosis, with a 90% or better 5-year survival rate, whereas those with high-risk disease—stage I high-grade

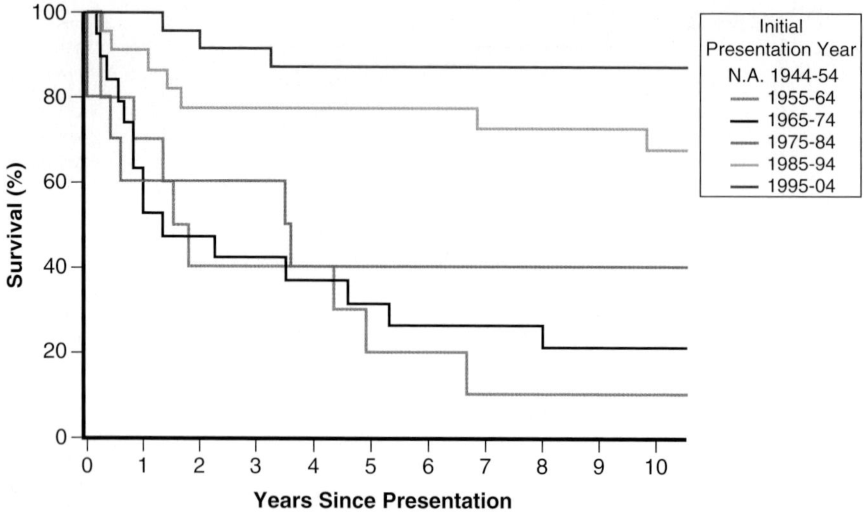

Fig. 9.3 Survival rates for patients with regional (SEER stage) ovarian cancer (1944–2004) ($P<0.0001$, log-rank test for trend). Because of the very small number of individuals with regional ovarian cancer seen from 1944 to 1954, data from this period were excluded. *N.A.* not applicable.

endometrioid or serous carcinomas, or clear cell carcinomas—have a 5-year survival of about 50%. Thus, such a heterogeneous group of tumors does not lend itself to a very meaningful analysis.

Survival in Women with Regional Disease

Survival outcome data for women with regional disease—presumably stage II—are presented in Fig. 9.3. It is apparent that overall survival improved markedly during the last two decades of the study period, with 5-year survival rates of 40% or less before the mid-1980s increasing to 77–87% after that. Similarly, 10-year survival rates of 40% or less increased to 68–87%. One possible explanation for this phenomenon is that surgical staging became increasingly accurate during the latter time frame because of better physician education and training. Conversely, in the earlier time frame, patients with apparent regional spread actually had more advanced disease that went undetected because of suboptimal surgical staging.

Survival in Women with Distant Disease

As expected, survival for women with distant or advanced-stage disease was uniformly poor throughout the entire study period (Fig 9.4). However, significant

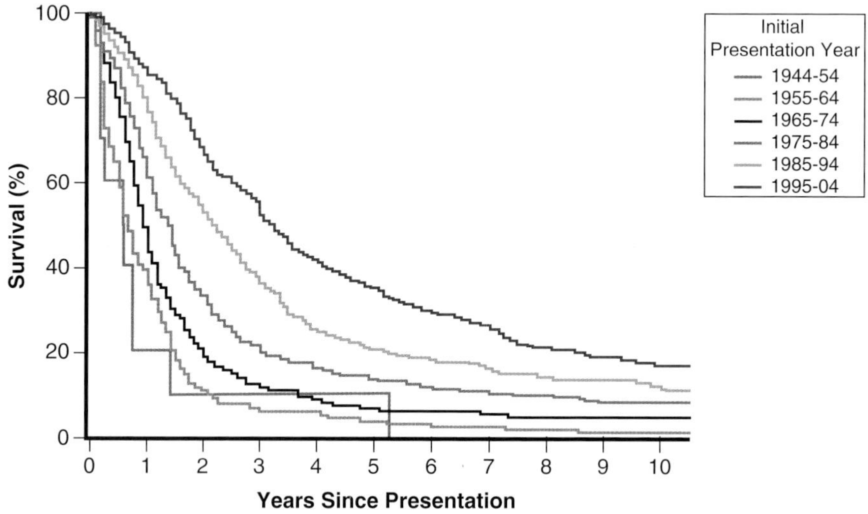

Fig. 9.4 Survival rates for patients with distant (SEER stage) ovarian cancer (1944–2004) ($P<0.0001$, log-rank test for trend).

improvement in survival occurred during the last two decades of the study period. Five-year survival rates significantly improved, from less than 14% in the mid-1980s to 21% in the 1985–1994 decade, and then to 35% in the 1995–2004 period. Likewise, 10-year survival rates essentially doubled between the mid-1980s and the last decade of the study period.

Possible explanations for this improvement in outcome for patients with advanced-stage disease include the more widespread practice of aggressive cytoreductive surgery beginning in the 1980s. Additionally, platinum-based combination chemotherapy became the standard postoperative therapy by the mid-1980s, and taxanes were introduced into standard chemotherapy regimens by the mid-1990s.

Current Management Approach

Standard treatment for epithelial ovarian cancer has improved over the past few decades, based on results from randomized trials combined with large-scale descriptive studies. For women with apparent early-stage disease (stages I and II), accurate surgical staging is a major treatment principle. Adjuvant therapy is generally recommended for patients with high-risk disease (stage I high-grade serous and endometrioid tumors, clear cell tumors, and stage II tumors) and consists of taxane/platinum chemotherapy. No postoperative therapy is recommended for those with low-risk disease (stage I low-grade serous and endometrioid tumors and mucinous tumors).

For women with advanced-stage disease, treatment principles consist of maximum primary cytoreductive surgery followed by chemotherapy. For selected patients with serious comorbidities, massive effusions, or extensive disease (e.g., hepatic metastases or extensive upper abdominal disease), neoadjuvant chemotherapy followed by interval cytoreductive surgery is generally recommended. This approach has recently been studied in a European randomized study.

Standard postoperative therapy for advanced-stage patients includes the combination of a taxane (paclitaxel or docetaxel) and carboplatin for six cycles. However, several alternate strategies have been, or are being, studied in randomized clinical trials and are usually considered potential treatment options. Three randomized trials conducted by the GOG have demonstrated enhanced outcome in women with optimal residual disease who received intraperitoneal chemotherapy compared with pure intravenous chemotherapy. Survival improvement was most pronounced in the most recent trial (GOG 172); however, only 42% of women in the intraperitoneal chemotherapy arm were able to complete six cycles, and the toxic effects in terms of neurotoxicity and neutropenia were substantial [6]. Another strategy that has been studied in two randomized trials is the addition of bevacizumab (both concomitantly with chemotherapy and as maintenance therapy); preliminary results appear to be positive, but final reports are not yet available.

For women with advanced-stage disease, maintenance therapy after completion of primary chemotherapy remains an option [7]. One randomized trial demonstrated a progression-free survival advantage for patients who received 12 vs. 3 monthly cycles of paclitaxel, and a follow-up randomized trial is in progress.

For women who develop recurrent disease, the current approach is to categorize them as either platinum-sensitive (treatment-free interval of ≥6 months) or platinum-resistant (treatment-free interval of <6 months). Options for women with platinum-sensitive recurrent disease include combinations of paclitaxel/carboplatin, gemcitabine/platinum, or pegylated liposomal doxorubicin. For those with platinum-resistant disease, treatment options include pegylated liposomal doxorubicin, topotecan, gemcitabine with or without platinum, capecitabine, oral etoposide, hormonal therapy (tamoxifen), docetaxel, or bevacizumab [8]. In addition, for women with platinum-sensitive recurrent disease, secondary cytoreductive surgery has been reported to be potentially beneficial in several retrospective studies and is being studied in multiple randomized clinical trials.

Targeted therapies are a major focus of clinical trials for women with recurrent ovarian cancer. Examples include the use of poly (ADP)-ribose polymerase (PARP) inhibitors in women with BRCA germline mutations, as well as phosphatidylinositol-3 kinase (PI3K)/AKT/mTOR inhibitors and inhibitors of the MAP kinase pathway in women with low-grade serous carcinomas [9, 10]. Concomitantly, separate trials are emerging for women with uncommon subtypes—BRCA germline mutations, low-grade serous carcinomas, clear cell carcinomas, and mucinous carcinomas.

For patients with uncommon histologic types—malignant germ cell tumors and sex cord-stromal tumors—contemporary treatment is quite different. Primary surgery is standard for all patients. For adult patients with all histologic subtypes of malignant germ cell tumors—except stage IA dysgerminoma and stage I, grade 1 immature teratoma—the standard for several years has been postoperative chemotherapy with BEP. However, in the pediatric population, surveillance is being studied as an alternative. Several reports already indicate favorable outcomes with close postoperative surveillance, but further study is warranted, especially for adults.

For patients with sex cord-stromal tumors, primary surgery remains the cornerstone of treatment. For postoperative management, no standard exists. For stage I granulosa cell tumor, no postoperative therapy is recommended. For women with metastatic disease, platinum-based chemotherapy is generally recommended, with BEP or paclitaxel/carboplatin being the two most popular regimens. In addition, patients with stage I poorly differentiated Sertoli–Leydig cell tumors appear to have a poor prognosis, with a relapse rate as high as 60%. Thus, adjuvant chemotherapy may be recommended, although sufficient data indicating a benefit of such are lacking.

Perspective and Future Directions

As the standards for care are methodically assessed, the overarching intent is to extend the lives of our patients. A report from the Surveillance, Epidemiology, and End Results (SEER) program suggests that steady progress is being made in this regard, with years of life gained from treatment nearly doubling between the early 1970s and the 2000s. However, closer examination of these data suggests that the proportion of patients cured of their disease contributes only a small fraction to this statistic, highlighting both the marginal improved efficacy of existing therapy and the urgent need for effective screening and early detection. Nevertheless, the contemporary investigative environment is challenging each of these areas aggressively and with greater statistical rigor.

One particularly promising development is the exponential growth in our understanding of the biological processes of this disease. Concerted efforts to ferret out critically linked processes driving the malignant phenotype have led to the incorporation of novel agents, used both alone and in combination with other agents, such as chemotherapy. The most mature of these currently in use in ovarian cancer is bevacizumab, a chimeric antibody targeting vascular endothelial growth factor A (VEGF-A), which has demonstrated clinical efficacy as a single agent and in combination with chemotherapy in both the recurrent and front-line settings. Several ongoing trials are evaluating its efficacy in combination with various chemotherapy backbones in recurrent disease and in combination with other biological agents. The clinical promise in targeting this pathway for ovarian cancer patients has ushered in a number of new agents that are also in clinical development, including those targeting the recently discovered mechanisms of resistance to VEGF antibody targeting and those focusing on important tumor growth and survivor factors, such as the PI3K family pathway.

Seemingly endless in potential possibilities, this emerging cache of information has enabled the consideration of personalizing treatment to individual tumor characteristics. Numerous challenges abide in this intuitive next step, but at least some inference into the possibility may be realized by reviewing the impact of agents targeting the single-strand DNA repair enzyme, PARP, in patients with germline mutation in BRCA. These patients who develop ovarian cancer generally harbor tumors in which the homologous recombination function from BRCA is impaired, placing greater responsibility on PARP for continued growth. Several PARP inhibitors have entered the clinic, and preliminary evidence supports the hypothesis that these agents are efficacious in this setting; this is because of the inhibitor's limited toxicity, which is due to the intact function of BRCA in unaffected tissues.

As outlined above, treatment standards for both epithelial and non-epithelial ovarian cancer continue to be refined. MD Anderson continues to play a pivotal role in this progress through its discovery and translation of new therapy options, including the emergence of the therapeutic delivery of non-coding RNA; its expertise in rare tumors of the ovary; its leadership in bringing a global audience to the clinical investigation of these diseases; and its investigative leadership and continued participation in a cooperative group mechanism of investigation.

References

1. Smith JP, Rutledge JP. Chemotherapy in the treatment of cancer of the ovary. Am J Obstet Gynecol. 1970;107:691–703.
2. Gershenson DM, Morris M, Cangir A, et al. Treatment of malignant germ cell tumors of the ovary with bleomycin, etoposide, and cisplatin. J Clin Oncol. 1990;8:715–20.
3. McGuire WP, Hoskins WJ, Brady MF, et al. Cyclophosphamide and cisplatin compared with paclitaxel and cisplatin in patients with stage III and stage IV ovarian cancer. N Engl J Med. 1996;334:1–6.
4. Brown J, Shvartsman HS, Deavers MT, et al. The activity of taxanes in the treatment of sex cord-stromal ovarian tumors. J Clin Oncol. 2004;22:3517–23.
5. Ozols RF, Bundy BN, Greer BE, et al. Phase III trial of carboplatin and paclitaxel compared with cisplatin and paclitaxel in patients with optimally resected stage III ovarian cancer: a Gynecologic Oncology Group study. J Clin Oncol. 2003;21:3194–200.
6. Armstrong DK, Bundy B, Wenzel L, et al. Intraperitoneal cisplatin and paclitaxel in ovarian cancer. N Engl J Med. 2006;354:34–43.
7. Herzog TJ, Coleman RL, Markman M, et al. The role of maintenance therapy and novel taxanes in ovarian cancer. Gynecol Oncol. 2006;102:218–25.
8. Burger RA, Sill MW, Monk BJ, et al. Phase II trial of bevacizumab in persistent or recurrent epithelial ovarian cancer or primary peritoneal cancer: a Gynecologic Oncology Group Study. J Clin Oncol. 2007;25:5165–71.
9. Fong PC, Boss DS, Yap TA, et al. Inhibition of poly(ADP-ribose) polymerase in tumors from BRCA mutation carriers. N Engl J Med. 2009;361:123–34.
10. Hennessy BT, Coleman RL, Markman M. Ovarian cancer. Lancet. 2009;374:1371–82.

Chapter 10
Cervical Cancer

Patricia J. Eifel and Charles Levenback

Introduction

Since its inception in 1948, MD Anderson Cancer Center has been at the forefront of innovative cervical cancer treatment. In the 1940s, cervical cancer was still a very important public health problem in the United States. Although cytologic screening and treatment of preinvasive disease subsequently led to a dramatic reduction in the incidence of invasive cervical cancer in the United States, this disease continues to affect about 11,000 women per year. In 2009, an estimated 4,070 women died of cervical cancer in the United States. Cervical cancer disproportionately affects medically underserved women in the United States and is still a leading cause of cancer death for women in many underdeveloped countries. During the past 60 years, innovations in treatment have substantially improved outcome and quality of life for many patients with this disease.

Historical Perspective

Fortunately, cervical cancer is usually confined locoregionally at presentation. Good outcome depends on appropriate selection and skilled delivery of locoregional treatments. For patients who have small cancers (usually ≤4 cm) confined to the

P.J. Eifel (✉)
Department of Radiation Oncology, The University of Texas MD Anderson Cancer Center, 1515 Holcombe Boulevard, Houston, TX 77030, USA
e-mail: peifel@mdanderson.org

C. Levenback
Department of Gynecologic and Reproductive Medicine, The University of Texas MD Anderson Cancer Center, Houston, TX, USA

M.A. Rodriguez et al. (eds.), *60 Years of Survival Outcomes at The University of Texas MD Anderson Cancer Center*, DOI 10.1007/978-1-4614-5197-6_10,

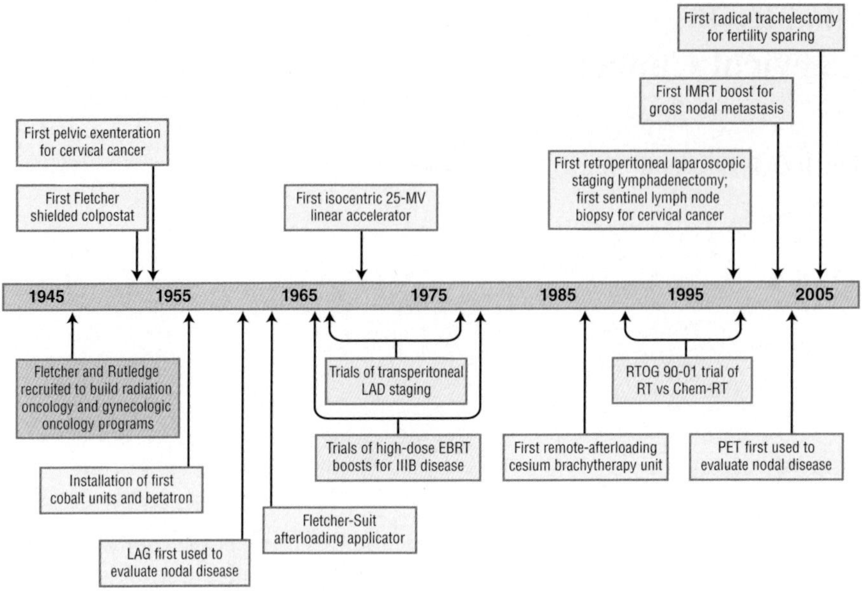

Fig. 10.1 Timeline of sentinel events in the treatment of cervical cancer at MD Anderson Cancer. *EBRT* external beam radiation therapy, *IMRT* intensity-modulated radiation therapy, *LAD* lymphadenectomy, *LAG* lymphangiography, *PET* positron emission tomography, *RT* radiation therapy, *RTOG* Radiation Therapy Oncology Group.

cervix, either radical hysterectomy or primary radiation therapy may be curative. For patients with more locally advanced cancers, radiation therapy is usually the treatment of choice. In the late 1990s, prospective randomized trials demonstrated improved local control and survival rates with use of radiation therapy and concurrent cisplatin-based chemotherapy, which has become standard for most patients with locoregionally advanced disease.

Despite the decreasing national incidence of invasive cervical cancer, MD Anderson's reputation as a center of excellence, its commitment to indigent patient care, and its proximity to Central America resulted in a steady flow of new patients referred for treatment of cervical cancer. From its earliest years, MD Anderson has reported some of the highest survival rates for women with locally advanced disease. The pioneering collaboration between Drs. Gilbert Fletcher (radiation oncologist) and Felix Rutledge (gynecologic oncologist), continued by several generations of radiation oncologists, gynecologic oncologists, imagers, pathologists, and other professionals, made the Gynecologic Oncology Center a model of successful multidisciplinary treatment. Technological innovation, as well as careful observational studies and prospective trials, has led to refinements in treatment that were built on early successes and led to the current high rates of cure, even for patients with locally advanced disease (Fig. 10.1).

The MD Anderson Cancer Center Experience

Between 1944 and December 2004, 21,346 patients with cancer of the cervix were seen at MD Anderson Cancer Center. Of these, 12,833 had received no previous treatment, and 11,442 subsequently received their definitive treatment at MD Anderson. Patients whose primary cancers had arisen in sites other than the cervix or superficial skin were excluded from the analyses. The remaining 10,269 patients were included in survival analyses.

The initial stages at presentation of women with cervical cancer treated at MD Anderson from 1944 through 2004 (Table 10.1) were classified according to the Surveillance, Epidemiology, and End Results (SEER) 1977 system (Table 10.2).

The overall survival of patients treated for cervical cancer between 1944 and 2004 is shown in Fig. 10.2 and Table 10.3. Significant improvement in overall survival was observed over the 60-year study period. Particularly marked improvements in overall survival were seen in the time intervals after 1955 and 1975, which correspond to periods of major change in the management of cervical cancer at MD Anderson.

Local Disease

As seen in Fig. 10.1, the first of these improvements in survival followed a period of dramatic technological innovation that, by the late 1950s, had put in place most of the tools that are central to the successful treatment of locally advanced disease. MD Anderson was one of the first medical centers in the world to embrace the use of megavoltage radiation. The beam of the 25 MV betatron, in particular, was ideally suited to the treatment of deep pelvic tumors and was used immediately after its introduction in 1956 to treat most patients with invasive cervical cancer at MD Anderson. Unfortunately, this expensive technology was not widely embraced in other centers; few units were produced, and it wasn't until the 1980s, with the production of

Table 10.1 Women with cervical cancer treated at MD Anderson, 1944–2004

	SEER stage at presentation					
	In situ	Local	Regional	Distant	Unstaged	Total
Decade	[No. (%) of patients]					
1944–1954	24 (3.9)	164 (26.8)	394 (64.3)	11 (1.8)	20 (3.3)	613 (100.0)
1955–1964	329 (14.4)	586 (25.6)	1,211 (52.9)	141 (6.2)	21 (0.9)	2,288 (100.0)
1965–1974	479 (21.2)	576 (25.5)	1,003 (44.4)	198 (8.8)	3 (0.1)	2,259 (100.0)
1975–1984	537 (25.5)	658 (31.2)	748 (35.5)	159 (7.5)	8 (0.4)	2,110 (100.0)
1985–1994	430 (22.4)	730 (38.0)	570 (29.6)	162 (8.4)	31 (1.6)	1,923 (100.0)
1995–2004	147 (13.7)	395 (36.7)	349 (32.4)	146 (13.6)	39 (3.6)	1,076 (100.0)
Total	*1,946 (19.0)*	*3,109 (30.3)*	*4,275 (41.6)*	*817 (8.0)*	*122 (1.2)*	*10,269 (100.0)*

SEER Surveillance, Epidemiology, and End Results program

Table 10.2 Surveillance, Epidemiology, and End Results (SEER) program staging groups[a]

In situ
Noninvasive, preinvasive, intraepithelial
Local
Minimal stromal invasion; "microinvasion"
Invasive cancer confined to the cervix
Regional (by direct extension or nodes)
Direct extension to:
Corpus uterus (body of the uterus)
Upper 2/3 of the vaginal wall including fornices
Parametrium (paracervical soft tissue)
Broad, cardinal or uterosacral ligaments
Lower 1/3 of the vagina
Bladder wall; bladder, NOS excluding mucosa;
Bullous edema of the bladder mucosa
Rectal wall; rectum, NOS excluding mucosa
Tumor causes hydronephrosis or nonfunctioning kidney (FIGO IIIB)
Cul de sac (rectouterine pouch)
Pelvic lymph nodes:
Hypogastric, iliac, obturator, paracervical, parametrial, sacral, or pelvic nodes, NOS
Distant (by direct extension, distant nodes, or metastasis)
Direct extension to:
Bladder or rectal mucosa
Ureter
Urethral
Sigmoid colon
Small intestine
Vulva
Ovary or fallopian tube
"Frozen pelvis"
Distant lymph nodes
Aortic, inguinal, other distant nodes
Distant metastases
Bone, brain, liver, lung

[a]From [1]

15–20 MV linear accelerators, that most other major centers began to have access to the deeply penetrating radiation beams that are best suited to pelvic treatment.

At about this same time, Dr. Gilbert Fletcher and his colleague, Dr. Herman Suit, began developing innovative vaginal brachytherapy applicators that markedly improved the safety and practicality of cervical cancer brachytherapy [2]. By the early 1960s, radiation oncologists at MD Anderson had leveraged these two elements—high-energy pelvic external beam therapy and high-quality intracavitary brachytherapy—to optimize treatment for most patients with localized cervical cancer [3, 4]. Meanwhile, Felix Rutledge developed surgical techniques that optimized treatment for patients with very early stage I disease, particularly for young women who would benefit from preserved ovarian function.

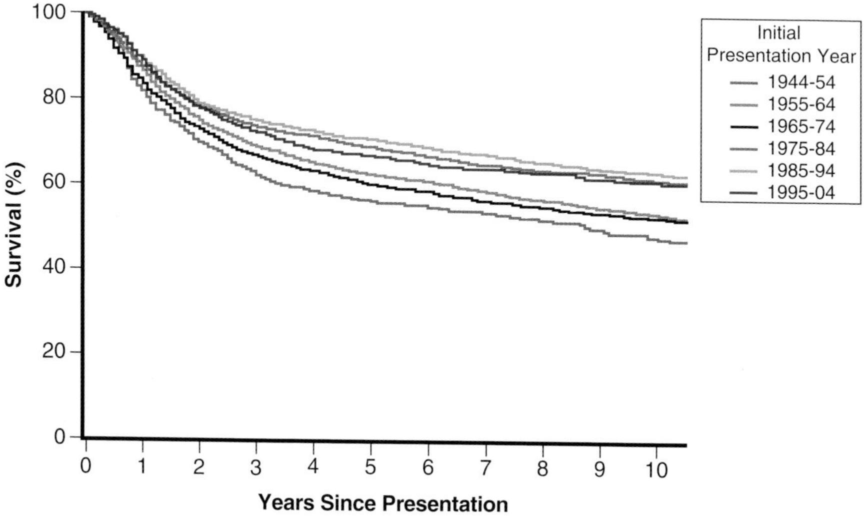

Fig. 10.2 Overall survival rates for patients with cervical cancer (1944–2004) ($P<0.0001$, log-rank test for trend).

Table 10.3 Overall survival according to years treated and SEER stage groups

	SEER stage (% survival)					
	Local		Regional		Distant	
Decade	5 years	10 years	5 years	10 years	5 years	10 years
1944–1954	74.9	63.2	49.2	42.6	9.1	9.1
1955–1964	79.8	70.9	52.8	42.8	7.8	5.0
1965–1974	84.1	76.4	41.9	32.5	6.7	2.6
1975–1984	82.5	73.6	50.4	41.7	8.6	4.2
1985–1994	83.0	73.2	53.6	45.4	13.3	9.5
1995–2004	82.6	78.3	57.3	51.8	16.9	12.7

SEER Surveillance, Epidemiology, and End Results program

With these innovations, outcome for patients with localized disease improved markedly, with cure rates in the 1970s that approached those achieved today (Fig. 10.3). Recurrences were rare for patients with early-stage disease treated with radical surgery or radiation therapy. Although some patients experienced treatment-related adverse effects, long-term follow-up studies indicated that major complications were uncommon, particularly in patients who were treated for early disease [5]. However, pelvic recurrence continued to be a problem for some patients with localized tumors that measured ≥5 cm in diameter [6]. Although local treatment with irradiation is still the mainstay of modern management, recent trials have demonstrated that outcome can be improved with use of concurrent cisplatin-based chemotherapy [7].

Recent research efforts have focused on reducing the adverse effects of treatment in patients with very early, localized, smaller tumors [International Federation of

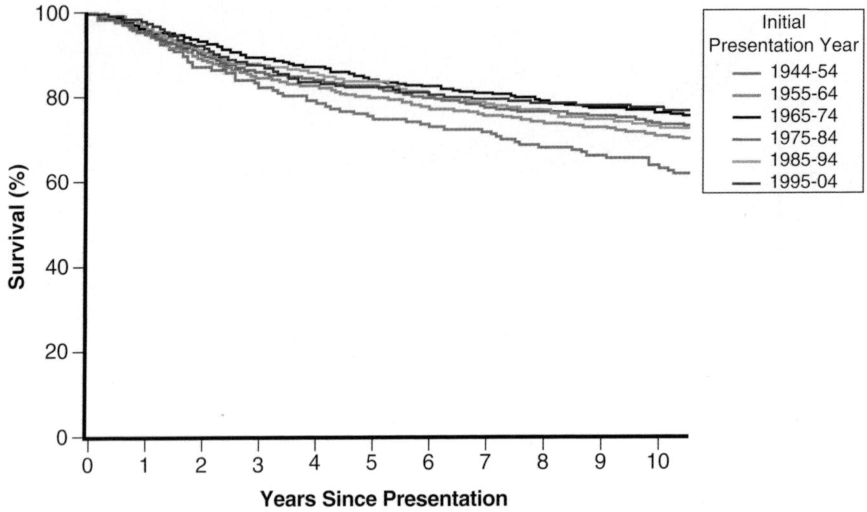

Fig. 10.3 Survival rates for patients with local (SEER stage) cervical cancer (1944–2004) ($P=0.044$, log-rank test for trend).

Gynecology and Obstetrics (FIGO) stage IB1]. Laparoscopic surgical techniques, including fertility-sparing radical hysterectomy, have improved the quality of life for appropriately selected women with early cervical cancers [8].

Surgical techniques for patients with localized disease have been rapidly developing in recent years. In 2005, the first radical trachelectomy was performed at MD Anderson [9]. Since then, multiple successful pregnancies have been reported among cervical cancer survivors treated with fertility-sparing surgery. MD Anderson investigators have pioneered sentinel lymph node biopsy in cervical cancer patients [10]. It is hoped that sentinel lymph node biopsy combined with minimally invasive surgical techniques will further reduce morbidity and mortality and preserve fertility in patients with small cervical cancers.

Regional Disease

Although the treatments available in the 1960s were excellent for patients with early disease, the 15-cm × 15-cm maximum field size of the betatron limited its utility for patients with regionally advanced disease; furthermore, the rapid dose gradient of intracavitary brachytherapy sometimes failed to sterilize tumor that had infiltrated the paracervical spaces. Although radiation therapy cured many patients with these more advanced, unresectable tumors, many others were still dying of uncontrolled regionally progressive cancer. In the 1970s, research at MD Anderson focused on improving outcome for these patients.

MD Anderson investigators recognized that regional nodal recurrence was an important element of treatment failure for patients with locally advanced disease. In the early 1960s, the only method of pelvic and nodal evaluation was exploratory laparotomy and lymphadenectomy. The first technique for imaging intra-abdominal lymph nodes, lymphangiography, was developed in the early 1960s. Previously, this technically demanding imaging method had been used primarily to stage lymphomas. However, in a series of carefully conducted correlative studies, Dr. Sidney Wallace and the gynecologic oncology team at MD Anderson demonstrated that lymphangiography permitted the detection of even sub-centimeter lymph node metastases in cervical cancer patients [11]. This was an important innovation that allowed clinicians to customize regional treatment of patients with nodal disease.

During this time, clinicians also studied the role of pretreatment lymphadenectomy in patients with locally advanced disease. Surgical staging was an accurate method for detecting nodal metastasis; however, by the late 1970s, it had become apparent that pretreatment transperitoneal staging markedly increased the incidence and severity of late radiation complications [12]. For this reason, surgical staging was abandoned until the late 1980s, when retroperitoneal staging was shown to prevent the intraperitoneal adhesions that escalated the morbidity of postoperative radiation therapy. The most recent advance in surgical staging is a retroperitoneal laparoscopic technique that was introduced at MD Anderson in 2003. This technique results in minimal treatment delay since the surgical incisions are limited to four puncture wounds.

By the early 1960s, 40 Gy of 25 MV pelvic external beam irradiation combined with low dose-rate intracavitary brachytherapy was yielding high 5-year survival rates for women with localized disease. However, pelvic recurrence rates were still high in patients with stage III disease. After MD Anderson acquired the deeply penetrating betatron beam, clinicians explored the differences in the balance of external beam and brachytherapy and hypothesized that the lateral parametrium might be more effectively treated with external beam boosts than with brachytherapy. Unfortunately, this approach resulted in a high incidence of major complications without improving the rate of local control [13]; in fact, during this period, the survival rate of patients with regional disease actually declined (Fig. 10.4). By the early 1980s, clinicians had come to realize that increases in the dose of external beam irradiation at the expense of brachytherapy had not improved outcome; brachytherapy was reemphasized in the treatment of stage IIIB disease with even greater weighting than in the early 1960s. With these modifications in treatment policy, survival rates for stage III disease approached 50%, exceeding those achieved at any previous time [13].

In 1990, MD Anderson physicians initiated a multi-institutional trial through the Radiation Therapy Oncology Group that compared treatment with irradiation alone with irradiation and concurrent cisplatin-based chemotherapy [7]. More than 40% of those enrolled in this trial were MD Anderson patients. This ground-breaking randomized trial demonstrated a 50% reduction in risk of recurrence with use of chemoradiation and stimulated a major change in the standard of care for locoregionally advanced cervical cancer. The introduction of concurrent cisplatin-based chemotherapy to standard management with irradiation corresponded with significant improvement in survival of patients with regional disease in 1995–2004 (Fig. 10.4).

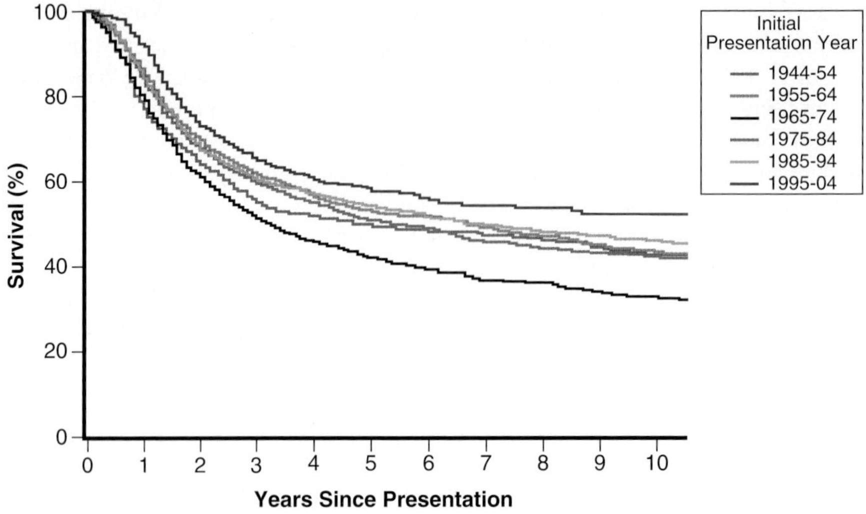

Fig. 10.4 Survival rates for patients with regional (SEER stage) cervical cancer (1944–2004) ($P<0.0001$, log-rank test for trend).

Metastatic Disease

The prognosis for most patients who present with distant disease is still poor. However, long-term survival rates have gradually improved, particularly during the most recent decade (1995–2004), when 17% of patients with distant disease survived at least 5 years (Fig. 10.5). Without more detailed analysis, it is hazardous to speculate on the reasons for this improvement. Certainly contributing to this improvement, however, were the advances made in diagnostic imaging and the selected use of retroperitoneal and laparoscopic surgical staging, which have permitted earlier detection of distant disease; some patients who benefitted from these advances, particularly those with para-aortic metastases, are now curable with conformal radiation therapy, which is often combined with concurrent cisplatin chemotherapy.

Although the prognosis of most patients with disease recurrence is poor, some with localized recurrence can be cured with radical radiation therapy or surgery [14, 15]. Dr. Rutledge was one of a handful of gynecologic oncologists who pioneered total pelvic exenteration for recurrent cervical cancer [15]. The essential indications for this operation have remained unchanged; however, diagnostic screening methods and surgical techniques have dramatically improved. Some of the surgical innovations that were developed to decrease the morbidity and improve the quality of life for patients undergoing pelvic exenteration, were continent urinary conduits, low rectal reanastomosis, and vertical rectus myocutaneous flap to construct a neovagina. As radiation therapy techniques have improved, the number of patients with central failure has declined; for selected patients, however, exenterative surgery is the only curative option. MD Anderson remains a referral center for these ultraradical procedures.

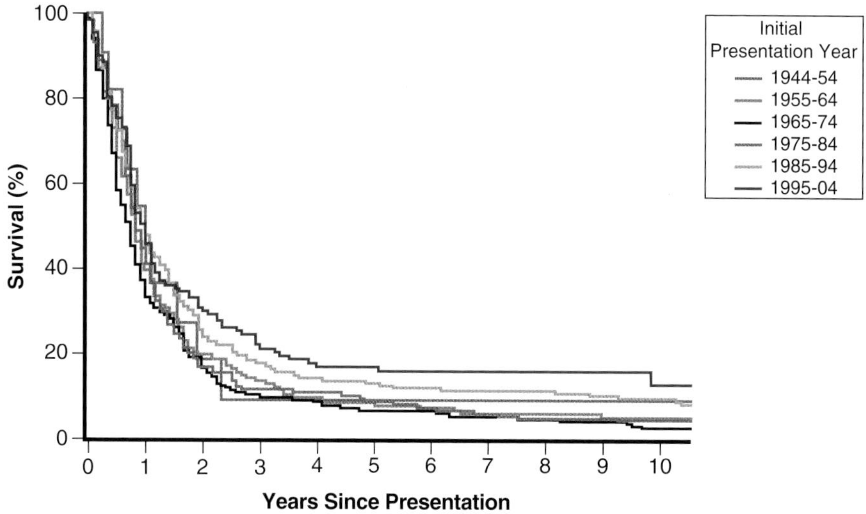

Fig. 10.5 Survival rates for patients with distant (SEER stage) cervical cancer (1944–2004) (P=0.003, log-rank test for trend).

Unfortunately, some patients still present with incurable distant metastatic disease. Improvements have been made in palliative multimodality therapy for these patients. However, progress with chemotherapy for advanced or recurrent squamous carcinomas has been very slow, and trials are considered successful if survival is increased by even a few months. New targeted therapies are becoming available for patients with advanced or recurrent disease and provide some hope for improved outcome for these patients in the future.

Supportive care, including improved pain management and spiritual support, has also been incorporated into the care of women who are dying of cervical cancer. Consultation services at MD Anderson, including the Pain Management Service, Palliative Care service, and Chaplaincy, have helped relieve the suffering of patients and families in these heartbreaking situations.

Discussion

Following the major technological advances in radiation therapy in the late 1950s, the elements were in place for a multidisciplinary team at MD Anderson to achieve remarkably high cure rates for most patients with locoregionally confined cervical cancer. During the three decades that followed, advances in imaging permitted more focused treatment of regional disease as clinicians learned to balance external beam therapy, brachytherapy, and surgical treatments to effect the highest therapeutic ratios. The survival rates achieved for these patients in the 1980s were among the highest reported in the clinical literature and were exceeded only when the value of concurrent chemotherapy was demonstrated in prospective randomized trials.

These trends are undoubtedly reflected in the evolving overall outcomes of our patients. However, the data need to be viewed with caution. During the past 60 years, many changes have taken place in tumor classification systems, methods of staging, patterns of referral, and other factors that could compromise the validity of historical comparisons. The clinical staging system is subjective and has been modified many times since 1948 [16]. For example, in the mid 1970s, FIGO added to the rules of staging an admonition that clinicians should choose the lesser stage whenever there was uncertainty about involvement of paracervical tissues; for the first time, they stated specifically that paracervical thickening that was not nodular should not be considered grounds for upstaging. Retrospective studies have shown that after this amendment to the rules of staging, a marked decline was noted in the proportion of patients diagnosed as having FIGO stage III disease on the basis of pelvic wall involvement at MD Anderson [13]. This and other changes were undoubtedly the source of stage migration that may have confounded historical comparisons.

Current Management Approach

In the current decade, advances in diagnostic imaging and treatment of cervical cancer are continuing that should lead to further improvements in outcome. The routine use of irradiation and concurrent chemotherapy, for example, beginning only in the last years of this review, should continue to improve outcome in future years.

Today, the definition of disease extent with magnetic resonance imaging and positron emission tomography is much more accurate than was possible using methods from the previous century. This permits more accurate selection of treatments for patients with various stages of disease. Radical hysterectomy continues to be the preferred treatment for small tumors, particularly in young women; however, this surgery is usually performed with use of laparoscopic or even robotic techniques that reduce postoperative recovery time and morbidity. In selected cases of young women who wish to preserve fertility, radical trachelectomy may be offered as a fertility-sparing option.

Today, irradiation and concurrent cisplatin-based chemotherapy (usually used weekly) is the standard treatment for most women with locally advanced disease. External beam therapy is always performed with use of three-dimensional image-guided techniques. Advances in the delivery of radiation, such as with use of intensity-modulated radiation therapy, permit clinicians to more accurately deliver tumoricidal doses of radiation to areas of gross regional involvement with less risk to adjacent critical structures than was possible with older techniques. Today, most brachytherapy is delivered with use of pulsed dose-rate or high dose-rate techniques that are safer than older brachytherapy delivery methods and permit greater individualization.

With these advances, however, the treatment of cervical cancer has become increasingly complex. The culture of close multidisciplinary collaboration that was initially fostered by Drs. Fletcher and Rutledge has never been more important. The integrated MD Anderson team of gynecologic oncologists, radiation oncologists, pathologists, diagnostic imagers, nurses, social workers, dieticians, physicists, therapists, and scientists is a model that must be considered one of the most important contributions to the curative treatment of women with this disease.

References

1. Young Jr JL, Roffers SD, Ries LAG, Fritz AG, Hurlbut AA, editors. SEER summary staging manual – 2000: codes and coding instructions. NIH Pub. No. 01-4969. Bethesda: National Cancer Institute; 2001.
2. Suit HD, Moore EB, Fletcher GH, et al. Modification of Fletcher ovoid system for afterloading, using standard-sized radium tubes (milligram and microgram). Radiology. 1963;81:126–31.
3. Fletcher GH, Rutledge FN, Chau PM. Policies of treatment in cancer of the cervix uteri. Am J Roentgenol Radium Ther Nucl Med. 1962;87:6–21.
4. Fletcher GH. Cancer of the uterine cervix. Janeway Lecture, 1970. Am J Roentgenol Radium Ther Nucl Med. 1971;3:225–42.
5. Eifel PJ, Levenback C, Wharton JT, et al. Time course and incidence of late complications in patients treated with radiation therapy for FIGO stage IB carcinoma of the uterine cervix. Int J Radiat Oncol Biol Phys. 1995;32:1289–300.
6. Eifel PJ, Morris M, Wharton JT, et al. The influence of tumor size and morphology on the outcome of patients with FIGO stage IB squamous cell carcinoma of the uterine cervix. Int J Radiat Oncol Biol Phys. 1994;29:9–16.
7. Eifel PJ, Winter K, Morris M, et al. Pelvic irradiation with concurrent chemotherapy versus pelvic and para-aortic irradiation for high-risk cervical cancer: an update of Radiation Therapy Oncology Group trial (RTOG) 90–01. J Clin Oncol. 2004;22:872–80.
8. Ramirez PT, Schmeler KM, Malpica A, et al. Safety and feasibility of robotic radical trachelectomy in patients with early-stage cervical cancer. Gynecol Oncol. 2010;116:512–5.
9. Ramirez PT, Schmeler KM, Soliman PT, et al. Fertility preservation in patients with early cervical cancer: radical trachelectomy. Gynecol Oncol. 2008;110:S25–8.
10. Levenback C, Coleman RL, Burke TW, et al. Lymphatic mapping and sentinel node identification in patients with cervix cancer undergoing radical hysterectomy and pelvic lymphadenectomy. J Clin Oncol. 2002;20:688–93.
11. Piver S, Wallace S, Castro JR. The accuracy of lymphangiography in carcinoma of the uterine cervix. Am J Roentgenol. 1971;111:97–101.
12. Wharton JT, Jones 3rd HW, Day Jr TG, et al. Preirradiation celiotomy and extended field irradiation for invasive carcinoma of the cervix. Obstet Gynecol. 1977;49:333–8.
13. Logsdon MD, Eifel PJ. FIGO IIIB squamous cell carcinoma of the cervix: an analysis of prognostic factors emphasizing the balance between external beam and intracavitary radiation therapy. Int J Radiat Oncol Biol Phys. 1999;43:763–75.
14. Ijaz T, Eifel PJ, Burke T, et al. Radiation therapy of pelvic recurrence after radical hysterectomy for cervical carcinoma. Gynecol Oncol. 1998;70:241–6.
15. Rutledge FN, Burns Jr BC. Pelvic exenteration. Am J Obstet Gynecol. 1965;91:692–708.
16. Eifel PJ. Problems with the clinical staging of carcinoma of the cervix. Semin Radiat Oncol. 1994;4:1–8.

Chapter 11
Endometrial Cancer

Thomas Burke, Anuja Jhingran, Karen Lu, and Russell Broaddus

Introduction

Endometrial cancers are the most common of the gynecologic malignancies, affecting an estimated 42,160 U.S. women in 2009 [1]. Both the incidence and the death rates associated with endometrial cancer have been gradually increasing. Carcinoma develops as a proliferation of epithelial cells lining the glands of the uterine cavity. Many endometrial tumors exhibit an indolent growth pattern and are contained within the uterus at the time of diagnosis. Spread to regional lymph nodes or distant metastatic sites such as the liver or lungs is less common. It is conceptually convenient to categorize endometrial tumors into two types: a hormonally driven well-differentiated lesion that is typically associated with a favorable prognosis, and an undifferentiated or variant group of histologic subtypes characterized by more aggressive clinical behavior and a poorer prognosis. Postmenopausal status, low parity, obesity, diabetes, and estrogen exposure have been epidemiologically associated

T. Burke (✉)
Department of Gynecologic Oncology, The University of Texas MD Anderson Cancer Center, 1400 Pressler Street, Unit 1485, Houston, TX 77030, USA
e-mail: tburke@mdanderson.org

A. Jhingran
Department of Radiation Oncology, The University of Texas MD Anderson Cancer Center, Houston, TX, USA

K. Lu
Department of Gynecologic Oncology and Reproductive Medicine, The University of Texas MD Anderson Cancer Center, Houston, TX, USA

R. Broaddus
Department of Pathology, The University of Texas MD Anderson Cancer Center, Houston, TX, USA

M.A. Rodriguez et al. (eds.), *60 Years of Survival Outcomes at The University of Texas MD Anderson Cancer Center*, DOI 10.1007/978-1-4614-5197-6_11,

with the well-differentiated lesions; the presence of identified oncogenes, overexpression of oncogenic proteins, or activation of aberrant signaling pathways have been more frequently associated with the aggressive variants of endometrial cancer.

Historical Perspective

Since most endometrial cancers are confined to the uterus, surgical treatment by hysterectomy and bilateral salpingo-oophorectomy has been the mainstay of therapy since the 1950s. Primary treatment with external and internal radiotherapy can be curative in a percentage of patients who are not believed to be suitable candidates for surgery [2]. However, cure rates for such therapy have been about 15% lower historically than rates achieved by resection. Throughout the 1950s and 1960s, endometrial cancer was clinically staged on the basis of physical examination, plain film radiography, and biopsy of the endometrium and cervix (Table 11.1). These clinical findings, however, correlated poorly with tumor findings identified at the time of surgical exploration. Consequently, a large national effort to define prognostic factors and spread patterns was undertaken in the 1970s and 1980s [3]. Data from surgical staging trials helped to define predictors of outcome. Specifically, uterine factors of major prognostic significance were found to include histologic grade, depth of myometrial penetration, and extension to the uterine cervix. Extrauterine prognostic features included positive peritoneal cytology, adnexal metastasis, lymph node metastasis to pelvic or para-aortic nodes, and spread to distant organs. This information led to the adoption of a surgical staging system in 1988 (Table 11.2).

Further clinical investigations, undertaken in the 1990s and 2000s, helped to refine treatment approaches and led to the application of minimally invasive surgical techniques, both laparoscopic and robotic; indications for adjuvant radiotherapy including whole pelvic, extended field, and vaginal brachytherapy; and identification of systemic agents with activity in metastatic disease.

Table 11.1 Clinical staging of uterine fundal tumors[a]

Stage	Description
I	The tumor is limited to the uterine fundus
IA	The uterine cavity measures ≤8 cm
IB	The length of the uterine cavity is >8 cm
II	The tumor extends to the uterine cervix
III	The tumor has spread to the adjacent pelvic structures
IV	There is bulky pelvic disease or distant spread
IVA	Tumor invades the mucosa of the bladder or rectosigmoid
IVB	Distant metastases are present

[a]International Federation of Gynecology and Obstetrics, 1988

Table 11.2 Surgical staging of uterine fundal tumors[a]

Stage	Description
I	The tumor is confined to the uterine fundus
IA	The tumor is limited to the endometrium
IB	The tumor invades less than one-half of the myometrial thickness
IC	The tumor invades more than one-half of the myometrial thickness
II	The tumor extends to the cervix
IIA	Cervical extension is limited to the endocervical glands
IIB	The tumor invades the cervical stroma
III	There is regional tumor spread
IIIA	The tumor invades the uterine serosa or adnexa, or there is positive peritoneal cytology
IIIB	Vaginal metastases are present
IIIC	The tumor has spread to pelvic or para-aortic lymph nodes
IV	There is bulky pelvic disease or distant spread
IVA	Tumor invades the mucosa of the bladder or rectosigmoid
IVB	Distant metastases are present

[a]International Federation of Gynecology and Obstetrics, 1988

Table 11.3 Women with endometrial cancer treated at MD Anderson, 1944–2004

	SEER stage at presentation				
	Local	Regional	Distant	Unstaged	Total
Decade	[No. (%) of patients]				
1944–1954	42 (56.8)	17 (23.0)	10 (13.5)	5 (6.8)	74 (100.0)
1955–1964	231 (66.2)	47 (13.5)	64 (18.3)	7 (2.0)	349 (100.0)
1965–1974	352 (68.0)	66 (12.7)	96 (18.5)	4 (0.8)	518 (100.0)
1975–1984	461 (60.2)	168 (21.9)	127 (16.6)	10 (1.3)	766 (100.0)
1985–1994	391 (57.9)	138 (20.4)	119 (17.6)	27 (4.0)	675 (100.0)
1995–2004	417 (59.0)	130 (18.4)	128 (18.1)	32 (4.5)	707 (100.0)
Total	*1,894 (61.3)*	*566 (18.3)*	*544 (17.6)*	*85 (2.8)*	*3,089 (100.0)*

SEER Surveillance, Epidemiology, and End Results program

The MD Anderson Cancer Center Experience

The MD Anderson Tumor Registry data set was derived from 10,182 women who were diagnosed as having endometrial cancer between 1944 and 2004. Of this group, 4,318 had received no previous treatment for their malignancy. After excluding patients with multiple primary cancers and those treated elsewhere, 3,089 women received definitive primary treatment at MD Anderson Cancer Center. The numbers of patients presenting by time interval and stage are summarized in Table 11.3. Sixty-one percent had disease confined to the uterus at diagnosis.

Prior assessment of a subset of stage I cases suggested that the MD Anderson experience was more heavily weighted toward women with high-risk subtypes than

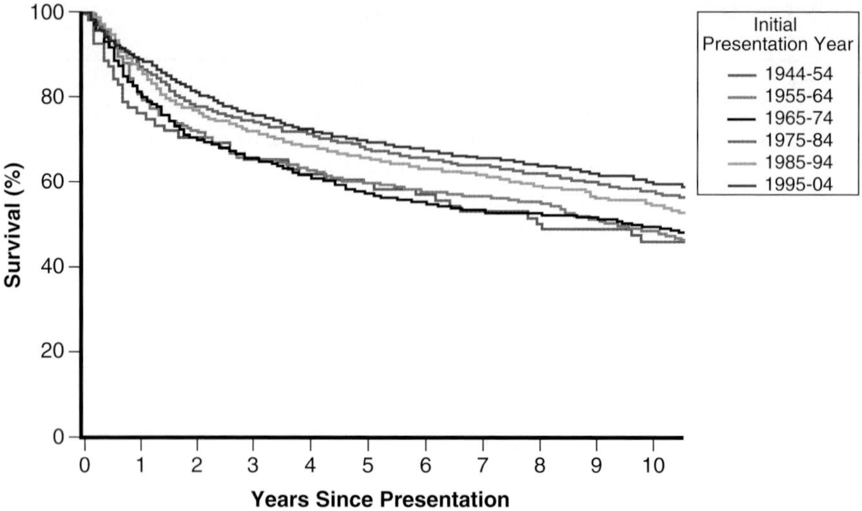

Fig. 11.1 Overall survival rates for patients with endometrial cancer (1944–2004) ($P<0.0001$, log-rank test for trend).

would be seen in the general population [4]. This would not be surprising, given the referral nature of the institution. Several of these aggressive subtypes of endometrial cancer, particularly the clear cell and papillary serous subtypes, were not clearly identified and defined until the 1980s. Consequently, no effort has been made to separate subsets by tumor histology.

The computed survival curves in this chapter represent clinical outcomes for all women who received definitive treatment at MD Anderson between 1944 and 2004. The overall survival curve shows incremental improvement in 5-year survival rates, from 59% to 69%, and in 10-year survival rates, from 46% to 60% (Fig. 11.1). The usual Tumor Registry methodology of describing disease extent under the headings of localized, regional, or distant has been used in the construction of survival curves by "stage." During the earlier years of this analysis, stage assignments were made on the basis of both clinical and limited surgical findings. Clinical findings typically would have been based on physical examination, limited plain film radiographs, and gross evidence of extrauterine disease. A defined surgical assessment and staging procedure would have been performed in most cases from the late 1970s forward. In addition, more recently treated women would have had a more extensive presurgical evaluation by computed tomography or magnetic resonance imaging, particularly when an aggressive histologic subtype was identified in the biopsy specimen. Consequently, stage assignment across the 60-year course of data recording was not uniform but would have been conducted with use of the best available information at the time of registration.

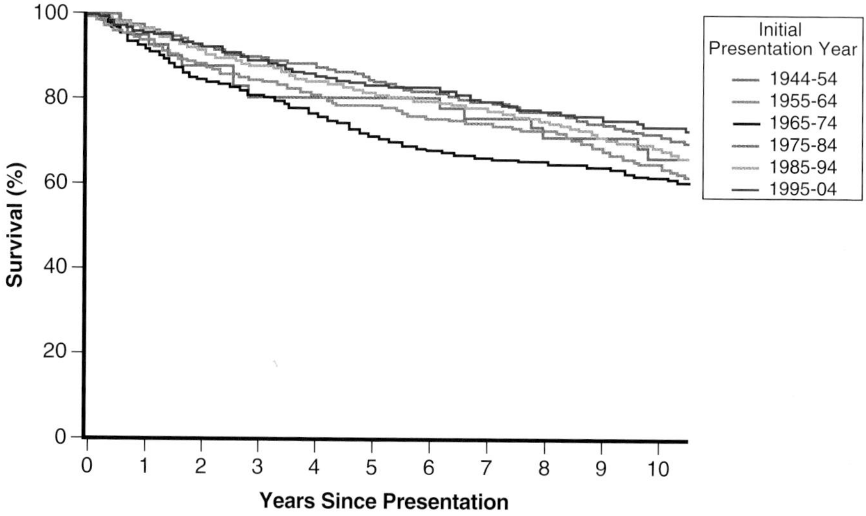

Fig. 11.2 Survival rates for patients with local (SEER stage) endometrial cancer (1944–2004) ($P=0.076$, log-rank test for trend).

Survival Outcome and Localized Tumors

The survival curves for women with localized tumors (Fig. 11.2) reveal significantly improved 5- and 10-year outcomes for women treated during the most recent time intervals (84% and 81%, respectively) compared with outcomes from earlier decades (74% and 64%, respectively) ($P<0.005$). However, since the surgical technique for hysterectomy has not changed substantively over the study period, women with tumor confined to the uterus might have been expected to have identical outcomes over the 60-year period. At least three possible explanations can be given for the observed differences in survival rates. First, surgical staging procedures that incorporated a systematic approach to the detection of extrauterine disease became common during the second half of the study interval. Surgical staging data from MD Anderson and other sources determined that peritoneal cytology, omental biopsy, biopsy of palpable abnormalities, and selective or complete pelvic lymphadenectomy were important in the identification of small volume extrauterine disease [3–5]. Detection of gross abdominal or retroperitoneal metastases would have been expected in the earlier time intervals, but some proportion of patients with microscopic tumor spread would have been classified as having local disease only. Such patients would have had a higher incidence of recurrence.

Second, the surgical staging experience led to the identification of high-risk prognostic features. Subsets of women with high-grade tumors, deep myometrial invasion, or extension to the cervix could be targeted for more aggressive adjuvant therapy after hysterectomy in hopes of diminishing the incidence of primary treatment failure. To date, several randomized phase three trials have failed to

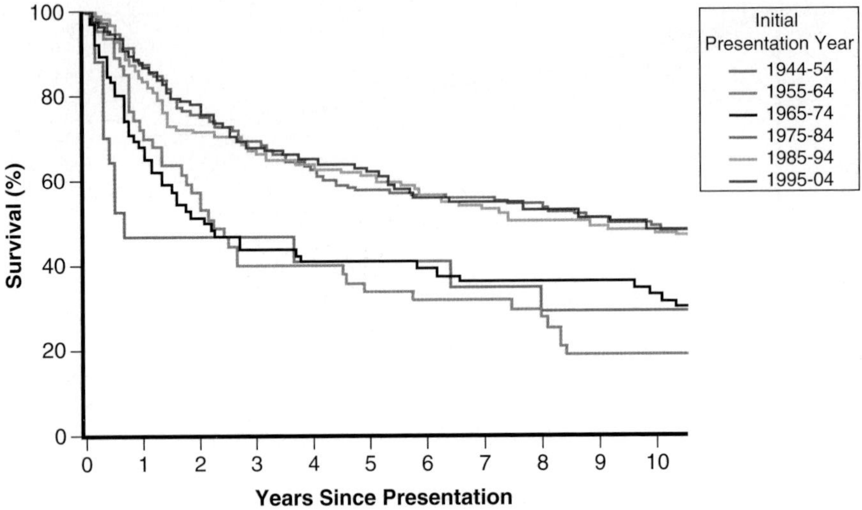

Fig. 11.3 Survival rates for patients with regional (SEER stage) endometrial cancer (1944–2004) (P<0.0001, log-rank test for trend).

demonstrate a survival advantage for women who received postoperative adjuvant pelvic irradiation or systemic progestin therapy [6–8]. Nevertheless, women with known risk for treatment failure are current candidates for clinical trials and are routinely treated more aggressively than are those without such features.

Third, women with endometrial carcinoma are frequently postmenopausal, obese, and afflicted with cardiovascular and metabolic comorbidities; they are also at significant risk of perioperative complications including death. General improvement in surgical and supportive care over the course of the study interval has likely contributed to reduced perioperative mortality from infection, stroke, myocardial infarction, and pulmonary embolus. Analysis of more than 800 women with endometrial cancer being treated surgically who underwent hysterectomy during the 2000s revealed no perioperative deaths within 30 days of surgery. This is remarkable, given the surgical risk profiles of these women. As a composite result of these changes in treatment approach (and perhaps in part resulting from other approaches yet to be identified), 5- and 10-year survival rates for women with localized endometrial cancer have improved over time and are now excellent.

Survival Outcome and Regional Tumors

The most dramatic change in decade-by-decade survival rates has been seen in women with regional disease. A sharp separation in curves can be seen beginning in 1975 (Fig. 11.3). The difference between the cluster of curves representing the first

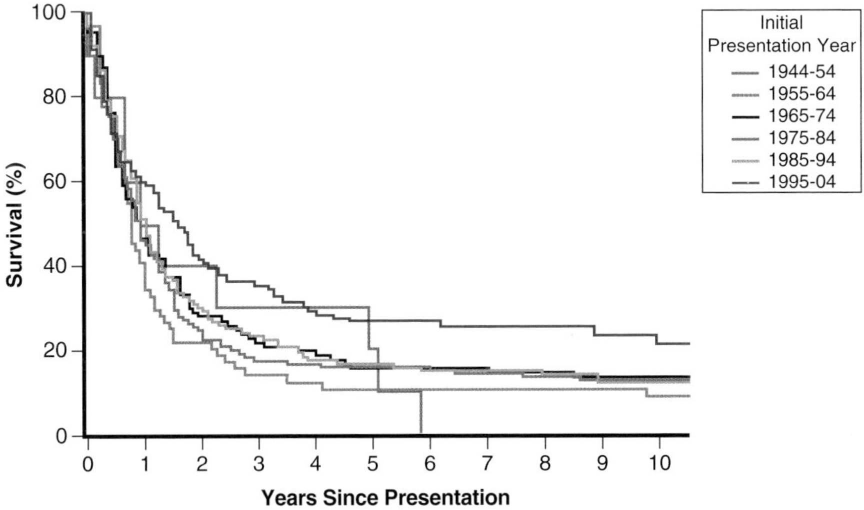

Fig. 11.4 Survival rates for patients with distant (SEER stage) endometrial cancer (1944–2004) ($P=0.048$, log-rank test for trend).

three decades and those representing the more recent three is highly significant ($P<0.0001$). Almost certainly some of these differences can be attributed to changes in the surgical management of uterine cancer. Before the widespread application of surgical staging procedures, the identification of regional disease was limited to visualization and palpation at the time of exploration. Therefore, most women in the regional disease category during the early decades of the study interval were likely to have grossly metastatic disease in the pelvic lymph nodes. Even with resection and postoperative radiotherapy, outcome for such women was limited.

Conversely, women assigned to the regional disease category during the second portion of the study included a mixture of those with gross disease and those with resected microscopic tumor. This latter group would be expected to have a much better outcome, especially when surgery was augmented by postoperative radiotherapy. The increasing sophistication of regional irradiation, which allowed doses capable of sterilizing small volume tumor to be safely delivered to pelvic and retroperitoneal lymph nodes, undoubtedly improved survival rates in this group. More recent information has also suggested that full pelvic lymphadenectomy may be associated with improved survival rates, presumably because of the removal of microscopic metastases [8].

Survival Outcome and Distant Tumors

As expected, outcome for women with distant disease has remained poor across the entire study period (Fig. 11.4). No statistically significant differences in survival rates were observed for any of the intervals evaluated. All are clustered near the 20% mark. Progestin therapy was the first widely used systemic treatment for metastatic endometrial cancer. Stimulation of the progesterone receptor was believed to be "antiestrogenic." Some patients with metastatic disease did respond to such treatment. However, receptor-positive tumors tend to be well differentiated and rarely metastatic, thus limiting the effectiveness of this treatment. Randomized trials were unable to demonstrate a survival benefit to adjuvant progestin therapy [9]. In fact, patients receiving hormonal treatment were more likely to experience thrombotic and cardiovascular complications than were controls.

Few cytotoxic agents produce lasting responses in metastatic disease. Doxorubicin, platinum agents, and taxanes are the most active chemotherapeutic agents. Single-agent or combination therapy has produced measurable responses in 30–60% of women. Most responses last less than 12 months. Survival benefit is therefore limited. The absence of effective long-lasting systemic therapy clearly explains the failure to affect outcome in these cases.

Current Management Approach

Our current approach to the management of endometrial carcinoma is stratified by surgical stage. After the initial diagnosis by outpatient biopsy or dilatation and curettage, a total abdominal hysterectomy with bilateral salpingo-oophorectomy is performed. Additional staging procedures performed at the time of exploration would include peritoneal cytology, omental biopsy, biopsy of palpable abnormalities within the peritoneal cavity, pelvic lymphadenectomy, and para-aortic lymph node biopsy or resection. A similar set of procedures performed via laparoscopy or robotics would be considered equivalent to an open procedure.

Women with low-risk disease require no further therapy. Those with intermediate-risk stage I tumors are offered vaginal cuff brachytherapy. Whole pelvic external beam irradiation is recommended for high-risk stage I/II patients and for those with regional lymph node metastases. Extended field irradiation is used in women with aortic nodal spread. Systemic therapy, either hormonal or cytotoxic, is appropriate for women with distant metastatic disease; these patients are ideal candidates for clinical trials since current standard treatment provides limited benefit.

Future improvements in survival outcome are likely to derive from three strategies: One, effective adjuvant therapy (regional or systemic, or a combination of both) for highest-risk stage I patients is needed. To date, no effective adjuvant treatment has been proven beneficial. Two, an aggressive approach to the management of regional pelvic disease must be defined and implemented. This will likely begin with cytoreduction of metastatic disease followed by radiotherapy, with or without chemotherapy. Three, a better understanding of the signaling pathways in endometrial tumors would permit a more targeted approach to metastatic disease that would build upon existing systemic treatment results.

References

1. Jemal A, Siegel R, Ward E, et al. Cancer statistics 2009. CA Cancer J Clin. 2009;59:225–49. doi:10.3322/caac.20006.
2. Kupelian PA, Eifel PJ, Tornos C, Burke TW, Delclos L, Oswald MJ. Treatment of endometrial carcinoma with radiation therapy alone. Int J Radiat Oncol Biol Phys. 1993;27:817–24.
3. Morrow C, Bundy B, Kurman R, et al. Relationship between surgical-pathological risk factors and outcome in clinical stage I and II carcinoma of the endometrium: a Gynecologic Oncology Group study. Gynecol Oncol. 1991;40:55–65.
4. Marino BD, Burke TW, Tornos C, et al. Staging laparotomy for endometrial carcinoma: assessment of peritoneal spread. Gynecol Oncol. 1995;56:34–8.
5. Chuang L, Burke TW, Tornos C, et al. Staging laparotomy for endometrial carcinoma: assessment of retroperitoneal lymph nodes. Gynecol Oncol. 1995;58(2):189–93.
6. Aalders J, Abeler V, Kolstad P, et al. Postoperative external irradiation and prognostic parameters in stage I endometrial carcinoma. Obstet Gynecol. 1980;56:419–27.
7. Creutzberg CL, van Putten WL, Koper PC, et al. Surgery and postoperative radiotherapy vs surgery alone for patients with stage-1 endometrial carcinoma: multicentre randomized trial. PORTEC Study Group, post operative radiation therapy in endometrial carcinoma. Lancet. 2000;355:1404–11.
8. Abu-Rustum NR, Iasonos A, Zhou Q, et al. Is there a therapeutic impact to regional lymphadenectomy in the surgical treatment of endometrial carcinoma? Am J Obstet Gynecol. 2008;198(4):457e1–e6.
9. Lewis GC, Slack N, Mortel R, et al. Adjuvant progestogen therapy in primary definitive treatment of endometrial cancer. Gynecol Oncol. 1974;2:368–76.

Chapter 12
Pancreatic Cancer (Exocrine)

Jason Fleming, Matthew Katz, Rosa Hwang, and Gauri Varadhachary

Introduction

There are two distinct types of pancreatic cancer, differentiated by whether they arise from exocrine or endocrine tissue. By far the most common (up to 95%) are neoplasms of the exocrine pancreas, and they are the focus of this discussion. Most exocrine pancreatic neoplasms (90%) are adenocarcinomas, and three quarters of them arise in the head of the pancreas. Neoplasms of the endocrine pancreas are relatively rare and differ both biologically and clinically from exocrine cancers. Because they affect endocrine tissue, they often cause recognizable hormonal symptoms; thus, they are often detected at early stages and are more successfully treated. Exocrine pancreatic cancers, in contrast, do not cause early symptoms, and when symptoms appear, they are often vague in nature. By the time significant pain, jaundice, or weight loss is evaluated, disease is usually advanced, and as many as 80% of patients present with disease defined as regionally advanced or metastatic on imaging studies.

Although there are factors associated with increased risk of pancreatic cancer, there is no method of widespread screening. Risk factors include smoking, obesity, age, and a personal or family history of pancreatitis or pancreatic cancer. This disease occurs more frequently in black persons than in white persons and is seen more in older age groups. More recently, genetic syndromes have been associated with

J. Fleming (✉) • M. Katz • R. Hwang
Department of Surgical Oncology, The University of Texas MD Anderson Cancer Center, 1400 Pressler Street, Houston, TX 77030, USA
e-mail: jbflemin@mdanderson.org

G. Varadhachary
Department of GI Medical Oncology, The University of Texas MD Anderson Cancer Center, Houston, TX, USA

M.A. Rodriguez et al. (eds.), *60 Years of Survival Outcomes at The University of Texas MD Anderson Cancer Center*, DOI 10.1007/978-1-4614-5197-6_12,

increased risk—familial aggregations of pancreatic cancer have been linked with known cancer-related mutations including BRCA, p16 (the FAMM syndrome), and STK11/LKB1 associated with Peutz–Jeghers syndrome. Patients who have relatives (including second degree) with a history of pancreatic cancer are considered at increased risk.

No specific tumor markers currently exist for pancreatic cancer. Although most patients with this disease have elevated CA19-9 levels, the specificity of this marker is too low to be of use as a screening tool because other conditions such as inflammation and pancreatitis also increase CA19-9 levels. This marker is currently used, however, to help gauge response to treatment and as one of several prognostic indicators. Currently, there is significant research interest in identifying biomarkers (in blood, pancreatic cysts, and cancer tissue) to help with early diagnosis of pancreatic cancer and for screening of high-risk individuals.

The survival curves for pancreatic cancer have not improved as significantly as they have for many other cancers. Although pancreatic cancer is the tenth most common cancer, it has become the fourth leading cause of cancer-related deaths. According to the American Cancer Society's 2009 estimates, 42,470 people were expected to be diagnosed with pancreatic cancer in that year, and overall (for all stages combined), only 5% of patients with exocrine pancreatic cancer will survive for 5 years [1]. The grim statistics for this cancer can be attributed to its biologic nature and to the fact that there is no screening measure for detection at early stages. This is a biologically aggressive cancer, which spreads quickly to adjacent tissues (invades the duodenum, the retropancreatic nerves, the portal and superior mesenteric veins, and regional lymph nodes) and to distant organs including the liver, peritoneum, omentum, and lungs—often before symptoms have heralded its presence.

The only curative treatment for pancreatic cancer is complete surgical resection of the tumor and surrounding pancreatic tissue. Unfortunately, only one in five patients present with disease that is considered resectable. Furthermore, to be successful, the resection must be considered complete, meaning that surgical margins are proven negative (R0) for disease by pathologic analysis of resected specimens. Studies have shown that anything less nullifies the value of the surgery; in fact, in cases in which even microscopic disease has been detected at the margins (R1), outcome has been comparable in terms of survival to having had only palliative treatment and no surgery [2].

The surgery—most commonly a pancreaticoduodenectomy—is a major operation with a significant risk of complications. Because the head of the pancreas is structurally tied to adjacent structures that share blood supply and ducts, the duodenum, part of the small intestine and common bile duct, the gallbladder, and often part of the stomach are removed along with it. The remaining pancreas body, stomach, and hepatic duct must then be reconstructed to accommodate digestive flow. The series of anastomoses required in this reconstruction is complex and is a source of potential complications such as leakage of enzyme-rich pancreatic fluid, biliary obstruction secondary to injury, or anastomotic stricture of the bile duct.

Dual phase computed tomography (CT) optimized for pancreatic imaging is the best tool for determining resectability; magnetic resonance imaging, magnetic resonance cholangiopancreatography, or CT angiography rarely offer any advantage over a dual-phase CT scan. On occasion, additional studies may be needed mainly to exclude extrapancreatic disease, but with multidetector CT scanning based on a pancreatic protocol, more than 90% of patients can be classified as having potentially resectable, borderline-resectable, locally advanced, or metastatic pancreatic cancer [3]. It is imperative that the decision regarding resectability be made preoperatively and when possible in a multidisciplinary forum in the presence of surgeons, radiologists, medical oncologists, and radiation oncologists. In patients with obstructive jaundice, it is imperative to obtain a good-quality pancreatic protocol CT scan before intervention with endoscopic retrograde cholangiopancreatography (ERCP). Occasionally, as a result of post-ERCP acute pancreatitis, inflammatory changes obscure the tissue planes between tumor and vessels, which makes it difficult to interpret imaging studies. Staging today relies upon diagnostic imaging, and gains seen in survival for this disease in the past two decades are largely due to advances in these technologies.

However, even under optimal conditions—small, organ-confined tumor with no evidence of lymph node involvement, and completely resected—the survival rate remains low: only 18–24% of patients who undergo surgery survive for 5 years [4]. It has become clear that even patients whose disease appears localized probably harbor microscopic disease and require systemic therapy; unfortunately, however, pancreatic cancer has proven to be resistant to chemotherapy agents.

Historical Perspective

Surgery has been and remains the definitive treatment for pancreatic cancer. Pancreaticoduodenectomy, the most commonly performed surgical procedure (for pancreatic head adenocarcinomas), was described as early as 1898 but was named for Allen O. Whipple after his description of this procedure in 1935. Since then, its use has not been without controversy because of its association with significant morbidity and mortality. During the 1970s, investigators began to question whether it should even be attempted. Over the decades, perioperative mortality associated with pancreatic cancer has dropped from a range of 25–40%, reported in various papers from the 1960s and 1970s, to today's rates of 4–5% overall; of note, however, is the fact that today's mortality rate is 1% or less in high-volume centers with surgeons experienced in the procedure but is up to 16% in small, low-volume hospitals or among surgeons who perform few procedures. Numerous studies have concluded that both hospital volume and surgeon experience affect operative morbidity and mortality [5]. In recognition of the technical challenges and presumed postoperative morbidity of pancreatic surgery, more patients over the past 10–15 years have been referred to tertiary cancer centers for this operation, which many believe has contributed to a mortality and morbidity reduction from the surgery.

Unfortunately, most patients present with unresectable disease. In the past, more patients underwent surgery for staging, some only to learn that their disease was not resectable. Today, preoperative staging relies on less invasive techniques, including endoscopic ultrasound and high-resolution diagnostic imaging such as helical CT and magnetic resonance imaging; this allows for better patient selection since only those who can benefit from surgery are selected, sparing those who likely would not benefit from an operation associated with significant morbidity.

By the early 1970s, it was clear that although surgery was necessary for eradication of pancreatic cancer, it was not sufficient, since surgery alone yielded a survival rate of less than 6%. Thus, identifying effective adjuvant therapies became a focus of research. Multiple trials during the next decades demonstrated a survival advantage for adjuvant chemotherapy, compared with controls who received no adjuvant therapy. Combination chemotherapies proved disappointing; trials of taxane and other agents in combination with 5-FU failed to produce significant improvements over 5-FU alone and led to additional toxic events.

At the same time, radiotherapy had been shown to have benefits, which led to the idea of combining chemotherapy and irradiation. The first major randomized group trial [the Gastro-Intestinal Study Group (GITSG) trial] was begun in the USA in 1973 to study concurrent chemotherapy and radiation therapy (CRT) as adjuvant therapy [6]. The study was slow to accrue, but by 1982, 43 patients had been randomized to receive either an adjuvant CRT regimen consisting of 5-FU and regional split course radiation therapy or no adjuvant treatment. The study was terminated at that time due to the large survival benefit seen with CRT (20 months vs. 11 months). The European Organisation for Research and Treatment of Cancer (EORTC) tried to replicate the results, which suggested a trend to better overall survival in the CRT arm, but its results were not statistically significant. Despite the fact that most of the following large phase III group trials were underpowered and did not yield consistent results, CRT became a standard option.

The next major milestone came in the 1990s with the addition of gemcitabine to the treatment regimen. Gemcitabine, classified as an antimetabolite, is a nucleoside analog that inhibits DNA replication. In a study done between 1992 and 1994 that compared gemcitabine with 5-FU in patients with advanced pancreatic cancer, significant benefits were seen in survival and in time to progression with gemcitabine [7]. This was the first time in 30 years that any agent had shown improvement over 5-FU. Moreover, a clinical benefit was noted, including improvements in pain, performance status, tumor-related symptoms, and weight, establishing the idea of a chemotherapy-induced palliative effect on disease-related symptoms and improvement in quality of life, all of which led to FDA approval of this agent in 1996. Single-agent gemcitabine became the standard to which other agents and combinations would be compared in the future. Gemcitabine has been studied in the adjuvant setting in several trials and is the current adjuvant therapy standard of care for resected pancreatic cancer. The role of radiation in this setting is controversial and is currently under study. In the past few years, another study compared gemcitabine plus erlotinib [an epidermal growth factor receptor (EGFR) tyrosine kinase inhibitor] to gemcitabine plus placebo. This study showed marginal clinical benefit but statistically significant improvement in the combination arm and led to FDA approval of erlotinib in 2005. A recent phase 3 study presented by Conroy and colleagues reported on FOLFIRINOX

(5-FU, oxaliplatin, and irinotecan) superiority over gemcitabine in the treatment of metastatic pancreatic cancer. The median overall survival was 11.1 months in the FOLFIRINOX group compared with 6.8 months in the gemcitabine group, and the authors concluded that FOLFIRINOX is an option for the treatment of patients with metastatic pancreatic cancer and a good performance status [8].

Improvements in surgical technique and in perioperative and supportive care over the past two decades are responsible for some of the gains in survival and for the better survival rates seen in high-volume centers—fewer people died of surgical complications. Of importance, these factors have also affected morbidity. Patients are therefore not just living longer, their quality of survival has been much improved. Ascites, bowel obstructions, and jaundice are examples of complications of this cancer that can be relieved with stents and decompression techniques. Advances in pain management have also contributed, with the addition of long-acting narcotics, pain pumps, and invasive procedures such as celiac axis neurolysis.

The MD Anderson Cancer Center Experience

The data set used for this discussion was derived from a total of 7,204 patients who presented to MD Anderson Cancer Center with pancreatic cancer between 1944 and 2004. Those with endocrine tumors or other primary cancers and patients who had been treated elsewhere were excluded, resulting in 2,079 patients who received definitive treatment at this institution for exocrine pancreatic cancer. Survival was calculated from initial presentation.

It should be noted that all data presented here are for exocrine pancreatic cancers. Most published survival statistics for pancreatic cancer include both endocrine and exocrine types. The 5-year overall Surveillance, Epidemiology, and End Results program (SEER) survival rate in the final decade of the timeframe (1995–2004) was 5% for all pancreatic cancers. At MD Anderson it was 15.3% for all pancreatic cancers and 10% for the exocrine type alone.

Presentation

Throughout the 60-year timespan, most patients presenting with exocrine pancreatic cancer had regional or distant disease (Table 12.1). The fact that there has been little change in the percentage of patients presenting with localized disease highlights the ongoing lack of a screening mechanism to identify early pancreatic cancers. For three decades (1955–1984), well over half of patients (58.8–67.5%) had metastatic disease on presentation, which also reflects, at least in some measure, referral trends.

Table 12.1 Patients with exocrine pancreatic cancer treated at MD Anderson, 1944–2004

	SEER stage at presentation				
	Local	Regional	Distant	Unstaged	Total
Decade	[No. (%) of patients]				
1944–1954	0 (0)	4 (57.1)	3 (42.9)	0 (0)	7 (100.0)
1955–1964	11 (12.9)	21 (24.7)	50 (58.8)	3 (3.5)	85 (100.0)
1965–1974	9 (7.1)	27 (21.4)	85 (67.5)	5 (4.0)	126 (100.0)
1975–1984	29 (11.3)	60 (23.3)	158 (61.5)	10 (3.9)	257 (100.0)
1985–1994	47 (8.8)	183 (34.1)	240 (44.8)	66 (12.3)	536 (100.0)
1995–2004	143 (13.4)	418 (39.1)	370 (34.6)	137 (12.8)	1,068 (100.0)
Total	*239 (11.5)*	*713 (34.3)*	*906 (43.6)*	*221 (10.6)*	*2,079 (100.0)*

SEER Surveillance, Epidemiology, and End Results program

Survival

The overall survival trend reflected in Fig. 12.1 indicates an improvement over the 60-year timespan, from 0% to 10% for 5-year survival and from 0% to 7.8% for 10-year survival.

With the exception of one decade, this increase was steady. The exception occurred during the 1975–1984 period, when overall survival rates were lower than those of the previous two decades (1955–1964 and 1965–1974); this finding was specific to patients presenting with local disease (Fig. 12.2).

These exceptions all involved single patients. There were 11 patients admitted with local disease between 1955 and 1964, 9 patients between 1965 and 1974, and 29 patients between 1975 and 1984. Among these patients, one in each decade survived longer than 5 years, and one in each of the latter two decades survived at least 10 years. Given the small number of patients, it is difficult to postulate causal factors; however, historically these periods predated many advancements in critical care and surgical technique that took place at MD Anderson Cancer Center since the early 1980s that have led to our current results.

The significant 5- and 10-year survival increases for patients presenting with local and regional disease occurred during the final two decades of the timeframe. For patients presenting with regional disease, we saw incrementally longer survival rates during each decade, but it is notable that 5-year survival rates were not seen until the past two decades (Fig. 12.3).

Metastatic pancreatic cancer. For patients presenting with distant metastases, gains in survival have been incremental; increases in the number of patients reaching the 5-year milestone have been small and have occurred only in the past two decades. Advances in palliative surgery, and more importantly, better supportive care measures, have improved the survival rates and the quality of survival for patients with metastatic disease (Fig. 12.4).

Localized pancreatic cancer. We do not attribute recent survival gains wholly to better treatments, but rather in large measure to advances in imaging technology that

a

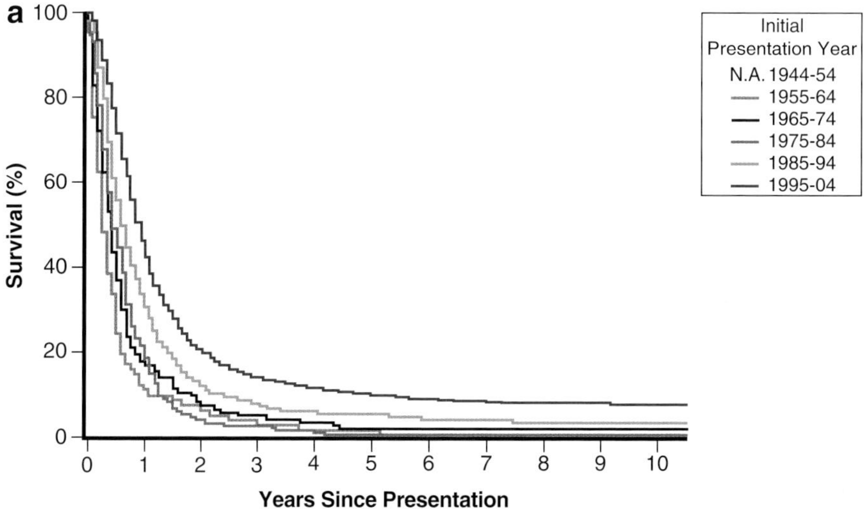

b

Year	Percent Survival	
	5 yr	10 yr
1944-54	0.0	0.0
1955-64	1.2	0.0
1965-74	1.6	1.6
1975-84	0.4	0.0
1985-94	5.0	3.4
1995-04	10.0	7.8

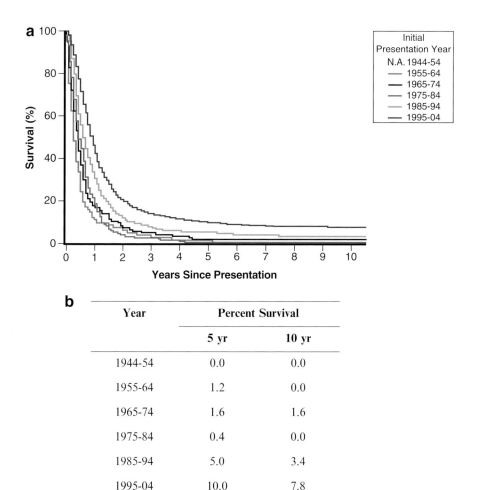

Fig. 12.1 (**a**) Overall survival rates for patients with exocrine pancreatic cancer (1944–2004) ($P<0.0001$, log-rank test for trend). Because of the very small number of individuals with exocrine pancreatic cancer seen from 1944 to 1954, data from this period were excluded. *N.A.* not applicable. (**b**) Kaplan–Meier survival table.

have allowed us to better stage disease preoperatively and to better select candidates for surgery. Specific refinements in the surgical approach to pancreatic cancer have been developed through our experience at MD Anderson Cancer Center; these include careful anatomic dissection of the tissues adjacent to the pancreas, the use of vascular resection in conjunction with pancreatectomy, and reduction in operative and postoperative complications. These improvements have resulted in low operative morbidity and mortality rates and a low rate of tumor recurrence at the site of surgical removal (local recurrence). We believe that these improvements and their associated results have contributed to the observed improvement in overall survival [9].

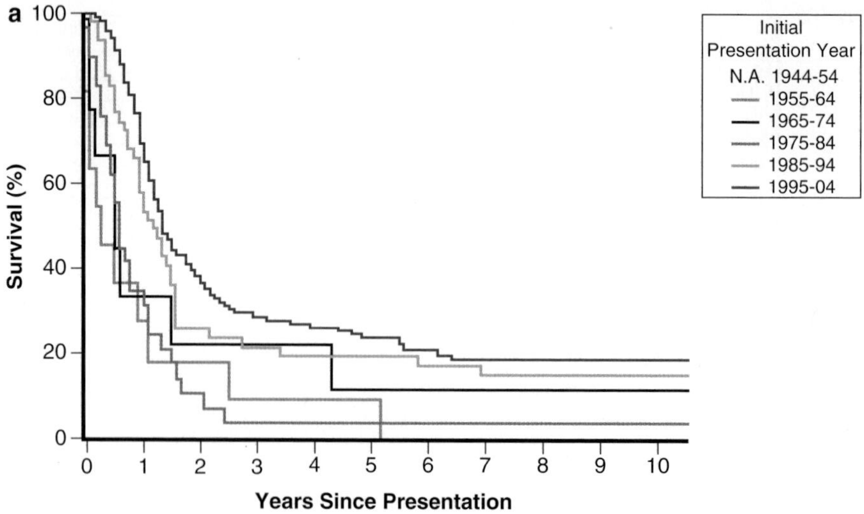

b

Year	Percent Survival	
	5 yr	10 yr
1944-54	0.0	0.0
1955-64	9.1	0.0
1965-74	11.1	11.1
1975-84	3.4	3.4
1985-94	19.1	14.9
1995-04	24.1	18.5

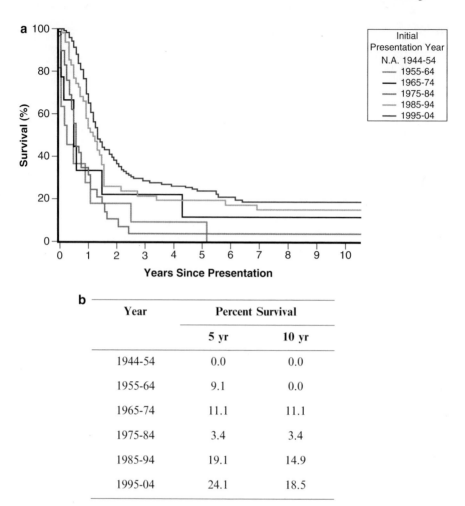

Fig. 12.2 (**a**) Survival rates for patients with local (SEER stage) exocrine pancreatic cancer (1944–2004) ($P<0.0001$, log-rank test for trend). Because of the very small number of individuals with local exocrine pancreatic cancer seen from 1944 to 1954, data from this period were excluded. *N.A.* not applicable. (**b**) Kaplan–Meier survival table.

Another significant treatment advance arose from our ability to resect the portal vein if necessary, which meant that more patients could receive potentially curative surgery; another benefit resulted from recognizing the importance of the retroperitoneal margin—the area between the tumor and the border of the superior mesenteric artery—which is frequently microscopically tumor-positive. Our approach is to take very thin serial sections of this tissue, from which we provide meticulously inked and oriented specimens for pathologic interpretation [10]. It is a technically challenging task to safely dissect tissue so close to the wall of the superior mesenteric artery, but it is a critical step because this is a site of frequent recurrence, even

a

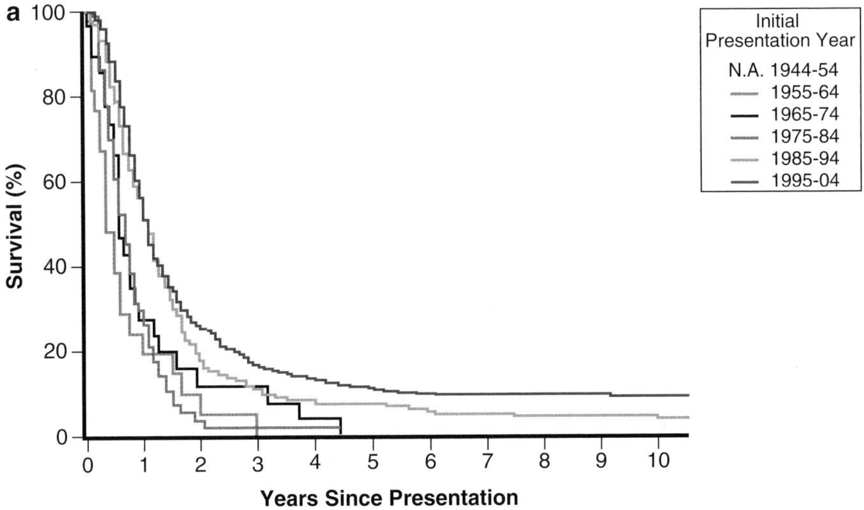

b

Year	Percent Survival	
	5 yr	10 yr
1944-54	0.0	0.0
1955-64	0.0	0.0
1965-74	0.0	0.0
1975-84	0.0	0.0
1985-94	7.4	4.0
1995-04	10.6	8.8

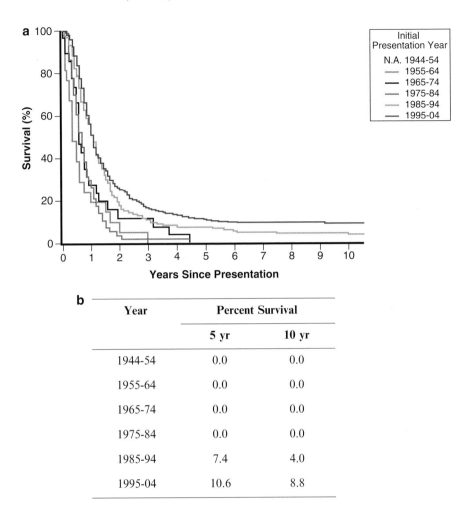

Fig. 12.3 (**a**) Survival rates for patients with regional (SEER stage) exocrine pancreatic cancer (1944–2004) ($P<0.0001$, log-rank test for trend). Because of the very small number of individuals with regional exocrine pancreatic cancer seen from 1944 to 1954, data from this period were excluded. *N.A.* not applicable. (**b**) Kaplan–Meier survival table.

after resections of margins believed to be negative. This may explain, at least in part, the high recurrence rates previously reported after resections of tissue believed to be complete. The cornerstone of this approach is preoperative imaging, which has only recently become refined enough to be able to assess this area, which is mere millimeters wide.

Another treatment milestone came in the mid to late 1990s, when we began to focus on preoperative therapy for disease at earlier stages than were previously considered. This is an approach we continue to favor.

a

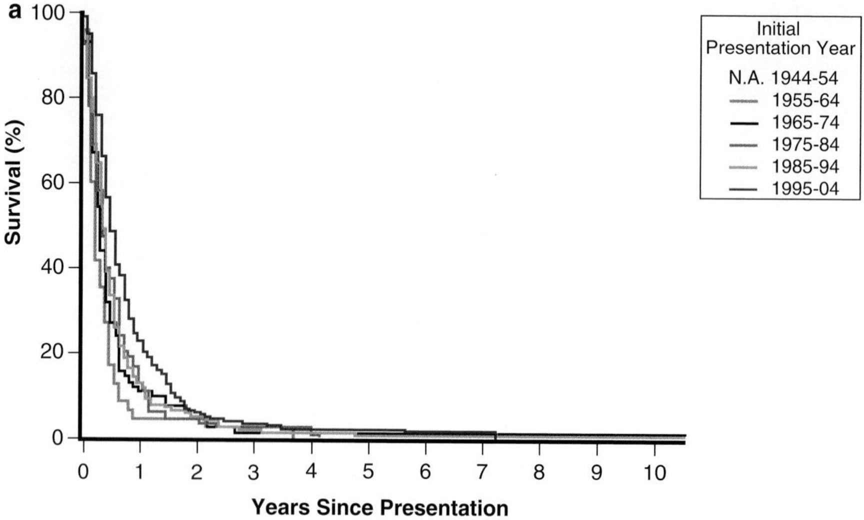

b

Year	Percent Survival	
	5 yr	10 yr
1944-54	0.0	0.0
1955-64	0.0	0.0
1965-74	1.2	1.2
1975-84	0.0	0.0
1985-94	0.6	0.6
1995-04	1.8	0.0

Fig. 12.4 (**a**) Survival rates for patients with distant (SEER stage) exocrine pancreatic cancer (1944–2004) ($P<0.0001$, log-rank test for trend). Because of the very small number of individuals with distant exocrine pancreatic cancer seen from 1944 to 1954, data from this period were excluded. *N.A.* not applicable. (**b**) Kaplan–Meier survival table.

Finally, there have been other advances in the treatment of pancreatic cancer that should not go unmentioned, advances that have not affected the length of survival but have impacted its quality. These include pain management and palliative radiologic and surgical techniques such as biliary decompression and relief from gastric outlet obstruction, causes of significant distress and morbidity associated with pancreatic cancer.

Current Management Approach

The hallmarks of the current approach to the management of pancreatic cancer at MD Anderson are thorough preoperative staging and a preference for preoperative (neoadjuvant) therapy (preferably on clinical trial when available) in earlier-stage disease than is considered standard.

Management begins with high-resolution imaging according to a defined pancreas protocol, beginning with multidetector helical CT imaging, which is optimal for evaluation of tumor and vessel orientation, para-pancreatic lymph nodes, and metastatic disease of the liver and peritoneum. Endoscopic ultrasound, which has higher sensitivity than CT has, is used to evaluate primary tumors and to guide fine-needle aspiration biopsy if a mass is present. If indicated, ERCP is used to relieve obstructive jaundice before preoperative therapy with the placement of a plastic or metal stent; the latter is preferred in patients receiving preoperative therapy for >8 weeks.

Preoperative therapy—chemotherapy followed by chemoradiation or chemoradiation alone—is favored at our institution, even in patients whose disease is initially considered resectable. There are several compelling reasons for this. First, given the high rates of recurrence after potentially curative resections, most agree that pancreatic cancer is a systemic disease in the majority of patients. Second, radiation-based preoperative therapy likely helps increase the chance of an R0 resection. A third rationale for preoperative therapy is that as many as 25% of patients who proceed with a surgery-first approach never receive postoperative therapy because of the prolonged recovery after surgery. Finally, preoperative therapy helps identify patients who will benefit from surgery. Patients receiving systemic therapy whose disease is rapidly progressive are likewise identified and spared the morbidity of the surgery.

Concerns about choosing preoperative therapy instead of upfront surgery in patients whose disease is considered resectable are related to losing a "window" in the setting of a rapidly progressive disease. However, recent trials at our institution have indicated that in most patients whose disease is deemed unresectable, distant metastatic disease is responsible for disease progression. In our single-institution trials of 170 total patients who received preoperative gemcitabine-based chemoradiation, survival duration among those who underwent resection was 32–36 months [9].

For disease that is considered "borderline resectable," preoperative therapy can render some cases operable. Currently, 30–40% of patients in this category progress to surgery at our institution. In many cases, vessel involvement by tumor was the determinant of nonresectability [9].

Future improvements in this disease depend on continued research in the following areas:

- Identification of more effective systemic agents.
- Identification of specific biomarkers that would help direct therapy in a targeted way and provide a mechanism with which to identify early disease.
- Better understanding of molecular and genetic characteristics unique to this cancer.

To those ends, current clinical trials are aimed at building on improvements seen by the introduction of gemcitabine and more recently FOLFIRINOX; we are keen to identify other novel agents and combinations that can improve current results and disease control. Similar studies are being designed to determine the mechanisms responsible for the relative chemoresistance of pancreatic tumors.

One hallmark characteristic of pancreatic cancer is the abundant dense stroma that surrounds the cancer. The stromal cells themselves have been shown to contribute toward disease growth and metastasis, as well as chemoresistance and radiation resistance of pancreatic cancer [11]. Moreover, the dense stroma might also impair delivery of drugs to tumor cells [12]. We are currently performing a novel clinical study that examines surgical tumor specimens to detect levels of drugs given preoperatively (gemcitabine) and even during surgery.

Current basic research studies focus on transgenic mouse models in order to better understand how specific gene expression is regulated by extracellular signals, how cell proliferation is controlled, and what mechanisms are involved in tumorigenesis and metastasis in pancreas cancer—all keys to developing targeted therapies and identifying predictive markers for screening. Acquiring a better understanding of not only the pancreatic cancer cells but also the tumor microenvironment, such as the stroma, is critical to developing novel effective therapies for this disease.

Tools that are essential for an effective basic and translational research program in pancreatic cancer are a well-established tissue bank and integrated clinical database. Because of its location deep in the peritoneum, pancreatic cancer is not accessible for serial biopsy, and therefore the tissue repository for study is less rich than it is for many other cancers. At our institution, we have established standard operating procedures for the collection of high-quality tissue with annotated clinical data for all patients with pancreatic cancer [13]. Novel methods of study developed from the biospecimen bank include our current tumor xenograft program, in which individual tumors surgically removed from patients at MD Anderson are grown in mice and used for genetic testing [14]. In the future, these methods will be used for individualized patient care.

Increasing awareness of this deadly disease may help attract more support for needed research. Currently, pancreatic cancer is the least funded of the major cancers. Research efforts directed at improved methods of detection, understanding the mechanisms of drug resistance, and development of novel therapeutic targets (on both cancer and stromal compartments) are needed to make any significant progress in this deadly disease.

References

1. Altekruse SF, Kosary CL, Krapcho M, et al., editors. SEER Cancer Statistics Review, 1975–2007. National Cancer Institute; 2010. http://seer.cancer.gov/csr/1975_2007/, based on November 2009 SEER data submission, posted to the SEER Web site. Accessed 23 May 2012.
2. Tempero MA, Arnoletti JP, Behrman SW. Pancreatic Adenocarcinoma, Version 2.2012 Updates to the NCCN Guidelines. J Natl Compr Canc Netw. 2012 Jun 1;10(6):703–13.

3. Varadhachary GR, Tamm EP, Abbruzzese JL, et al. Borderline resectable pancreatic cancer: definitions, management, and role of preoperative therapy. Ann Surg Oncol. 2006;13(8): 1035–46.
4. National Cancer Institute Pancreatic Cancer Treatment (PDQ®), Health Professional Version. http://www.cancer.gov. Updated 5 March 2010. Accessed 22 May 2012.
5. Fernández-del Castillo C, Rattner DW, Warshaw AL. Standards for pancreatic resection in the 1990s. Arch Surg. 1995 Mar;130(3):295–9; discussion 299–300.
6. Kalser MH, Ellenberg SS. Pancreatic cancer: adjuvant combined radiation and chemotherapy following curative resection. Arch Surg. 1985;120:899–903.
7. Burris III HA, Moore MJ, Andersen J, et al. Improvements in survival and clinical benefit with gemcitabine as first-line therapy for patients with advanced pancreas cancer: a randomized trial. J Clin Oncol. 1997;15:2403–13.
8. Gourgou-Bourgade S, de la Fouchardière C, Bennouna J, et al. Groupe Tumeurs Digestives of Unicancer; PRODIGE Intergroup. FOLFIRINOX versus gemcitabine for metastatic pancreatic cancer. N Engl J Med. 2011;364(19):1817–25.
9. Katz MH, Wang H, Fleming JB, et al. Long-term survival after multidisciplinary management of resected pancreatic adenocarcinoma. Ann Surg Oncol. 2009;16(4):836–47.
10. Raut CP, Tseng JF, Sun CC, et al. Impact of resection status on pattern of failure and survival after pancreaticoduodenectomy for pancreatic adenocarcinoma. Ann Surg. 2007;246(1): 52–60.
11. Hwang RF, Moore T, Arumugam T, et al. Cancer-associated stromal fibroblasts promote pancreatic tumor progression. Cancer Res. 2008;68(3):918–26.
12. Olive KP, Jacobetz MA, Davidson CJ, et al. Inhibition of Hedgehog signaling enhances delivery of chemotherapy in a mouse model of pancreatic cancer. Science. 2009; 324(5933):1457–61.
13. Hwang RF, Wang H, Lara A, et al. Development of an integrated biospecimen bank and multidisciplinary clinical database for pancreatic cancer. Ann Surg Oncol. 2008;15(5):1356–66.
14. Kim MP, Evans DB, Wang H, Abbruzzese JL, Fleming JB, Gallick GE. Generation of orthotopic and heterotopic human pancreatic cancer xenografts in immunodeficient mice. Nat Protoc. 2009;4(11):1670–80.

Chapter 13
Kidney Cancer

Scott E. Delacroix Jr., Surena F. Matin, John Araujo, and Christopher G. Wood

Introduction

Approximately 58,000 people in the United States were diagnosed with kidney cancer in 2011, and an estimated 13,000 people will die as a result of the disease [1]. Cancer of the kidney represents 3.9% of all U.S. cancers and 2% of all cancer deaths. During their lifetime, 1 in 70 men and women will be diagnosed with cancer of the kidney or renal pelvis [2]. Worldwide, the mortality from renal cell carcinoma (RCC) is estimated to exceed 100,000 per year [3].

Kidney cancer is subdivided into two major histologic subtypes: RCC and transitional cell carcinoma. RCC arises within the renal parenchyma and accounts for about 85% of all primary renal neoplasms. RCC is further subdivided into multiple subtypes that exhibit differential biologic and prognostic features. Transitional cell carcinoma arising from the renal pelvis accounts for 7% of primary renal neoplasms, and its biology is similar to that of transitional cell carcinoma of the bladder. Several other rare parenchymal epithelial tumors, such as oncocytomas, collecting duct tumors, and renal sarcomas, account for the remaining tumors. Herein, we will review the advances and treatment of RCC at The University of Texas MD Anderson Cancer Center.

S.E. Delacroix Jr. • S.F. Matin • C.G. Wood (✉)
Department of Urology, The University of Texas MD Anderson Cancer Center, 1515 Holcombe Boulevard, Unit 1373, Houston, TX 77030, USA
e-mail: cgwood@mdanderson.org

J. Araujo
Department of Genitourinary Medical Oncology, The University of Texas MD Anderson Cancer Center, 1515 Holcombe Boulevard, Unit 1374, Houston, TX 77030, USA

M.A. Rodriguez et al. (eds.), *60 Years of Survival Outcomes at The University of Texas MD Anderson Cancer Center*, DOI 10.1007/978-1-4614-5197-6_13,

Historical Perspective

For localized disease, the mainstay of treatment for RCC has been surgical excision. In the 1960s, radical nephrectomy became the procedure of choice, with a reported 66% 5-year survival rate, which compared favorably with that of simple nephrectomy at 48%. For almost 35 years, the procedure was relatively static, with only slight modifications associated with the excision of the ipsilateral adrenal gland and the management of regional lymph nodes. In the 1990s, minimally invasive surgical techniques (laparoscopy) were heralded, followed by the adoption of partial nephrectomy techniques (nephron-sparing surgery). In properly selected patients, partial nephrectomy has yielded equivalent oncologic outcomes and has become the standard of care for many patients with small renal masses [4]. Although initially used only to perform radical nephrectomy, the laparoscopic approach is now used for some nephron-sparing surgeries.

In the 2000s, further advances in technology have spawned ablative technologies (cryotherapy and radiofrequency ablation) for small renal masses as well as robotic extirpative and reconstructive techniques. The durability of oncologic outcomes with the use of ablative techniques remains to be proven.

Even more recently, active surveillance of the small (less than 4 cm) renal mass has gained increasing popularity for those with a reduced life expectancy due to age, severe medical conditions, or a high surgical risk. The use of partial nephrectomy for small renal masses has an equivalent cancer-specific survival rate and possibly an improved overall survival rate compared with radical nephrectomy [4]. The increased overall survival is purported to be due to a decrease in the comorbid chronic medical conditions associated with the development of chronic renal insufficiency. As in many aspects of oncologic treatment, surgical therapy for RCC is best modified for each individual patient. Systemic agents are also tailored to the individual patient with use of a multifaceted analysis of histologic subtype, patient comorbid medical conditions, burden of disease, and other characteristics.

Risk Factors

Numerous environmental and clinical factors have been implicated in the etiology of RCC [5]: tobacco use; occupational exposure to toxic compounds such as cadmium, asbestos, and petroleum by-products; obesity; acquired polycystic disease of the kidney (typically associated with dialysis); and analgesic abuse nephropathy. Cigarette smoking doubles the likelihood of RCC and contributes to as many as one-third of all cases [6–8]. The risk of developing RCC in patients with acquired polycystic disease of the kidney has been estimated to be 30 times greater than in the general population [9].

Although most RCCs are sporadic (>90%), factors suggesting a hereditary cause include first-degree relatives with the disease [10–13], onset before age 40, and bilateral or multifocal disease [14]. An enhanced risk of RCC has been observed in patients with certain inherited disorders (von Hippel–Lindau disease, hereditary papillary renal cancer, hereditary leiomyomatosis renal cancer syndrome, and Birt–Hogg–Dube syndrome), thereby implicating various genetic abnormalities in its etiology. In addition, patients with tuberous sclerosis and hereditary polycystic kidney disease, although not having a substantially increased incidence of renal cancer, can have cancers with unique features.

Staging

Approximately 75% of patients present with clinically localized disease amenable to surgical treatment. Despite the initial presentation, up to 40% of these patients will experience recurrence of disease after the primary lesion is treated. In RCC, the most consistent predictor of patient outcome is stage. Multiple modifications to the American Joint Committee on Cancer (AJCC) staging system have occurred to further improve the prognostic accuracy of the staging system. In 2002, the T1 stage was further subdivided into T1a and T1b [15]. In 2009, the T2 and T3 staging categories were modified and the nodal stage simplified to better reflect outcome in patients with advanced-stage disease (Table 13.1) [16].

The overall incidence of RCC in the United States for all races has been increasing and is now three times higher than the mortality rate. Since 1950, there has been a 126% increase in the incidence of RCC, accompanied by a 37% increase in annual mortality [17, 18]. Moreover, the 5-year survival rate of patients diagnosed with RCC has improved, from 34% for those diagnosed in 1954 to 67% for those diagnosed in 2004 [19].

With the widespread introduction of cross-sectional imaging in the mid-1980s, the incidence of low-stage tumors increased substantially. Incidental discovery of RCC increased from approximately 10% in the 1970s to 60% in 1998, and the mortality rate between 1990 and 2005 decreased by approximately 5% [18, 20].

Stage migration has been continuous: the incidence of stage I disease has continued to increase, whereas that of stages II and III disease has shown a statistically significant decline. The incidence of stage IV disease has remained stable over the past two decades [20]. Stage grouping (Table 13.2) shows the poor 5-year survival rates in patients with locally advanced and metastatic disease.

Although the decrease in mortality during the past 20 years is most likely a result of the increased incidence of lower-stage tumors (stage migration), multiple advances in understanding the biology of RCC have led to novel targeted treatments for patients with advanced/metastatic disease. Although complete responses are anecdotal, these targeted agents are providing extended survival in a large percentage of stage IV patients—survival times not previously seen in the recorded history of the disease.

Table 13.1 AJCC Version 7.0 staging of renal cell carcinoma

Primary tumor (T)	
TX	Primary tumor cannot be assessed
T0	No evidence of primary tumor
T1	Tumor 7 cm or less in greatest dimension, limited to the kidney
T1a	Tumor 4 cm or less in greatest dimension, limited to the kidney
T1b	Tumor more than 4 cm but not more than 7 cm in greatest dimension limited to the kidney
T2	Tumor more than 7 cm in greatest dimension, limited to the kidney
T2a	Tumor more than 7 cm but less than or equal to 10 cm in greatest dimension, limited to the kidney
T2b	Tumor more than 10 cm, limited to the kidney
T3	Tumor extends into major veins or perinephric tissues but not into the ipsilateral adrenal gland and not beyond Gerota's fascia
T3a	Tumor grossly extends into the renal vein or its segmental (muscle containing) branches, or tumor invades perirenal and/or renal sinus fat but not beyond Gerota's fascia
T3b	Tumor grossly extends into the vena cava below the diaphragm
T3c	Tumor grossly extends into the vena cava above the diaphragm or invades the wall of the vena cava
T4	Tumor invades beyond Gerota's fascia (including contiguous extension into the ipsilateral adrenal gland)
Regional lymph nodes (N)	
NX	Regional lymph nodes cannot be assessed
N0	No regional lymph node metastasis
N1	Regional lymph node metastasis
Distant metastasis (M)	
M0	No distant metastasis (no pathologic M0; use clinical M to complete stage group)
M1	Distant metastasis

Used with the permission of the American Joint Committee on Cancer (AJCC), Chicago, Illinois. The original source for this material is the *AJCC Cancer Staging Manual*, Seventh Edition (2010) published by Springer Science and Business Media LLC, www.springer.com [16]

Table 13.2 Correlation of stage grouping with survival in patients with renal cell cancer

Cancer stage	Tumor category	Node category	Metastasis category	5-year survival rates
I	T1	N0	M0	90–95
II	T2	N0	M0	70–85
III	T3a	N0	M0	50–65
	T3b	N0	M0	50–65
	T3c	N0	M0	45–50
	T1	N1	M0	25–30
	T2	N1	M0	25–30
	T3	N1	M0	15–20
IV	T4	Any N	M0	10

The MD Anderson Cancer Center Experience

The MD Anderson Tumor Registry data set was derived from 10,308 patients diagnosed with kidney cancer between 1944 and 2004. Of this total group, 4,601 received no prior treatments. After excluding patients with other primary noncutaneous malignancies and those previously treated at other institutions, survival data were calculated from the remaining 2,839 patients. The number of patients presenting by time interval is summarized in Table 13.3.

Until the early 1990s, there were no FDA-approved treatments for metastatic RCC, represented by the high percentage of new referrals for patients with distant metastatic disease. With the approval of high-dose interleukin 2 (HD IL-2) in 1992 and more recently with the approval of multiple targeted agents for the treatment of metastatic RCC (2005–present), the percentage of referrals for advanced disease may plateau.

The Kaplan–Meier survival curves for patients with RCC reveal significantly improved 5- and 10-year outcomes over the 60-year analysis period (Fig. 13.1). Equally apparent is the stage migration, noted since the mid-1980s with the prevalent use of cross-sectional imaging; analyzing outcome on the basis of stage provides better insight into the historical improvements in the treatment of this disease. Significant improvements in the treatment of localized and regional disease have increased survival rates, as shown in Figs. 13.2 and 13.3, respectively.

Unfortunately, up to 40% of patients with localized/regional disease will experience recurrence of disease after treatment of the primary lesion; however, no adjuvant treatments have been approved for these patients at high risk of recurrence. Since the approval of the first targeted agent in 2005, overall survival rates for patients with metastatic disease have increased significantly. As shown in Fig. 13.4, survival rates for those with distant disease have not substantially improved over the analysis period, but these data do not include the survival rates achieved since the introduction of newer effective agents. For the time periods surveyed, the only

Table 13.3 Patients with kidney cancer treated at MD Anderson, 1944–2004

	SEER stage at presentation				
	Local	Regional	Distant	Unstaged	Total
Decade	[No. (%) of patients]				
1944–1954	3 (50.0)	0 (0)	2 (33.3)	1 (16.7)	6 (100.0)
1955–1964	15 (21.1)	12 (16.9)	43 (60.6)	1 (1.4)	71 (100.0)
1965–1974	35 (19.1)	18 (9.8)	126 (68.9)	4 (2.2)	183 (100.0)
1975–1984	74 (18.2)	65 (16.0)	262 (64.5)	5 (1.2)	406 (100.0)
1985–1994	167 (22.3)	130 (17.4)	444 (59.4)	7 (0.9)	748 (100.0)
1995–2004	513 (36.0)	232 (16.3)	651 (45.7)	29 (2.0)	1,425 (100.0)
Total	807 (28.4)	457 (16.1)	1,528 (53.8)	47 (1.7)	2,839 (100.0)

SEER Surveillance, Epidemiology, and End Results program

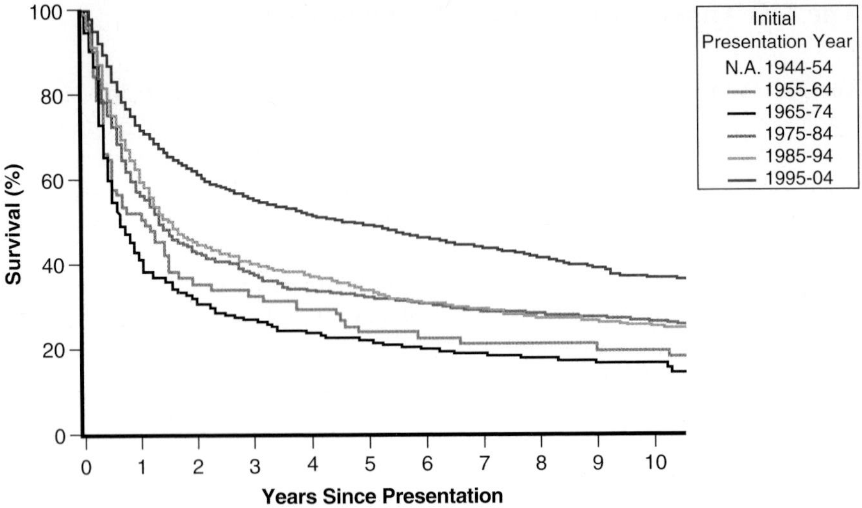

Fig. 13.1 Overall survival rates for patients with kidney cancer (1944–2004) ($P<0.0001$, log-rank test for trend). Because of the very small number of individuals with kidney cancer seen from 1944 to 1954, data from this period were excluded. *N.A.* not applicable.

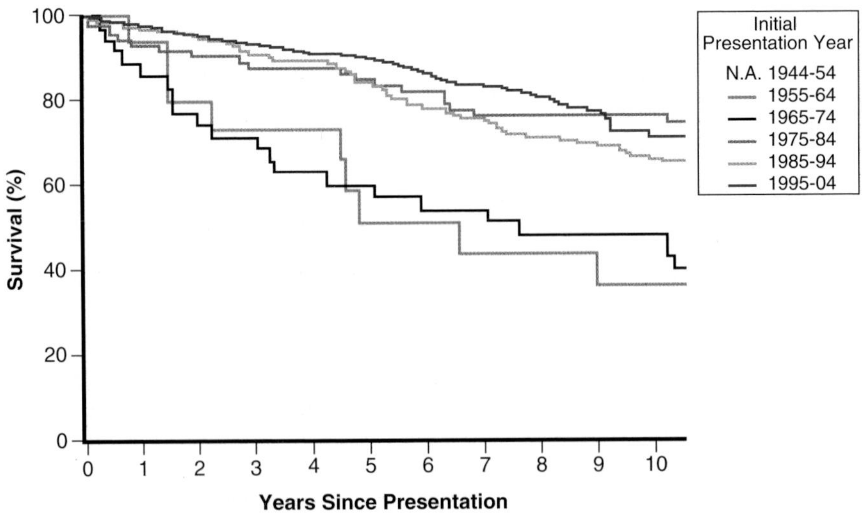

Fig. 13.2 Survival rates for patients with local (SEER stage) kidney cancer (1944–2004) ($P<0.0001$, log-rank test for trend). Because of the very small number of individuals with local kidney cancer seen from 1944 to 1954, data from this period were excluded. *N.A.* not applicable.

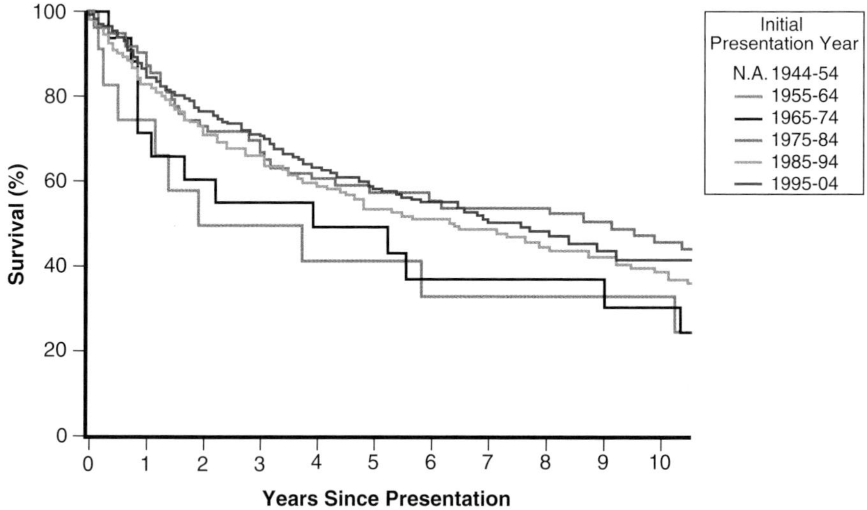

Fig. 13.3 Survival rates for patients with regional (SEER stage) kidney cancer (1955–2004) ($P=0.56$, log-rank test for trend). Because no individuals with regional kidney cancer were seen from 1944 to 1954, data from this period were excluded. *N.A.* not applicable.

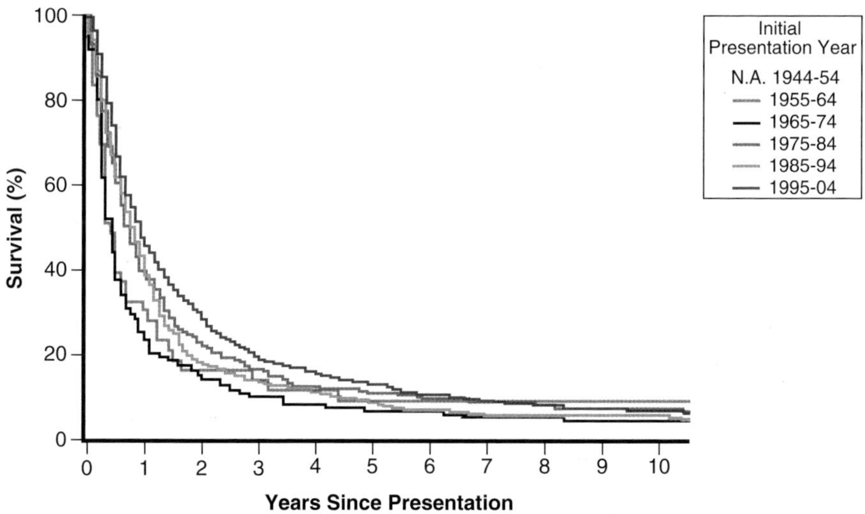

Fig. 13.4 Survival rates for patients with distant (SEER stage) kidney cancer (1944–2004) ($P<0.0001$, log-rank test for trend). Because of the very small number of individuals with distant kidney cancer seen from 1944 to 1954, data from this period were excluded. *N.A.* not applicable.

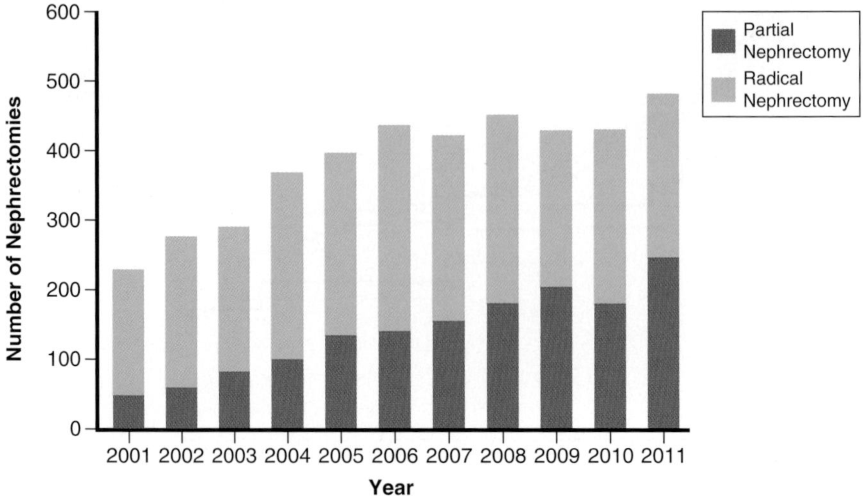

Fig. 13.5 Number of patients treated with partial versus radical nephrectomies at MD Anderson Cancer Center between 2001 and 2011.

effective treatment for metastatic RCC (outside of a clinical trial) has been HD IL-2 therapy [21]. Although associated with the highest durable long-term survival (7% complete durable responders), this treatment is difficult to tolerate and therefore cannot be used by most patients with metastatic disease. Multiple agents targeted at the angiogenesis pathway have been widely used since the first agent was approved in December 2005. At MD Anderson Cancer Center, many of these same targeted agents used for metastatic disease are currently being tested in the adjuvant setting for high-risk patients, and results are forthcoming.

The use of partial nephrectomy rather than radical nephrectomy for treatment of small localized lesions has provided an overall survival benefit by decreasing the comorbidities associated with the development of chronic renal insufficiency [4]. Figure 13.5 shows the relative number of partial to radical nephrectomies performed at MD Anderson Cancer Center between 2001 and 2011. The increasing number of partial nephrectomies is due to both the ever-increasing number of small renal masses (resulting from earlier detection) and improvements in technique allowing more complex masses to be removed while sparing the remaining renal parenchyma.

Oncologic outcomes with the use of partial and radical nephrectomy are equivalent in properly selected patients. The technique of partial nephrectomy is now the standard of care for many patients with tumors amenable to this procedure. Application and adoption of minimally invasive techniques (robotic and laparoscopic) has further augmented the surgical treatment of RCC.

Current Management Approach

Our current approach to the management of RCC is stratified by clinical and pathologic stage. For systemic disease, histologic subtyping of RCC is particularly important since the biologic mechanisms, and therefore the response rates to targeted agents, are varied. For tumors with a predominance of sarcomatoid dedifferentiation, traditional cytotoxic agents are also offered on the basis of multiple small single-institution studies and an ongoing study at MD Anderson Cancer Center.

Future improvements in survival for patients with metastatic disease will likely come from several strategies. First, development of an effective adjuvant treatment for patients with a high risk of recurrence after primary treatment could significantly affect the overall survival of the 40% of patients whose disease is destined to recur. Second, delineation of the biologic pathways involved in the development of resistance to targeted and standard chemotherapeutics could enable the design of agents specific to resistant tumors or of agents to be used up front to prevent resistance. Third, further advances in surgical technology and techniques with appreciation for surgical morbidity as well as oncologic outcome will aid patients diagnosed with this disease. Historic advances have been achieved in the past 20 years, and with continued research, we hope to continue to advance the treatment of patients with all stages of RCC.

References

1. Jemal A, Siegel R, Xu J, Ward E. Cancer statistics 2010. CA Cancer J Clin. 2010;60(5): 277–300.
2. Horner M, Ries L, Krapcho M, Neyman N, Aminou R. SEER cancer statistics review 1975–2006. Bethesda, MD 2009;(11):11.1–28. http://seer.cancer.gov/csr/1975_2006/. Accessed 1 Dec 2009.
3. Ferlay J, Shin HR, Bray F, Forman D, Mathers C, Parkin DM. GLOBOCAN 2008, cancer incidence and mortality worldwide: IARC CancerBase No. 10 [Internet]. Lyon: International Agency for Research on Cancer; 2010. http://globocan.iarc.fr. Accessed 1 Dec 2009.
4. Thompson RH, Boorjian SA, Lohse CM, et al. Radical nephrectomy for pT1a renal masses may be associated with decreased overall survival compared with partial nephrectomy. J Urol. 2008;179(2):468–71 [discussion 72–3].
5. Mandel JS, McLaughlin JK, Schlehofer B, et al. International renal-cell cancer study. IV. Occupation. Int J Cancer. 1995;61(5):601–5.
6. La Vecchia C, Negri E, D'Avanzo B, Franceschi S. Smoking and renal cell carcinoma. Cancer Res. 1990;50(17):5231–3.
7. Yu MC, Mack TM, Hanisch R, Cicioni C, Henderson BE. Cigarette smoking, obesity, diuretic use, and coffee consumption as risk factors for renal cell carcinoma. J Natl Cancer Inst. 1986;77(2):351–6.
8. Hunt JD, van der Hel OL, McMillan GP, Boffetta P, Brennan P. Renal cell carcinoma in relation to cigarette smoking: meta-analysis of 24 studies. Int J Cancer. 2005;114(1):101–8.
9. Brennan JF, Stilmant MM, Babayan RK, Siroky MB. Acquired renal cystic disease: implications for the urologist. Br J Urol. 1991;67(4):342–8.

10. Gago-Dominguez M, Yuan JM, Castelao JE, Ross RK, Yu MC. Family history and risk of renal cell carcinoma. Cancer Epidemiol Biomarkers Prev. 2001;10(9):1001–4.
11. Schlehofer B, Pommer W, Mellemgaard A, et al. International renal-cell-cancer study. VI. the role of medical and family history. Int J Cancer. 1996;66(6):723–6.
12. McLaughlin JK, Mandel JS, Blot WJ, Schuman LM, Mehl ES, Fraumeni Jr JF. A population–based case–control study of renal cell carcinoma. J Natl Cancer Inst. 1984;72(2):275–84.
13. Mellemgaard A, Engholm G, McLaughlin JK, Olsen JH. Occupational risk factors for renal-cell carcinoma in Denmark. Scand J Work Environ Health. 1994;20(3):160–5.
14. Gnarra JR, Glenn GM, Latif F, et al. Molecular genetic studies of sporadic and familial renal cell carcinoma. Urol Clin North Am. 1993;20(2):207–16.
15. Green FL, Blach CM, Haller DG, Morrow M. AJCC cancer staging manual. 6th ed. New York: Springer; 2002.
16. Edge SB, Byrd DR, Compton CA, editors. AJCC cancer staging manual. 7th ed. New York: Springer; 2010.
17. Jemal A, Siegel R, Ward E, et al. Cancer statistics, 2006. CA Cancer J Clin. 2006;56(2): 106–30.
18. Pantuck AJ, Zisman A, Belldegrun AS. The changing natural history of renal cell carcinoma. J Urol. 2001;166(5):1611–23.
19. Jemal A, Siegel R, Ward E, Hao Y, Xu J. Cancer statistics 2009. CA Cancer J Clin. 2009;59: 225–49.
20. Kane CJ, Mallin K, Ritchey J, Cooperberg MR, Carroll PR. Renal cell cancer stage migration: analysis of the National Cancer Data Base. Cancer. 2008;113(1):78–83.
21. Fisher RI, Rosenberg SA, Sznol M, Parkinson DR, Fyfe G. High-dose aldesleukin in renal cell carcinoma: long-term survival update. Cancer J Sci Am. 1997;3 Suppl 1:S70–2.

Chapter 14
Bladder Cancer

Robert S. Svatek, Ashish M. Kamat, Arlene Siefker-Radtke, and Colin P.N. Dinney

Introduction

About 70,980 new cases of bladder cancer were diagnosed in 2009 [1]. Bladder cancer, the fourth most common cancer in U.S. men, is three times more common in men than in women [1]. The number of bladder cancer cases diagnosed annually in the USA has increased more than 50% between 1985 and 2005 [2], which can be explained only in part by the aging U.S. population [3]. In addition, this increased incidence cannot be explained by changes in health care screening practices or improved diagnostics because the means by which bladder cancer is diagnosed (cystoscopy and biopsy) have remained constant since the 1930s.

The aggressiveness and metastatic potential of bladder cancer are heterogeneous but depend largely on disease grade. At presentation, 55–60% of tumors are well- or moderately differentiated and confined to the layers of the bladder superficial to the muscularis propria—the urothelium or the lamina propria [3]. The vast majority of patients with tumors at this stage of differentiation can be treated with endoscopic resection; however, in approximately 20% of these cases, the disease ultimately progresses to a higher grade or stage. On the other hand, of the 40–45% of patients who present with high-grade disease, more than half have muscle invasion or metastatic disease [3]. The standard of care for patients with invasive, high-grade disease

R.S. Svatek
Department of Urology, The University of Texas Health Science Center, San Antonio, TX, USA

A.M. Kamat • C.P.N. Dinney (✉)
Department of Urology, The University of Texas MD Anderson Cancer Center, 1515 Holcombe Boulevard, Unit 1373, Houston, TX 77030, USA
e-mail: cdinney@mdanderson.org

A. Siefker-Radtke
Department of Genitourinary Medical Oncology, The University of Texas MD Anderson Cancer Center, Houston, TX, USA

M.A. Rodriguez et al. (eds.), *60 Years of Survival Outcomes at The University of Texas MD Anderson Cancer Center*, DOI 10.1007/978-1-4614-5197-6_14,

is radical cystectomy, chemotherapy, or a combination of these modalities. In addition to disease grade and stage, aggressive variants have been identified on the basis of histologic features, loss of tumor suppression proteins, overexpression of oncogenic proteins, or aberrant signaling pathways [4, 5]. Current strategies are focused on determining the aberrant signaling pathways associated with this cancer, in hopes of yielding specific targets that may be modulated by the large cadre of targeting agents under development [6, 7].

Historical Perspective

Urothelial cancer is unique among noncutaneous carcinomas in that it is the only common epithelial neoplasm that usually presents at a superficial stage. At this stage, the lesions can be readily examined visually and cytologically for diagnostic and follow-up studies. In fact, 80–85% of urothelial cancers are exophytic papillary lesions that tend to recur but only rarely evolve into a higher-grade invasive cancer. The remaining urothelial cancers are nonpapillary and invasive at diagnosis and arise from severe dysplasia or carcinoma in situ. The vast majority of invasive bladder cancers occur in patients without a prior history of papillary tumors.

Transurethral resection (TUR) is adequate therapy for most low-grade noninvasive lesions, but the majority of these lesions recur within 5 years; however, they rarely invade or result in death from bladder cancer. The recurrence rate of low-grade bladder cancer is decreased by a single post-TUR intravesical instillation of chemotherapy. Although various intravesical therapies (chemotherapy and immunotherapy) are used for higher-risk noninvasive tumors, bacillus Calmette–Guerin remains the most effective intravesical treatment. Patients with muscle invasion have a potentially life-threatening disease, but those with pathologically confirmed organ-confined bladder cancer have an 80–85% long-term disease-free survival rate with radical cystectomy and pelvic lymphadenectomy. Outcome is improved in patients presenting with locally advanced cancers by the addition of multiagent chemotherapy. For patients with grossly metastatic disease, contemporary chemotherapy regimens produce reliable symptom palliation and median survival ranging from 13 to 18 months. Although few responses are durable, large trials consistently show a 10–15% long-term disease-free survival rate after multiagent chemotherapy.

The MD Anderson Cancer Center Experience

The MD Anderson Tumor Registry data set was derived from 10,950 men and women who were seen for a diagnosis of bladder cancer between 1944 and 2004. Of this group, 2,811 had no previous treatment for their malignancy and received definitive primary treatment at MD Anderson. After excluding patients with multiple primary cancers, except for superficial skin cancers and those treated elsewhere,

Table 14.1 Clinical staging of bladder cancer[a]

Stage	Description
Tx	Primary tumor cannot be assessed
T0	No evidence of primary tumor
Ta	Noninvasive papillary carcinoma
Tis	Carcinoma in situ
T1	Tumor invades subepithelial connective tissue
T2	Tumor invades detrusor muscle
T3b	Palpable three-dimensional mass on examination under anesthesia after endoscopic resection of tumor
T4a	Tumor invades prostate, uterus, or vagina
T4b	Tumor invades pelvic wall or abdominal wall

[a]According to the 1997 American Joint Committee on Cancer and the International Union Against Cancer (AJCC-UICC) primary tumor, regional nodes, and metastasis (TNM) staging system

Table 14.2 Pathologic staging of bladder cancer[a]

Stage	Description
Tx	Primary tumor cannot be assessed
Ta	Noninvasive papillary carcinoma
Tis	Carcinoma in situ
T1	Tumor invades subepithelial connective tissue
T2	Tumor invades detrusor muscle
T3b	Tumor invades perivesical tissue macroscopically
T4a	Tumor invades prostate, uterus, or vagina
T4b	Tumor invades pelvic wall or abdominal wall

[a]According to the 1997 American Joint Committee on Cancer and the International Union Against Cancer (AJCC-UICC) primary tumor, regional nodes, and metastasis (TNM) staging system

1,564 patients remained and formed the basis of this report, including 1,112 (71.1%) men and 452 (28.9%) women. The large majority of patients presented with local (50.1%) or regional (34.9%) disease, whereas 12% presented with distant disease (see Tables 14.1, 14.2, and 14.3 for staging definitions). This distribution of cases by stage has changed slightly over time (Fig. 14.1). In particular, there was a decrease in the number of regional disease stage presentations from the 1950s to 2004, and the number of patients seen for distant disease has steadily increased over time. These changes may be in part related to time-dependent stage classification changes, improvement in imaging techniques, and changes in referral patterns over time.

The Kaplan–Meier survival estimates reveal incremental improvement in overall survival over time for patients presenting to MD Anderson with bladder cancer (Fig. 14.2). The 10-year overall survival rate was 19.4–24.1% during the years 1944–1974 and 34.8–44.5% during 1975–2004. The survival rate for patients with local disease significantly improved over time (Fig. 14.3). For patients with localized disease, the average 5-year and 10-year overall survival rates within the first three decades vs. the most recent three decades were 52.2% vs.73.9% and 28.1% vs. 56.4%, respectively (Fig. 14.3). Similarly, for patients with regional disease, the

Table 14.3 SEER summary staging 2000

Stage	Description	TNM
In situ	Tumor is only in the layer of cells in which it began	Ta–Tis and N−
Local	Tumor is confined to the primary site	T1–T2 and N−
Regional	Tumor has spread to regional lymph nodes or beyond primary site	T3–T4a or Regional N+[a]
Distant	Tumor has metastasized to nonregional lymph nodes, visceral organs, abdominal wall, or pelvic wall	T4b, nonregional N+[b], or M+

[a]Includes perivesical, internal iliac (hypogastric), external iliac, obturator, and sacral
[b]Includes common iliac and above. However, common iliac was considered regional in the 1977 Surveillance, Epidemiology, and Ends Results (SEER) summary staging guide

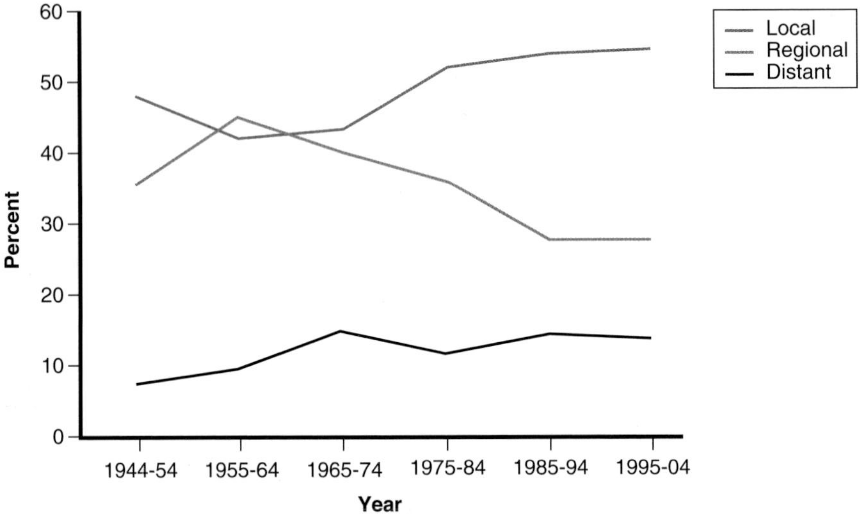

Fig. 14.1 Trends in stage presentation over time.

average 5-year and 10-year overall survival rates within the first three decades vs. the most recent three decades were 15.5% vs. 39.9% and 13.4% vs. 30.3%, respectively (Fig. 14.4).

The improved survival estimates for patients with local and regional disease across the study period are likely attributable to several factors. Whereas refinements in surgical technique have remained relatively constant, the frequency of surgical removal of regional lymph nodes has increased over time, with growing recognition of the survival benefit afforded with extended pelvic nodal dissection compared with limited pelvic dissection. Several major medical centers reported improved outcome for patients undergoing extended vs. limited nodal dissections. As a result, the extent of nodal dissection changed considerably during the study period. It is expected that a proportion of patients presumed to be node-negative were actually

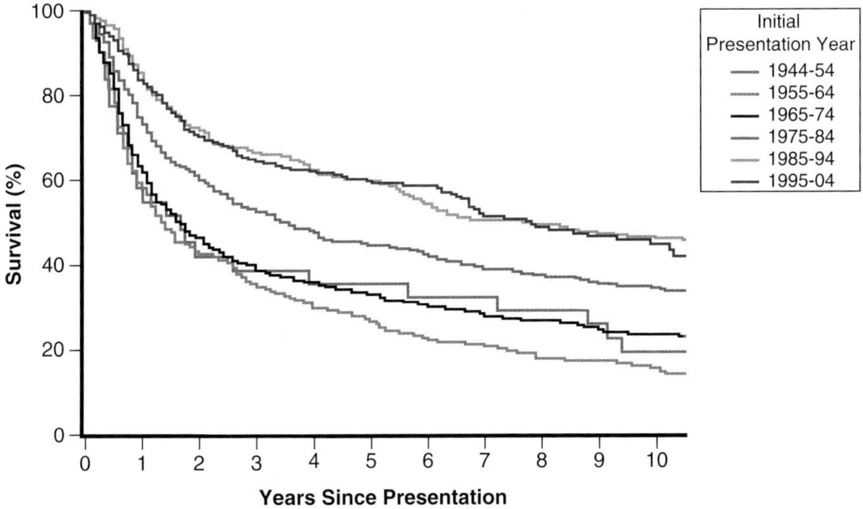

Fig. 14.2 Overall survival rates for patients with bladder cancer (1944–2004) ($P<0.0001$, log-rank test for trend).

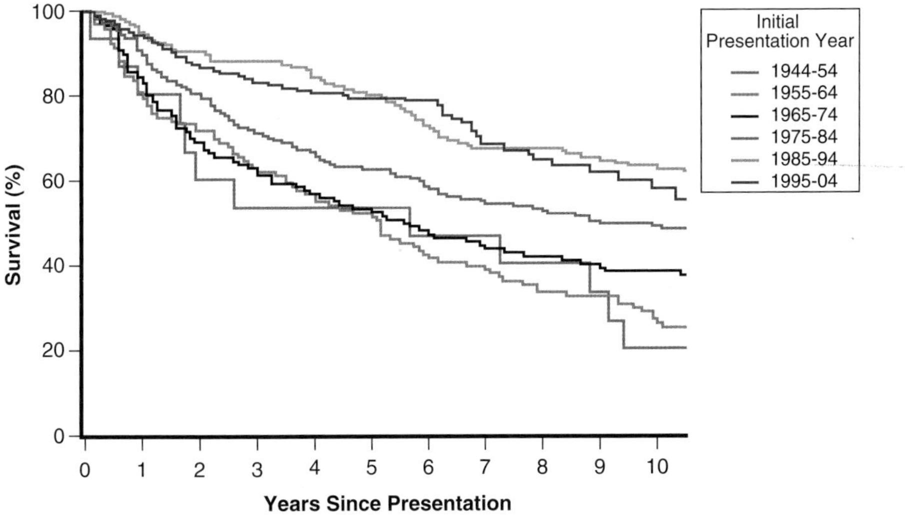

Fig. 14.3 Survival rates for patients with local (SEER stage) bladder cancer (1944–2004) ($P<0.0001$, log-rank test for trend).

node-positive in the early part of the study period because they underwent limited nodal dissection. Improvements in staging accuracy, identification of aggressive tumors, use of selective adjuvant chemotherapy, and the application of surgical consolidation for patients with initial node-positive disease have also been important.

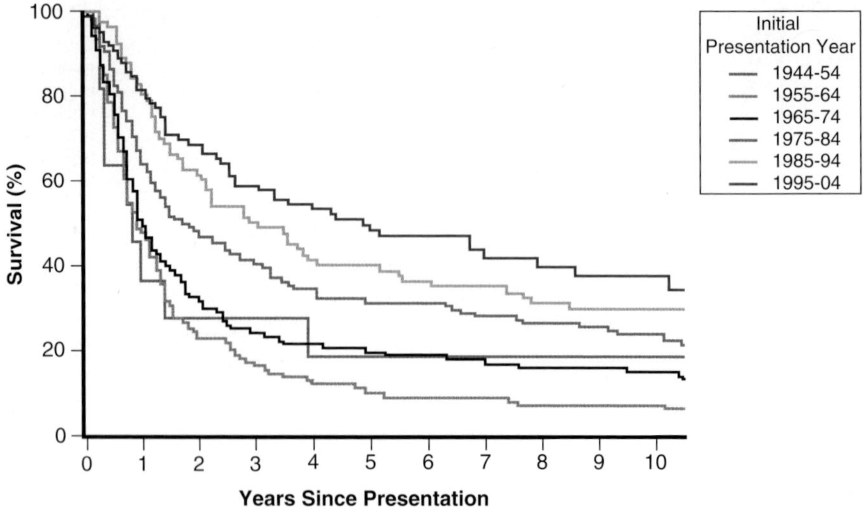

Fig. 14.4 Survival rates for patients with regional (SEER stage) bladder cancer (1944–2004) ($P<0.0001$, log-rank test for trend).

Surgical staging in bladder cancer with use of computed tomography or magnetic resonance imaging became routine during the second half of the study interval, and refinements in these imaging modalities have improved staging accuracy.

Another explanation for the improvements in overall survival for patients with local and regional disease over time is the identification of high-risk tumors based on variant histology or clinical prognostic features. For example, identification of the micropapillary variant of urothelial cell carcinoma of the bladder as a particularly aggressive subtype by researchers at our institution led to a more aggressive surgical approach (i.e., extirpative surgery even at early stages) for patients with these tumor subtypes [8, 9]. In addition, chemotherapy is now routinely recommended for patients with adverse variant histologic subtypes such as small cell carcinoma [10, 11] and on protocol for selected patients with other variants such as micropapillary urothelial cell carcinoma [10, 12, 13]. In addition, the use of routine re-resection for all patients with cT1 disease has improved staging accuracy and has identified patients more likely to experience disease progression, thereby prompting recommendations to undergo immediate cystectomy.

An additional explanation for the improvements in overall survival during the study period may be the improvements that have been made in supportive care. Bladder cancer is strongly associated with tobacco exposure, and patients with bladder cancer frequently experience additional medical conditions such as chronic obstructive pulmonary disease, emphysema, coronary artery disease, vascular disease, obesity, and metabolic comorbidities. Indeed, these patients are at significant risk for perioperative complications, including mortality. Improvements in supportive care, frequent use of supportive services such as specialized preoperative assessment

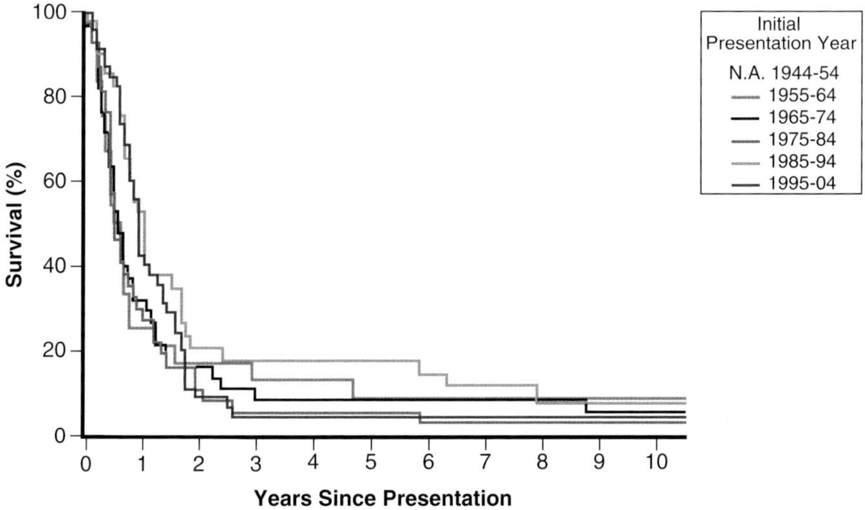

Fig. 14.5 Survival rates for patients with distant (SEER stage) bladder cancer (1944–2004) ($P=0.109$, log-rank test for trend). Because of the very small number of individuals with distant bladder cancer seen from 1944 to 1954, data from this period were excluded. *N.A.* not applicable.

centers, and improved nursing and infrastructure have likely resulted in fewer deaths due to perioperative mortality or from other diseases.

Unlike patients with local and regional disease, overall survival in patients with distant disease has remained poor across the study period (Fig. 14.5). No statistically significant differences or trends in survival estimates were observed at the 10-year increments evaluated ($P=0.109$). Although bladder cancer is considered a chemosensitive tumor, with response rates up to 60% with use of cisplastin-based regimens, the response is invariably transient, and patients usually succumb to their disease within 2 years of a diagnosis of metastatic disease. Unfortunately, no major improvements have been made in chemotherapeutic regimens for bladder cancer since the 1980s, and the treatment of metastatic disease remains largely incurable except for selected groups of patients with nodal metastasis [14, 15]. However, recent data support the utility of neoadjuvant chemotherapy in the setting of muscle-invasive surgically resectable cancer [16]. It is hoped that the identification of targeted therapies based on the aberrant pathway(s) of tumors will lead to new therapies that will improve outcome for patients with distant disease.

Current Management Approach

Our current approach to the management of bladder cancer is dependent on grade, stage, and variant histology (Fig. 14.6). In general, most patients presenting to MD Anderson with a diagnosis of bladder cancer undergo immediate cystoscopic

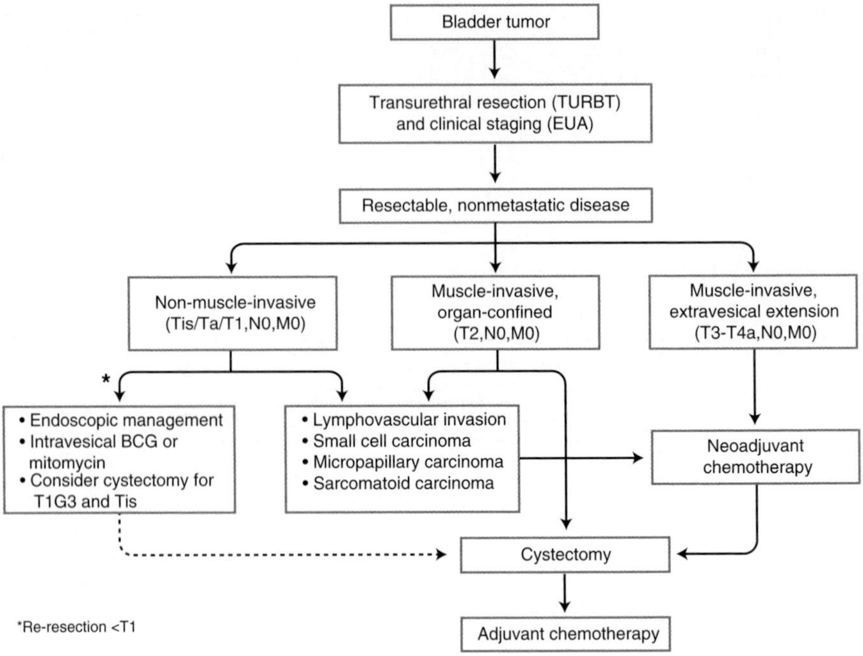

Fig. 14.6 Our current approach to the management of bladder cancer, based on grade, stage, and variant histology. *BCG* bacillus Calmette–Guerin, *EUA* examination under anesthesia, *TURBT* transurethral resection of bladder tumor.

examination under anesthesia as well as transurethral re-resection of the tumor or scarred area of the resected tumor. Re-resection is important not only to confirm that the tumor was removed by the referring urologist but also to gain biologic insight into the behavior of the tumor. For example, patients with T1 disease who have residual/recurrent tumor on re-resection performed at 4–6 weeks after initial TUR are at increased risk of disease progression and should be counseled as patients with T2 disease. This approach provides a uniform assessment of disease stage and enables us to counsel patients toward a treatment approach based on all clinicopathologic features of their disease.

Patients with low-grade disease are treated with endoscopic resection and routine surveillance, with or without intravesical chemotherapy. Patients with intermediate-stage disease (Tis and T1) are counseled to undergo endoscopic resection, intravesical bacillus Calmette–Guerin, or immediate cystectomy on the basis of clinicopathologic features. Patients with advanced-stage disease but without evidence of high-risk features for micrometastasis are counseled to undergo immediate radical cystoprostatectomy with urinary diversion. Our group previously identified high-risk features associated with increased likelihood of pathologic upstaging, including the presence of lymphovascular invasion, hydronephrosis, a three-dimensional mass on examination under anesthesia, and variant adverse histology. Patients with any of these high-risk features are counseled to receive aggressive neoadjuvant cytotoxic chemotherapy [12, 17].

Although the advent of neoadjuvant cisplatin-based combination chemotherapy has had an impact in the treatment of urothelial cancer, the overall outcome in the setting of visceral metastases remains poor. Recent improvements in supportive care with antiemetics and growth factor support have improved the tolerability of chemotherapy. However, gemcitabine plus cisplatin (GC), as well as methotrexate, vinblastine, adriamycin, and cisplatin (M-VAC), remain the standards against which newer chemotherapy will be judged [18]. The use of a dose-dense form of M-VAC, in which all four of the treatment's agents are repeated every 2 weeks, has resulted in an improved toxicity profile and an improved response rate in bladder cancer patients [19], although improvement in survival rate was not seen in this small phase II trial. In light of the improved toxicity profile with dose-dense M-VAC, this combination of drugs has become our preferred treatment.

Conclusion

In this review of the MD Anderson cancer experience between 1944 and 2004, we have observed significant stage migration as the number of patients presenting with regional disease decreased while those presenting with local and distant disease increased. These changes are likely associated with time-dependent stage classification changes, improvement in imaging techniques, and changes in referral patterns. In addition, we observed improvement in the overall survival rates for patients presenting to MD Anderson with bladder cancer. This improvement may be explained by the refinements made in surgical approaches with more complete nodal dissections, improved staging accuracy, and identification of high-risk features, which enabled proper selection of patients for perioperative chemotherapy, as well as improved infrastructure and support systems.

References

1. Jemal A, Siegel R, Ward E, et al. Cancer statistics, 2009. CA Cancer J Clin. 2009;59:225–49.
2. Jemal A, Murray T, Ward E, et al. Cancer statistics, 2005. CA Cancer J Clin. 2005;55:10–30.
3. Messing E. Campbell-Walsh urology. 9th ed. St. Louis: W.B. Saunders; 2007.
4. Black PC, Brown GA, Dinney CP. The impact of variant histology on the outcome of bladder cancer treated with curative intent. Urol Oncol. 2009;27:3–7.
5. Black PC, Dinney CP. Growth factors and receptors as prognostic markers in urothelial carcinoma. Curr Urol Rep. 2008;9:55–61.
6. Adam L, Kassouf W, Dinney CP. Clinical applications for targeted therapy in bladder cancer. Urol Clin North Am. 2005;32:239–46. vii.
7. Svatek RS, Kamat AM, Dinney CP. Novel therapeutics for patients with non-muscle-invasive bladder cancer. Expert Rev Anticancer Ther. 2009;9:807–13.

8. Kamat AM, Dinney CP, Gee JR, et al. Micropapillary bladder cancer: a review of the University of Texas MD. Anderson Cancer Center experience with 100 consecutive patients. Cancer. 2007;110:62–7.
9. Kamat AM, Gee JR, Dinney CP, et al. The case for early cystectomy in the treatment of nonmuscle invasive micropapillary bladder carcinoma. J Urol. 2006;175:881–5.
10. Siefker-Radtke AO, Dinney CP, Abrahams NA, et al. Evidence supporting preoperative chemotherapy for small cell carcinoma of the bladder: a retrospective review of the M.D. Anderson cancer experience. J Urol. 2004;172:481–4.
11. Siefker-Radtke AO, Kamat AM, Grossman HB, et al. Phase II clinical trial of neoadjuvant alternating doublet chemotherapy with ifosfamide/doxorubicin and etoposide/cisplatin in small-cell urothelial cancer. J Clin Oncol. 2009;27:2592–7.
12. Siefker-Radtke A, Millikan RE, Kamat AM, et al. A phase II trial of sequential neoadjuvant chemotherapy with ifosfamide, doxorubicin, and gemcitabine (IAG), followed by cisplatin, gemcitabine, and ifosfamide (CGI) in locally advanced urothelial cancer: Final results from the MD Anderson Cancer Center. J Clin Oncol. 2008;26:269s.
13. Abrahams NA, Moran C, Reyes AO, et al. Small cell carcinoma of the bladder: a contemporary clinicopathological study of 51 cases. Histopathology. 2005;46:57–63.
14. Sweeney P, Millikan R, Donat M, et al. Is there a therapeutic role for post-chemotherapy retroperitoneal lymph node dissection in metastatic transitional cell carcinoma of the bladder? J Urol. 2003;169:2113–7.
15. Siefker-Radtke A. Systemic chemotherapy options for metastatic bladder cancer. Expert Rev Anticancer Ther. 2006;6:877–85.
16. Grossman HB, Natale RB, Tangen CM, et al. Neoadjuvant chemotherapy plus cystectomy compared with cystectomy alone for locally advanced bladder cancer. N Engl J Med. 2003;349:859–66.
17. Millikan R, Dinney C, Swanson D, et al. Integrated therapy for locally advanced bladder cancer: final report of a randomized trial of cystectomy plus adjuvant M-VAC versus cystectomy with both preoperative and postoperative M-VAC. J Clin Oncol. 2001;19:4005–13.
18. von der Maase H, Hansen SW, Roberts JT, et al. Gemcitabine and cisplatin versus methotrexate, vinblastine, doxorubicin, and cisplatin in advanced or metastatic bladder cancer: results of a large, randomized, multinational, multicenter, phase III study. J Clin Oncol. 2000;18:3068–77.
19. Sternberg CN, de Mulder PH, Schornagel JH, et al. Randomized phase III trial of high-dose-intensity methotrexate, vinblastine, doxorubicin, and cisplatin (MVAC) chemotherapy and recombinant human granulocyte colony-stimulating factor versus classic MVAC in advanced urothelial tract tumors: European Organization for Research and Treatment of Cancer Protocol no. 30924. J Clin Oncol. 2001;19:2638–46.

Chapter 15
Cutaneous Melanoma

Jeffrey E. Gershenwald, Geoffrey G. Giacco, and Jeffrey E. Lee

Introduction

According to the American Cancer Society, melanoma represents the sixth most commonly diagnosed cancer in the USA; approximately 76,250 individuals are expected to be diagnosed with invasive melanoma in 2012 [1]. Between 1975 and 2005, the annual incidence of invasive cutaneous melanoma in the USA rose by an average of 3.1% per year, faster than that of nearly all other cancers [2, 3]. The estimated lifetime risk of developing cutaneous melanoma will be 1 in 50 by 2015 [2]. Moreover, recent data showed a real increase in incidence for both males and females, including young women. Also concerning is the finding that although the incidence of most cancers monitored by the surveillance, epidemiology, and end results (SEER) program has been decreasing, the incidence of melanoma has been increasing; in fact, the increase in the incidence of melanoma is the highest of all cancers, even among the subset of cancers that showed increasing incidence between 1995 and 2006 [2].

Melanoma of the skin, known as cutaneous melanoma, arises from melanocytes, the neural crest-derived pigment-producing cells found at the dermal–epidermal junction of the skin. Historically, melanoma has been subtyped on the basis of histopathologic factors, anatomic site, and degree of sun damage, and conventionally further classified as superficial spreading melanoma, nodular melanoma, lentigo maligna melanoma, acral lentiginous melanoma, or desmoplastic melanoma [4].

J.E. Gershenwald (✉) • J.E. Lee
Department of Surgical Oncology, The University of Texas MD Anderson Cancer Center, 1400 Pressler Street, FCT 17.6000, Houston, TX 77030, USA
e-mail: jgershen@mdanderson.org

G.G. Giacco
Department of Tumor Registry, The University of Texas MD Anderson Cancer Center, Houston, TX, USA

M.A. Rodriguez et al. (eds.), *60 Years of Survival Outcomes at The University of Texas MD Anderson Cancer Center*, DOI 10.1007/978-1-4614-5197-6_15,

Despite the longevity of the classic "histogenetic" classification system for melanoma, evidence has been rapidly accumulating showing that distinct categories of melanoma do exist and that underlying genetic alterations drive observed morphologic differences among melanomas. This so-called morphogenetic classification has very recently gained popularity along with the appreciation that specific activating mutations in melanomas that result in aberrant signaling pathways are also correlated with morphology. Examples of important mutations in melanoma include BRAF [5], NRAS, and c-KIT [6]. Although the vast majority of patients with invasive primary cutaneous melanoma present with clinically localized disease (stage I or II), a subset of these patients actually harbor occult regional lymph node disease [7, 8]. In fact, regional lymph node spread represents the most common first site of metastasis in patients with cutaneous melanoma. Unfortunately, in some patients, spread to distant metastatic sites such as liver, lung, or brain occurs.

Historical Perspective

Cutaneous melanoma can occur anywhere on the body; typically, it is found on the lower extremities in women and on the trunk in men. When a patient presents with a suspicious (generally pigmented) lesion suggestive of melanoma, performing a biopsy and histological assessment of the findings is required in order to make a definitive diagnosis and to obtain essential information about the primary tumor, the latter of which is of critical importance in staging, prognosis, and treatment decision-making.

Since the vast majority of patients with invasive primary cutaneous melanoma present with early-stage disease, surgical resection, known as wide excision, with margins appropriate for tumor thickness, is the mainstay of clinical management for most patients. Historically, melanomas were excised with extensive margins (i.e., 3–5 cm), but these excision margins have since narrowed. Current recommendations for excision margin for invasive melanomas range from 1 to 2 cm, depending on tumor thickness of the primary lesion.

Refinements in staging and prognosis—including the important concept of primary melanoma microstaging—were based on landmark attempts to define melanoma-specific prognostic factors in the 1970s and 1980s [9]; such refinements led to the development of important clinical trials that have helped define predictors of outcome, including Breslow tumor thickness (the measured "depth" of invasion of the melanoma using an ocular micrometer), Clark level of invasion, primary tumor ulceration, and regional node involvement. This information, in turn, led to the establishment of the first American Joint Committee on Cancer (AJCC) melanoma staging system in 1977 [10, 11], itself representing the first formal integration of microstaging into the staging criteria. Multiple evidence-based refinements in staging have subsequently occurred, for which MD Anderson has played an important contributory role, up to and including the most recent AJCC melanoma staging system in 2010 (Tables 15.1 and 15.2) [12–15].

Table 15.1 TNM staging categories for cutaneous melanoma [12]

Classification	Thickness (mm)	Ulceration status/mitoses
T		
Tis	NA	NA
T1	≤1.00	(a) Without ulceration and mitosis <1/mm^2 (b) With ulceration or mitoses ≥1/mm^2
T2	1.01–2.00	(a) Without ulceration (b) With ulceration
T3	2.01–4.00	(a) Without ulceration (b) With ulceration
T4	>4.00	(a) Without ulceration (b) With ulceration
N	**No. of metastatic nodes**	**Nodal metastatic burden**
N0	0	NA
N1	1	(a) Micrometastasis[a] (b) Macrometastasis[b]
N2	2–3	(a) Micrometastasis[a] (b) Macrometastasis[b] (c) In transit metastases/satellites without metastatic nodes
N3	4+ metastatic nodes, or matted nodes, or in transit metastases/ satellites with metastatic nodes	
M	**Site**	**Serum LDH**
M0	No distant metastases	NA
M1a	Distant skin, subcutaneous, or nodal metastases	Normal
M1b	Lung metastases	Normal
M1c	All other visceral metastases	Normal
	Any distant metastasis	Elevated

NA not applicable, *LDH* lactate dehydrogenase
[a]Micrometastases are diagnosed after sentinel lymph node biopsy
[b]Macrometastases are defined as clinically detectable nodal metastases confirmed pathologically

Historically, wide excision of the primary tumor and nodal observation were the standard of care, although regional lymph node metastasis, the most common first site of recurrence in patients with primary melanoma, occurred in a significant minority of patients, many of whom ultimately developed distant metastases and/or whose disease relapsed in the treated nodal basin. Although an approach known as *elective lymph node dissection* was popularized as an early intervention for "at-risk" clinically node-negative patients as part of the initial surgical management, since approximately 20% of such patients harbored occult nodal disease, a consequence was that 80% of patients without any evidence of nodal disease were exposed to the risks of surgery with no potential for benefit [16].

Stemming from this controversy, the "revolutionary" technique of lymphatic mapping and sentinel node biopsy (SLNB) was introduced in 1990 [7, 17, 18] and

Table 15.2 AJCC anatomic stage groupings for cutaneous melanoma [12]

	Clinical staging[a]				Pathologic staging[b]		
	T	N	M		T	N	M
0	Tis	N0	M0	0	Tis	N0	M0
IA	T1a	N0	M0	IA	T1a	N0	M0
IB	T1b	N0	M0	IB	T1b	N0	M0
	T2a	N0	M0		T2a	N0	M0
IIA	T2b	N0	M0	IIA	T2b	N0	M0
	T3a	N0	M0		T3a	N0	M0
IIB	T3b	N0	M0	IIB	T3b	N0	M0
	T4a	N0	M0		T4a	N0	M0
IIC	T4b	N0	M0	IIC	T4b	N0	M0
III	Any T	N>N0	M0	IIIA	T1-4a	N1a	M0
					T1-4a	N2a	M0
				IIIB	T1-4b	N1a	M0
					T1-4b	N2a	M0
					T1-4a	N1b	M0
					T1-4a	N2b	M0
					T1-4a	N2c	M0
				IIIC	T1-4b	N1b	M0
					T1-4b	N2b	M0
					T1-4b	N2c	M0
					Any T	N3	M0
IV	Any T	Any N	M1	IV	Any T	Any N	M1

[a]Clinical staging includes microstaging of the primary melanoma and clinical/radiologic evaluation for metastases. By convention, it should be used after complete excision of the primary melanoma with clinical assessment for regional and distant metastases

[b]Pathologic staging includes microstaging of the primary melanoma and pathologic information about the regional lymph nodes after partial (i.e., sentinel node biopsy) or complete lymphadenectomy. Pathologic stage 0 or stage 1A patients are the exception; they do not require pathologic evaluation of their lymph nodes

was soon adopted at MD Anderson as a surgical staging strategy to identify a subset of patients with primary melanoma who actually harbor occult regional lymph node metastasis and to potentially facilitate the management of regional nodal metastases [7, 19]. More than 20 years later, it is evident that this technique has become a standard of care for patients with melanoma and has already had a remarkable and durable impact on melanoma staging and prognosis [8, 20].

Clinical investigations since the 1970s have helped to refine treatment, including evidence-based approaches to excision margins and the approach to the regional nodal basin in patients with melanoma [20, 21]. Other techniques (including the use of adjuvant radiotherapy for certain high-risk primary tumors and bulky nodal disease), refinements in surgical technique (such as lymphatic mapping and SLNB), and the use of metastasectomy in patients with distant metastasis [22] have also played a major role in improving treatment approaches.

Although a multitude of systemic approaches spanning conventional chemotherapeutic, immunologic, and biologic arenas have been used over the past several decades in an attempt to treat patients with distant melanoma metastases, some of which resulted in improved response rates compared with prior treatment regimens (e.g., biochemotherapy) [23], few of these approaches have been associated with clear-cut survival benefit or widespread adoption in the melanoma community. Nonetheless, despite these significant challenges and the overall poor prognosis that continue to be associated with distant metastatic disease, some patients have clearly responded to such systemic approaches in a clinically meaningful way. In addition, two very recent therapeutic developments have sent a wave of enthusiasm throughout the global melanoma community. Very recent clinical trial data have provided new hope for treatments that capitalize on molecularly defined targeted approaches for patients with particular mutations (so-called personalized or targeted therapy) [24]; results from targeted intervention of the immune system (e.g., anti-CTLA-4, adoptive cell transfer) [25, 26] have been encouraging as well. Based on recently published randomized clinical trials demonstrating a survival benefit, the FDA has very recently approved two new therapies for metastatic melanoma—ipilimumab (an anti-CTLA-4 monoclonal antibody) [26] and vemurafenib (a small molecular inhibitor of V600E mutant BRAF for patients with unresectable or distant metastases and whose tumor has the mutation) [24, 27].

The MD Anderson Cancer Center Experience

The MD Anderson data set used for this monograph was derived from 21,434 patients with melanoma of the skin (cutaneous melanoma) initially presenting at MD Anderson between 1 March 1944, and 31 December 2004. It is important to note, however, that only 2,516 (11.7%) met inclusion criteria for this analysis (i.e., no previous treatment before presenting at MD Anderson, including after excisional diagnostic biopsy alone); when an additional 810 patients who did not have definitive treatment at MD Anderson and/or had at least one other primary malignancy (except superficial non-melanoma skin cancer) were excluded, only 1,692 (7.9%) of the 21,434 patients were included in the current data set.

Specifically, from a tumor registry standpoint, the structured approach to the definition of an "analytic" case—which dictated inclusion or exclusion of a particular patient in this data set—was not melanoma-specific, yet had tremendous impact on the population included in this analysis, not only with respect to the overall fraction of total patients included (only 7.9% overall), but also to stage distribution. For example, since the tumor registry specifically excluded from entry those patients with melanoma who had undergone complete "excision" as a component of their treatment (even if their "treatment" was subsequently performed at MD Anderson), it is likely that nearly all patients with in situ melanoma and a significant minority of patients with diminutive invasive melanoma (i.e., a substantial fraction of patients with "local" disease) were excluded from this analysis. It also follows that since patients with regional and/or distant disease would be less likely to have all diseases removed during treatment after the initial diagnosis (and hence more likely to present

Table 15.3 Initial presentation year by SEER stage

	SEER stage at presentation[a,b]				
	Local	Regional	Distant	Unstaged	Total
Decade	[No. (%) of patients]				
1944–1954	24 (54.5)	7 (15.9)	7 (15.9)	6 (13.6)	44 (100.0)
1955–1964	88 (47.8)	39 (21.2)	26 (14.1)	31 (16.8)	184 (100.0)
1965–1974	120 (37.5)	58 (18.1)	63 (19.7)	79 (24.7)	320 (100.0)
1975–1984	273 (67.4)	67 (16.5)	54 (13.3)	11 (2.7)	405 (100.0)
1985–1994	224 (67.7)	62 (18.7)	41 (12.4)	4 (1.2)	331 (100.0)
1995–2004	260 (63.7)	115 (28.2)	30 (7.4)	3 (0.7)	408 (100.0)
Total	*989 (58.5)*	*348 (20.6)*	*221 (13.1)*	*134 (7.9)*	*1,692 (100.0)*

SEER Surveillance, Epidemiology, and End Results program
[a]Because of registry-based methodologies used to define “analytic” cases included in the Tumor Registry (and this table), only 7.9% of patients with cutaneous melanoma initially presenting to MD Anderson through 2004 (1,692 of 21,434 patients) are included in this table. As such, data do not accurately reflect clinical breadth of patients or accurately represent distribution of patients by clinical SEER stage seen at MD Anderson
[b]Insufficient analytic Tumor Registry data to include in situ melanoma

to MD Anderson with some disease remaining) and before definitive treatment, these patients were likely overrepresented in this data set. Although these observations very significantly limit the utility of some aspects of this data presentation (and interpretation), selected observations are nonetheless noteworthy and represent the framework for this monograph.

With these limitations noted, the number of patients presenting by time interval and SEER stage is summarized in Table 15.3. As anticipated, the number of patients with localized disease generally increased over time, whereas the fraction of patients who presented with regional or distant disease decreased. The computed survival curves (Figs. 15.1, 15.2, 15.3, and 15.4) represent clinical outcomes for the 1,706 analytic patients with melanoma described above who received definitive treatment at MD Anderson and who were not excluded for reasons already noted. The usual tumor registry methodology of describing disease extent under the headings of local, regional, and distant has been used in the construction of survival curves by “stage.” Since most histologic parameters and nearly all pathology-based stage groupings did not enter the clinical melanoma arena until the 1970s and 1980s, no attempts were made to stratify patients according to the AJCC melanoma staging system, itself a leader in evidence-based prognostic factors assessment since the late 1970s [28].

Despite these significant limitations, it is noteworthy that the overall survival curve (analytic patients only) documents significant incremental improvement in 5-year survival over the 60-year period ($P<0.0001$ for log-rank test for trend) (Fig. 15.1). The overall survival curves for patients (Fig. 15.1) demonstrate significantly improved 5-year and 10-year survival for patients treated during the most recent time interval compared with the earliest strata (68% vs. 39% and 57% vs. 25%, respectively). During the earlier decades of this analysis, stage assignments were based primarily on clinical staging. Over time, however, both primary tumor microstaging (based on histologic assessment of the primary tumor introduced

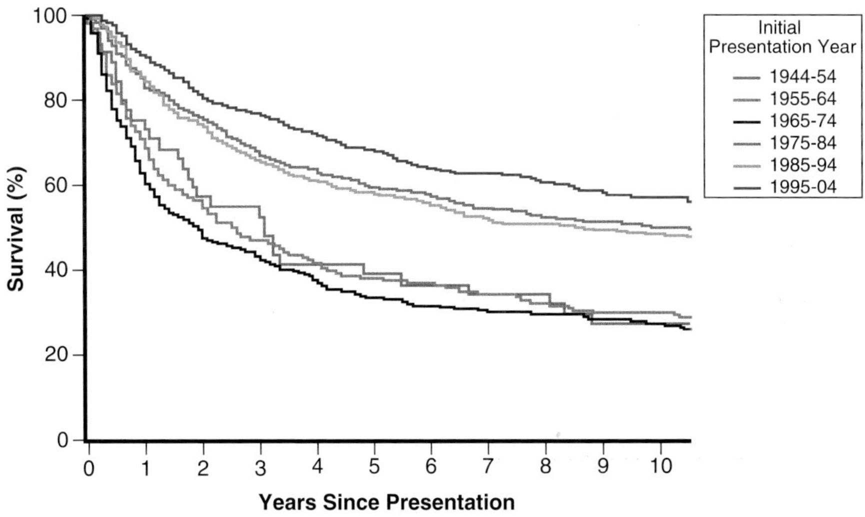

Fig. 15.1 Overall survival rates for patients with cutaneous melanoma (1944–2004) ($P < 0.0001$, log-rank test for trend).

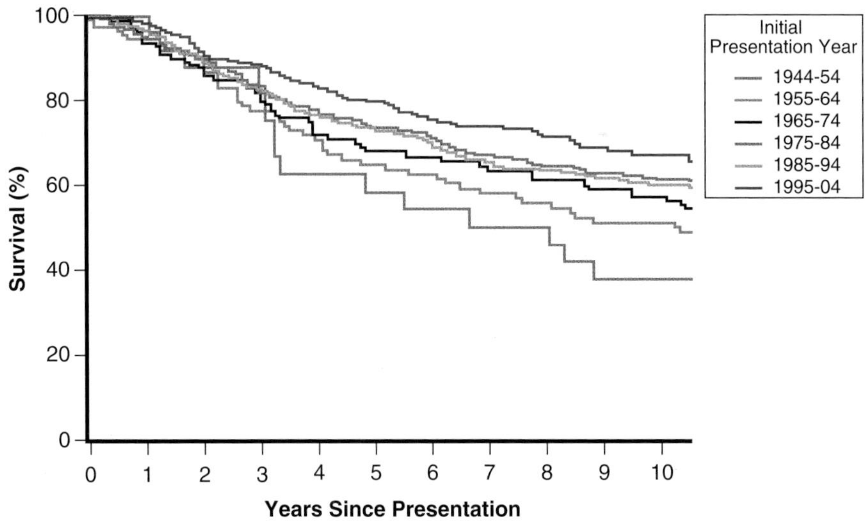

Fig. 15.2 Overall survival rates for patients with local (SEER stage) cutaneous melanoma (1944–2004) ($P < 0.0001$, log-rank test for trend).

in the 1970s) and regional node pathological staging (i.e., elective lymph node dissection for patients with clinically negative regional nodes predominantly in the 1970s and 1980s, and therapeutic lymph node dissection in the setting of clinically involved regional nodes throughout this overall experience) began to define the concept of pathological staging in melanoma. Moreover, over the past 20 years,

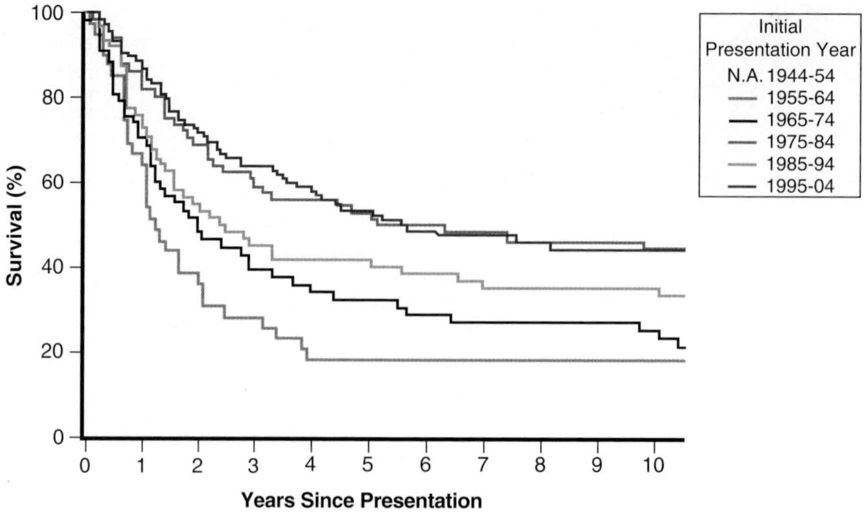

Fig. 15.3 Overall survival rates for patients with regional (SEER stage) cutaneous melanoma (1944–2004) ($P<0.0001$, log-rank test for trend). Because of the very small number of individuals with regional cutaneous melanoma seen from 1944 to 1954, data from this period were excluded. *N.A.* not applicable.

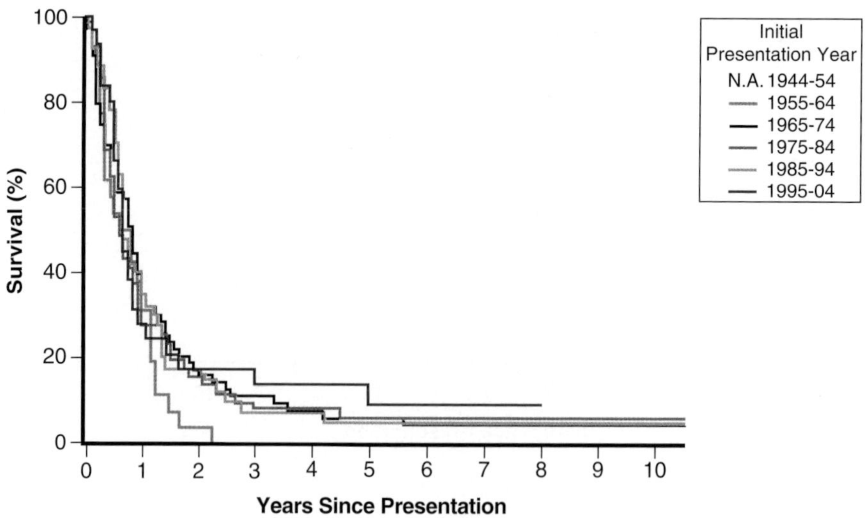

Fig. 15.4 Overall survival rates for patients with distant (SEER stage) cutaneous melanoma (1944–2004) ($P=0.79$, log-rank test for trend). Because of the very small number of individuals with distant cutaneous melanoma seen from 1944 to 1954, data from this period were excluded. *N.A.* not applicable.

surgical staging of regional nodes has been based on lymphatic mapping and SLNB for many patients with clinically negative nodes, further refining pathological regional node staging for patients with early-stage melanoma. Additionally, stage-appropriate evaluation by computed tomography, magnetic resonance imaging, and other modalities became more common among recently treated patients with melanoma. As such, it is evident that assignment of stage across the spectrum of the 60-year course of data was anything but uniform, and although clearly made with use of the best available information at the time of registration, has been subject to tremendous evolution, with more accurate definitions of local, regional, and distant disease emerging over time.

The survival curves for patients with localized tumors (Fig. 15.2) demonstrate significantly improved 5-year and 10-year survival outcomes for patients treated during the most recent time interval compared with the earliest strata (80% vs. 58% and 67% vs. 38%, respectively). During these decades, surgical treatment of the primary tumor—known as wide excision—evolved as a result of a cadre of clinical trials conducted since the 1970s that assessed excision margins on the basis of histologic parameters of the primary; these trials resulted in a relative "narrowing" of excision margins that has favorably affected surgical morbidity rates while not negatively impacting overall survival rates.

Relative improvements in survival among patients with localized disease may also be associated with improved awareness of melanoma, resulting in at least some patients diagnosed with "early" disease. Also likely relevant was the appreciation that regional nodes are the first and most important site of metastasis; accordingly, patients with clinical evidence of regional disease would be more likely to be identified (and thus included as "regional"). Furthermore, adoption of surgical strategies, including elective node dissection from a historical standpoint and more recently lymphatic mapping and SLNB, has contributed to "early" identification of microscopic regional node disease. These patients' disease was therefore appropriately coded as regional and *excluded* from the localized patient cohort. Because of the incorporation of SLNB, a surgical staging method to evaluate regional nodal basins at risk for microscopic regional node disease, into the melanoma management algorithm in the early 1990s, it is likely that our enhanced ability to identify small-volume regional microscopic disease will continue to contribute to a more homogenous "local" group (by excluding node-positive patients) and associated improved survival over time.

It is important to emphasize that due to the registry-based procedures in documenting what constitutes an analytic case (and thus included in these survival curves), many patients with very early stage primary melanoma were likely excluded from this analysis. Accordingly, even though survival improved over time during the past 60 years, absolute survival estimates for patients with localized disease were likely *underestimated*. As an example of this phenomenon, after interrogation of the MD Anderson Tumor Registry for patients diagnosed with melanoma between 1995 and 2004 whose only previous treatment before coming to MD Anderson was surgery (including surgical excision for diagnosis and primary tumor microstaging only) during the prior 3 months and whose biopsy and/or surgical treatment removed

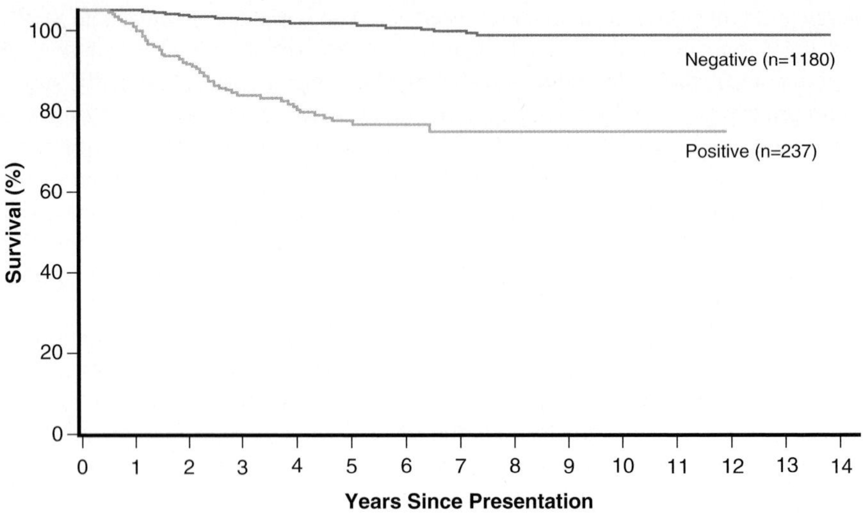

Fig. 15.5 Melanoma-specific survival of patients with stage I or II disease according to sentinel lymph node status.

all melanoma upon pathologic review, 1,899 patients were identified. Most of these patients had localized disease: 5-year and 10-year survival rates were 93% and 85.3%, respectively. This was significantly better than the associated 5-year and 10-year survival rates estimates for analytic patients with localized disease diagnosed during the same interval (80% and 67%, respectively) (Fig. 15.2); the mixed cohort actually included many patients excluded from the analytic component of this analysis who had early-stage low-risk primary melanoma.

Relatively dramatic improvement in survival is noted in patients with regional disease over the 60 years of data recording (Fig. 15.3), ranging from few, if any, long-term survivors in 1944–1954 to a 54% 5-year survival rate among patients with regional disease during 1995–2004. It is noteworthy that over time, particularly within the past 10–20 years, the way in which regional melanoma is diagnosed has evolved. Specifically, more than 30 years ago, nearly all patients who were diagnosed with regional disease at presentation had clinical disease at presentation, due in large part to tremendous strides in surgical-based staging of the regional node basins at risk in patients with primary melanomas; the overwhelming majority of patients currently diagnosed with regional metastasis have microscopic disease only, most commonly identified by lymphatic mapping and SLNB in those with clinically negative nodes [13].

An example of the prognostic significance of SLNB from a well-characterized clinical research database is shown in Fig. 15.5, in which patients with primary melanoma treated at MD Anderson who had had clinically negative nodes and had undergone SLNB between approximately 1991 and 2004 had remarkably differing survival outcomes when stratified by the histologic status of the sentinel lymph nodes (SLNs), the most likely nodes to contain disease if any are involved. Note in particular the favorable survival profile among the SLN-negative cohorts (Fig. 15.5, upper curve) compared with historical "local" patients (Fig. 15.2) and a similar observation among SLN-positive patients (Fig. 15.5, lower curve) compared with historical "regional" patients (Fig. 15.3).

Numerous studies, including comprehensive analyses of patients with regional disease conducted by the AJCC melanoma staging committee that included patients from MD Anderson, revealed tremendous heterogeneity among all patients with regional melanoma and the fact that patients with microscopic regional node disease (diagnosed by SLNB, for example) had more favorable survival rates than did patients with macroscopic (i.e., clinically or radiographically evident) regional disease [13]. In addition, overall better classification of patients with regional disease, achieved by excluding patients with synchronous distant disease, particularly among patients with clinically documented regional disease, has improved over the years with the advent of computed tomography, magnetic resonance imaging, and more recently, positron emission tomography/computed tomography—patients with documented yet asymptomatic distant metastasis would be classified as having distant, not regional, disease.

It is not surprising that survival outcomes for patients with melanoma who have distant disease have generally remained poor across the entire study spectrum (Fig. 15.4), with no statistically significant differences observed. During the 60-year period through 2004, although some patients undoubtedly responded to systemic treatment—including conventional chemotherapy with cytotoxic agents such as dacarbazine (DTIC), vinblastine, and cisplatin; chemotherapy combined with biologic agents such as interleukin-2 and interferon alpha-2b (known as biochemotherapy); biologic agents such as high-dose interleukin-2; immunologic approaches such as adoptive cell transfer; and surgical approaches for isolated or oligometastatic distant disease—durable responses were nonetheless difficult to achieve, which likely explains the failure to notably improve outcome in these patients with advanced disease. Along these lines, no randomized trial has demonstrated a survival benefit using any of these approaches during this 60-year period. Although these challenges are significant, very recent promising data have begun to shine light on the future for patients with distant metastatic disease. As noted above, two recent therapeutic approaches—ipilimumab and vemurafenib—received FDA approval in 2011 [24, 26, 27].

Current Management Approach

Current management of melanoma is stage-specific. For patients with primary cutaneous melanoma, treatment is based predominantly on primary tumor microstaging (i.e., tumor thickness, presence of ulceration, mitotic rate); comprehensive multimodality extent of disease imaging is rarely indicated for the asymptomatic patient with newly diagnosed melanoma due to the infrequent observation of synchronous radiographically evident distant metastasis. The mainstay of treatment of the primary tumor site is wide excision with margins based on tumor thickness. The approach to the regional nodal basin has been the subject of intense debate over the past several decades, although the surgery-based approach to pathologic staging of regional node basins (lymphatic mapping and SLNB) for patients with tumor thickness considered intermediate (i.e., 1–4 mm), thick (>4 mm), or as potentially high-risk thin invasive primary melanoma, identifies patient-specific afferent lymphatics leading to regional nodes (SLNs) and has revolutionized our ability to document early regional metastasis and to identify patients who may benefit from additional nodal surgery and adjuvant systemic therapy. Radiotherapy has also been identified as a way to enhance regional control among patients with extensive clinical regional metastasis.

Although the overwhelming majority of patients with early-stage *localized* melanoma require no additional treatment after surgery, patients with regional metastasis may be offered high-dose interferon alpha-2b, observation, or participation in a clinical trial. For patients with distant metastasis, surgery (for isolated or oligometastatic disease), systemic chemotherapy, biochemotherapy, biologic therapy (e.g., IL-2), or immunologic approaches such as adoptive cell transfer, preferably in the context of participation in a clinical trial, may be considered. Importantly, the treatment landscape for patients with metastatic melanoma has very recently changed with the approval of both ipilimumab and vemurafenib (both in 2011); as our understanding of mutations commonly found in melanoma has expanded, explosive interest in developing new anti-melanoma therapeutics by interrogating aberrantly active tumor-specific pathways has yielded an exciting new therapeutic (i.e., vemurafenib) and more broadly, has ushered in a new era of targeted therapy and personalized medicine.

Future improvements with melanoma survival outcomes are likely to be derived from multiple strategies: earlier diagnosis of patients with primary melanoma (i.e., thinner primary melanomas), more effective adjuvant therapies for patients with regional metastasis, and better multimodality approaches to distant metastasis. Although much has been learned recently regarding the nature of aberrant signaling pathways in melanoma resulting from various activating mutations (e.g., BRAF, NRAS, and cKIT), a better understanding of these pathways as they relate to specific cancer types will likely facilitate development of more targeted approaches to metastatic disease (e.g., combinatorial approaches) and hopefully improve existing systemic treatment results and options for our patients.

References

1. American Cancer Society. Cancer facts and figures 2012. Atlanta: American Cancer Society; 2012. http://www.cancer.org/acs/groups/content/@epidemiologysurveilance/documents/document/acspc-031941.pdf. Accessed 13 Mar 2012.
2. Ries LAG, Melbert D, Krapcho M, et al. SEER cancer statistics review, 1975–2005. Bethesda: National Cancer Institute; 2008.
3. Linos E, Swetter SM, Cockburn MG, Colditz GA, Clarke CA. Increasing burden of melanoma in the United States. J Invest Dermatol. 2009;129:1666–74.

4. Gershenwald JE, Hwu P. Melanoma. In: Hong WK, Bast RC, Hait WN, et al., editors. Cancer medicine. 8th ed. Shelton: People's Medical Publishing House; 2010. p. 1459–86.
5. Davies H, Bignell GR, Cox C, et al. Mutations of the BRAF gene in human cancer. Nature. 2002;417:949–54.
6. Curtin JA, Busam K, Pinkel D, Bastian BC. Somatic activation of KIT in distinct subtypes of melanoma. J Clin Oncol. 2006;24:4340–6.
7. Gershenwald JE, Thompson W, Mansfield PF, et al. Multi-institutional melanoma lymphatic mapping experience: the prognostic value of sentinel lymph node status in 612 stage I or II melanoma patients. J Clin Oncol. 1999;17:976–83.
8. Gershenwald JE, Ross MI. Sentinel-lymph-node biopsy for cutaneous melanoma. N Engl J Med. 2011;364:1738–45.
9. Breslow A. Thickness, cross-sectional areas and depth of invasion in the prognosis of cutaneous melanoma. Ann Surg. 1970;172:902–8.
10. Staging of malignant melanoma. In: Manual for staging of cancer, 1st (revised) ed. Chicago: American Joint Committee on Cancer; 1978. p. 131–40.
11. Staging of malignant melanoma. In: Manual for staging of cancer, 1st ed. Chicago: American Joint Committee on Cancer; 1977. p. 131–6.
12. Balch CM, Gershenwald JE, Soong SJ, et al. Final version of 2009 AJCC melanoma staging and classification. J Clin Oncol. 2009;27:6199–206.
13. Balch CM, Gershenwald JE, Soong SJ, et al. Multivariate analysis of prognostic factors among 2,313 patients with stage III melanoma: comparison of nodal micrometastases versus macrometastases. J Clin Oncol. 2010;28:2452–9.
14. Balch CM. Melanoma of the skin. In: Edge SB, Byrd DR, Compton CC, Fritz AG, Greene FL, Trotti III A, editors. AJCC cancer staging manual. 7th ed. New York: Springer; 2009.
15. Balch CM, Buzaid AC, Soong SJ, et al. Final version of the American Joint Committee on cancer staging system for cutaneous melanoma. J Clin Oncol. 2001;19:3635–48.
16. Ross MI. Surgery and other local-regional modalities for all stages of melanoma. Curr Opin Oncol. 1994;6:197–203.
17. Morton DL, Wen DR, Wong JH, et al. Technical details of intraoperative lymphatic mapping for early stage melanoma. Arch Surg. 1992;127:392–9.
18. Ross M, Reintgen D, Balch C. Selective lymphadenectomy: emerging role for lymphatic mapping and sentinel lymph node biopsy in the management of early stage melanoma. Semin Surg Oncol. 1993;9:219–23.
19. Gershenwald JE, Colome MI, Lee JE, et al. Patterns of recurrence following a negative sentinel lymph node biopsy in 243 patients with stage I or II melanoma. J Clin Oncol. 1998;16:2253–60.
20. Ross MI, Thompson JF, Gershenwald JE. Sentinel lymph node biopsy for melanoma: critical assessment at its twentieth anniversay. Surg Oncol Clin N Am. 2011;20(1):57–78.
21. Ross MI, Gershenwald JE. Evidence-based treatment of early-stage melanoma. J Surg Oncol. 2011;104(4):341–53.
22. Caudle AS, Ross MI. Metastasectomy for stage IV melanoma: for whom and how much? Surg Oncol Clin N Am. 2011;20(1):133–44.
23. Bedikian AY, Johnson MM, Warneke CL, et al. Systemic therapy for unresectable metastatic melanoma: impact of biochemotherapy on long-term survival. J Immunotoxicol. 2008;5:201–7.
24. Flaherty KT, Puzanov I, Kim KB, et al. Inhibition of mutated, activated BRAF in metastatic melanoma. N Engl J Med. 2010;363:809–19.
25. Dudley ME, Wunderlich JR, Yang JC, et al. Adoptive cell transfer therapy following non-myeloablative but lymphodepleting chemotherapy for the treatment of patients with refractory metastatic melanoma. J Clin Oncol. 2005;23:2346–57.
26. Hodi FS, O'Day SJ, McDermott DF, et al. Improved survival with ipilimumab in patients with metastatic melanoma. N Engl J Med. 2010;363:711–23.
27. Chapman PB, Hauschild A, Robert C, et al. BRIM-3 Study Group. Improved survival with vemurafenib in melanoma with BRAF V600E mutation. N Engl J Med. 2011;364:2507–16.
28. Gershenwald JE, Buzaid AC, Ross MI. Classification and staging of melanoma. Hematol Oncol Clin North Am. 1998;12:737–65.

Chapter 16
Liver Cancer

Evan S. Glazer and Steven A. Curley

Introduction

Primary malignancies of the liver typically include hepatocellular carcinoma (HCC) and biliary carcinoma (cholangiocarcinoma, CC). Although there are other primary cancers of the liver, such as hepatoblastoma, their rarity makes description and analysis of them difficult. An estimated 30,000 people in the USA developed liver cancer in 2008, and the incidence is increasing [1]. Nearly 20,000 people die of primary liver cancer each year [1]. Despite improved treatments for HCC, the overall 5-year survival rate in the USA for patients with this disease remains less than 10% [2]. Furthermore, in the USA, the most rapid increase in cancer-related deaths among men has been seen in those with HCC [3]. The standard of care remains multimodality therapy, but very few patients are candidates for curative resection or liver transplantation [4]. Intra-arterial chemoembolization is one component of multidisciplinary therapy, but it does not usually offer a cure. Even sorafenib, the most recently approved systemic (oral) drug for treatment of HCC, increased median survival length by less than 3 months compared with controls, to a total of 10.7 months [5].

The major risk factors for HCC include viral infections (hepatitis B and hepatitis C) and cirrhosis from any cause [6]. Other rare etiologies include inherited disorders, such as hemochromatosis and Wilson's disease. Of note, there is a growing, albeit poorly defined, association between nonalcoholic fatty liver disease, metabolic syndrome, diabetes, and HCC [6]. Even if this association increases the risk of HCC only slightly, the sheer number of people in the USA who are at risk

E.S. Glazer
Department of Surgery, The University of Arizona Medical Center, Tucson, AZ, USA

S.A. Curley (✉)
Department of Surgical Oncology, The University of Texas MD Anderson Cancer Center, 1400 Pressler Street, Unit 1447, Houston, TX 77030, USA
e-mail: scurley@mdanderson.org

M.A. Rodriguez et al. (eds.), *60 Years of Survival Outcomes at The University of Texas MD Anderson Cancer Center*, DOI 10.1007/978-1-4614-5197-6_16,

for developing nonalcoholic steatosis or steatohepatitis may greatly increase the number of patients with HCC.

Unfortunately, despite some evidence that hepatitis C virus may be associated with CC, there are no definitive predisposing risk factors for CC [6], which makes effective and efficient screening for CC nearly impossible. Patients often present with nonspecific findings such as fever, weight loss, and a dull upper abdominal or flank pain. Jaundice may be present, especially in advanced disease.

Screening of patients for HCC, typically cirrhotic patients, is highly recommended [based on National Comprehensive Cancer Network (NCCN) 2009 guidelines; see guidelines for the complete algorithm] [6]. Usually, patients have known risk factors such as chronic hepatitis C virus infection. It has been demonstrated that screening based on high-risk patients' serum alpha-fetoprotein (AFP) and transabdominal hepatic ultrasonography decreased HCC mortality by more than 37% [7]. Ideally, screening begins early in the disease course to evaluate changes in AFP or new findings on hepatic ultrasonography. Since both of these screening studies are relatively inexpensive and nearly risk-free, the clinical benefit is potentially significant.

Prognosis is associated with tumor characteristics, patient characteristics, and the treatment received. Tumor characteristics include stage/location, aggressiveness, vascular invasion, and growth rate. Larger, more aggressive, and faster-growing tumors are all associated with worse outcomes. Patient characteristics include overall health and liver function, as measured by one of the clinically validated scoring systems [i.e., Child-Pugh or Model End Stage Liver Disease (MELD) score] [6]. As expected, healthier people with normal liver function tend to have better outcomes with improved survival and decreased morbidity. The type of treatment that can be offered is based on the stage of disease and liver function (resection, thermal ablation, other local therapy, or systemic) and is directly related to survival. Tumors that can be completely resected are associated with a greater chance of long-term survival, whereas ablative therapies typically do not result in cure rates as high.

The diagnosis of HCC is typically made in a cirrhotic patient who either is symptomatic (dull/vague upper abdominal pain, anorexia/weight loss, or even occasionally a palpable mass) or has undergone screening as described. The most important imaging study is triphasic computed tomography (CT) to evaluate for the presence of lesions with significant arterial enhancement followed by contrast washout on the venous phase [6]. If a patient cannot undergo contrast CT, magnetic resonance imaging (MRI) may be a reasonable alternative. CC, however, is often best visualized on delayed phase CT or MRI, but there are no pathognomonic radiologic findings.

Historical Perspective

Most of the currently available surgical options/techniques or therapies for advanced disease, such as sorafenib, were developed in recent years. Historically, regional disease was nearly as fatal as distant metastatic disease. Although conformal radiotherapy is now an option in selected cases, the use of nontargeted ionizing radiation often results in devastating hepatic complications without major oncologic benefit. Likewise, modern techniques for hemostasis during liver resection have reduced the major perioperative morbidity and mortality combined rate from historically greater than 50% to currently less than 10% with experienced surgeons at high-volume centers. Cytotoxic chemotherapeutics used in patients with HCC or CC are neither targeted nor very effective, and as such, they do not typically offer significant benefits as first-line agents.

The MD Anderson Cancer Center Experience

Survival rates improved for non-metastatic primary liver cancer based on Kaplan–Meier analyses of the MD Anderson Cancer Center patient population over a 50-year study period (Table 16.1; Fig. 16.1). Because of the very small number of liver cancer patients who presented to MD Anderson during the first decade of its existence, this analysis focused on the period from 1955 to 2004. Improvements in surgical techniques, critical care, and earlier diagnosis all contributed to the increased survival seen in the latter two decades.

By 2004, patients with liver cancer limited to the liver had a 5-year survival rate of nearly 40%, whereas 50 years earlier, that rate was less than 20%. Moreover, the rate of 10-year survival in patients who presented with local [Surveillance, Epidemiology, and End Results (SEER) stage] disease nearly doubled over this 50-year study period (Table 16.1). In fact, some patients have even been cured of their disease, as seen in the small but significant 10-year survival rate ($P<0.0001$) (Fig. 16.2).

Just 20 years before the end of the study period, patients with regional spread (regional lymph nodes) and those with distant spread of liver cancer had the same survival rates of 0%. However, recent advancements in surgical technique and modest improvements in chemotherapeutic and multidisciplinary treatment options improved the 5-year and 10-year survival rates significantly (Fig. 16.3; $P=0.008$).

Table 16.1 Survival rate improvement for early-stage liver cancer based on Kaplan–Meier analyses of the MD Anderson Cancer Center patient population over a 50-year period[a]

	Percent survival by disease stage					
	Local		Regional		Distant	
Decade	5 years	10 years	5 years	10 years	5 years	10 years
1944–1954	–	–	–	–	–	–
1955–1964	18.2	18.2	0	0	0	0
1965–1974	16.1	12.9	0	0	4.2	4.2
1975–1984	15.6	10.4	0	0	0	0
1985–1994	27.8	19.5	8.3	4.1	6.1	4.9
1995–2004	38.6	25.9	10.1	3.4	2.4	2.4

[a]Because so few patients with hepatocellular carcinoma or cholangiocarcinoma presented to MD Anderson from 1944 to 1954 with clear diagnostic information, this analysis focused on the period from 1955 to 2004.

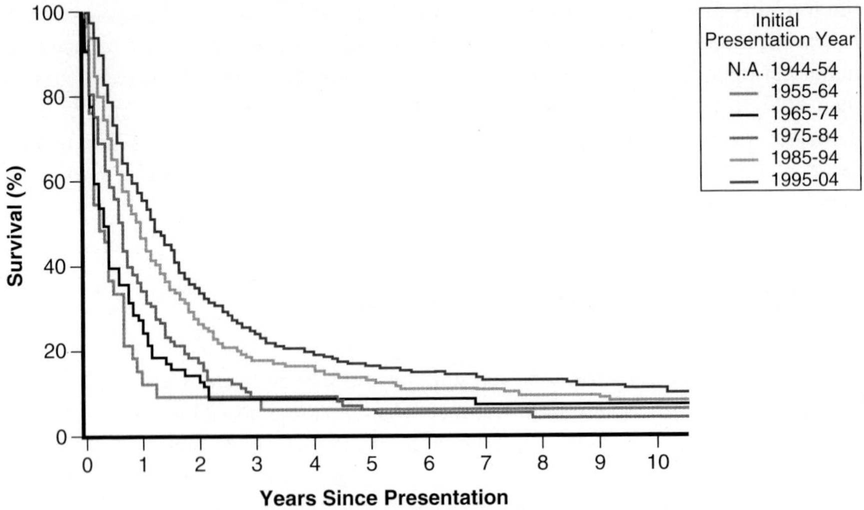

Fig. 16.1 Overall survival rates for patients who presented with liver cancer from 1955 to 2004 ($P<0.0001$, log-rank test for trend). Because of the very small number of individuals with liver cancer who were seen from 1944 to 1954, data from this period were excluded. *N.A.* not applicable.

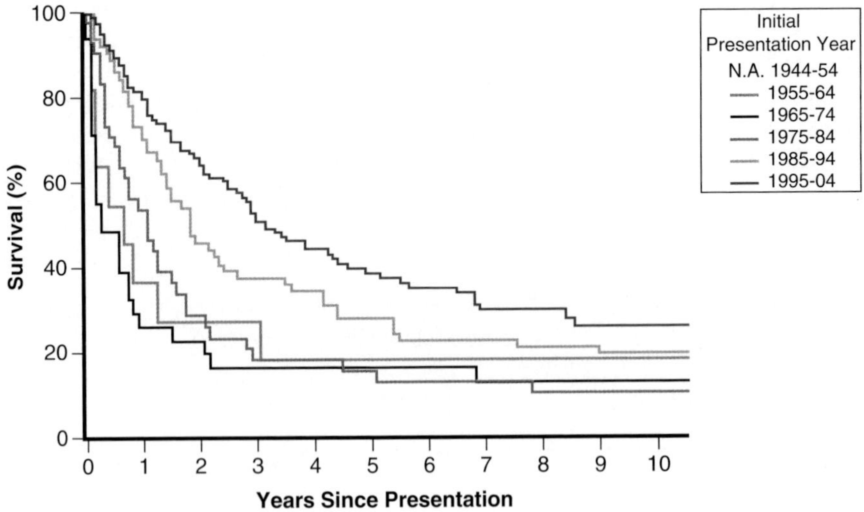

Fig. 16.2 Survival rates for patients who presented with liver cancer confined to the liver (local SEER stage) from 1955 to 2004 ($P<0.0001$, log-rank test for trend). Because of the very small number of individuals with liver cancer confined to the liver who were seen from 1944 to 1954, data from this period were excluded. *N.A.* not applicable.

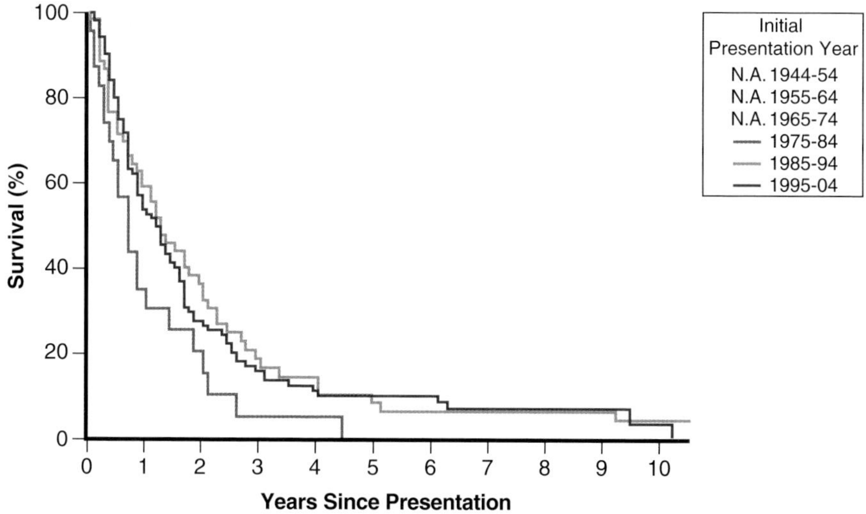

Fig. 16.3 Survival rates for patients with liver cancer who presented with regional (lymph node) disease (regional SEER stage) from 1955 to 2004 ($P=0.008$, log-rank test for trend). Because of the very small number of individuals with regional (lymph node) disease who were seen from 1944 to 1954, from 1955 to 1964, and from 1965 to 1974, data from these periods were excluded. *N.A.* not applicable.

In fact, a very small cohort of patients with advanced disease (2.4%) achieved significant long-term survival during the last decade of the analysis, as seen in the similar rates of 5-year and 10-year survivors (Figs. 16.2 and 16.3).

Although significant improvements have been made in the survival rates of patients with liver cancer limited to the liver and lymph nodes (regional), the same cannot be said about those with distant spread (stage 4 disease) at the time of presentation (Fig. 16.4). There is no clinical or statistical difference in 5-year or 10-year survival rates in patients with metastatic liver cancer. However, short-term (less than 3 years) survival has significantly increased over the past 50 years ($P<0.0001$). The clinical and personal (patient) significance of this added survival time to patients should not be ignored.

Current Management Approach

Screening

The most important step in the management of HCC is active screening to detect early-stage disease. Fortunately, development of the two major etiologies of HCC—cirrhosis and inherited disorders—can often be predicted well before the development of HCC. Specifically, we recommend that all high-risk cirrhotic patients (and

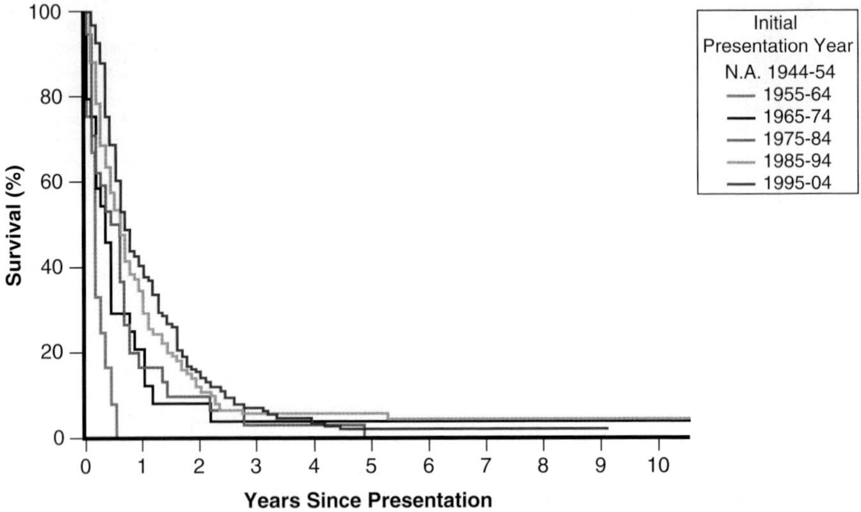

Fig. 16.4 Survival rates for patients with metastatic liver cancer (distant SEER stage) from 1955 to 2004 ($P<0.0001$, log-rank test for trend). Because of the very small number of individuals with metastatic liver cancer who were seen from 1944 to 1954, data from this period were excluded. *N.A.* not applicable.

patients with known inherited disorders involving liver metabolism) undergo screening every 6 months with transabdominal ultrasound and testing for serum AFP levels. In addition, contrast-enhanced ultrasonography should be used if available. Unfortunately, since there are no confirmed predisposing risk factors for CC, the precise population to screen remains unknown.

Diagnosis

As mentioned, the imaging modality of choice to suggest a diagnosis of HCC (and CC) is noninvasive, triphasic CT imaging. However, if the classic CT pattern is not seen, other imaging modalities may be used. Because of its high resolution, MRI is an excellent confirmatory tool. Ultrasound, if not already performed, is an option if it can be performed with intravenous microbubble contrast enhancement.

If noninvasive imaging does not confirm HCC, another option is diagnostic biopsy, typically performed as percutaneous fine-needle biopsy. Finally, surgical biopsy, preferably performed laparoscopically, is an option of last resort to confirm the histological diagnosis. Often, a nondiagnostic fine-needle or core biopsy is repeated before a surgical procedure is performed.

Serum biomarkers also play an important diagnostic role in HCC, but less so in CC [6, 7]. AFP, already mentioned as a screening tool, is used more importantly as a diagnostic tool. Any significant increase in serum AFP level should be considered evidence of HCC unless proven otherwise in high-risk patients undergoing screening. Furthermore, any serum AFP level above 200 ng/mL needs to be addressed as probable HCC, especially in conjunction with any finding on liver imaging studies.

Surgical Resection

Although complete tumor resection or liver transplantation is the optimal curative treatment option currently available, only a small subset of patients with primary liver cancer are candidates for these surgical approaches. Current treatment planning focuses on determining whether a given patient can have the entire lesion(s) safely removed. Although this is a very complex decision, the subsequent treatment is rather straightforward: some combination of resection, ablation, regional treatment, or systemic therapy. If a lesion can be resected, it should be. If a lesion cannot be resected but can be ablated, the patient should be informed of the risk of recurrence and offered aggressive ablation. If neither resection nor ablation is feasible, the patient may choose to undergo regional or systemic therapy based on the stage of disease and severity of concomitant chronic liver disease. Radiotherapy benefits some patients in a few very specific circumstances [8].

When considering resection, the function of the liver needs to be addressed in the context of the planned resection. Moderately cirrhotic patients should have at least 40% of their liver remaining after resection; very mildly cirrhotic patients should have 30% remaining; and noncirrhotic patients should have at least 20% [9]. Severely cirrhotic patients typically do not tolerate major operations such as hepatic resection [10]. Finally, before performing any procedure, the patient's health should be maximized from a cardiac, pulmonary, and renal perspective whenever possible.

Radiotherapy

Controlled, specific, and localized ionizing radiotherapy can be used to treat unresectable HCC in patients who are not candidates for transplantation or other appropriate locoregional therapies [6, 8]. Both electron beam and proton conformal external beam are reasonable options for some patients, albeit for a highly selected population. Radiotherapy is not recommended for treatment of distant metastatic disease except for palliation for bone metastases. Use of radiation is recommended as part of conformal external beam therapy to prevent injury to surrounding nonmalignant liver tissue [8]. Although the exact benefit is unknown, conformal radiotherapy is associated with improved outcomes [8]. Furthermore, conformal external beam proton radiotherapy is becoming more effective, with 5-year survival rates of 25–50% in unresectable patients [8]. Late-phase clinical trials may soon demonstrate reasonable effectiveness of this therapy in selected patients if results from early-phase trials are confirmed.

Unresectable Disease

Other local therapeutic options for unresectable HCC include radiofrequency or microwave thermal ablation and transarterial chemoembolization (TACE) [6]. These procedures may occasionally offer a chance for cure, but randomized studies to assess long-term survival have not yet been completed. Adverse events from these procedures, compared with those from resection, are infrequent, but the event rate varies significantly from study to study. The best use of TACE or ablative therapies seems to be as an adjunct for smaller HCC tumors in patients awaiting transplantation or to prolong survival and control symptoms in patients with large or multifocal tumors.

Systemic therapy is given to most patients with HCC since advanced disease is often diagnosed. Most chemotherapies are ineffective. Currently, the standard of care, based on multiple randomized placebo-controlled trials, is for patients to receive sorafenib [6]. It is generally recommended that patients receiving any treatment other than sorafenib be treated in the context of a clinical trial. The authors, however, feel strongly that nearly all eligible patients should be offered a clinical trial because the small 3-month survival benefit from sorafenib is not clinically sufficient to truly describe this drug as the "gold standard" for HCC treatment.

There is even less of a role for chemotherapy in patients with CC who are unable to undergo resection or who have recurrence of disease. This is because of the minimal benefit of chemotherapy in these patients, established with randomized controlled trials. However, cisplatin- and gemcitabine-based treatment protocols are beginning to show promising results. The authors, again, highly recommend that patients be referred to clinical trials for the best chance of treatment with an active systemic agent when resection is not possible or has failed.

Future Options

The outlook for patients with cancers of the liver is not entirely bleak. The recent approval of sorafenib has opened the door to other small-molecule inhibitors that may improve survival. In addition, other systemic treatments for unresectable HCC are in early-phase clinical trials. Over our 50-year analysis period, incremental improvements have taken place, and we look forward to further improvements over the next 50 years.

References

1. Jemal A, Siegel R, Ward E, et al. Cancer statistics 2008. CA Cancer J Clin. 2008;58:71–96.
2. Capocaccia R, Sant M, Berrino F, Simonetti A, Santi V, Trevisani F. Hepatocellular carcinoma: trends of incidence and survival in Europe and the United States at the end of the 20th century. Am J Gastroenterol. 2007;102:1661–70 [quiz 0, 71].

3. El-Serag HB, Rudolph KL. Hepatocellular carcinoma: epidemiology and molecular carcinogenesis. Gastroenterology. 2007;132:2557–76.
4. El-Serag HB, Marrero JA, Rudolph L, Reddy KR. Diagnosis and treatment of hepatocellular carcinoma. Gastroenterology. 2008;134:1752–63.
5. Llovet JM, Ricci S, Mazzaferro V, et al. Sorafenib in advanced hepatocellular carcinoma. N Engl J Med. 2008;359:378–90.
6. Benson III AB, Abrams TA, Ben-Josef E, et al. NCCN clinical practice guidelines in oncology: hepatobiliary cancers. J Natl Compr Canc Netw. 2009;7:350–91.
7. Zhang BH, Yang BH, Tang ZY. Randomized controlled trial of screening for hepatocellular carcinoma. J Cancer Res Clin Oncol. 2004;130:417–22.
8. Krishnan S, Dawson LA, Seong J, et al. Radiotherapy for hepatocellular carcinoma: an overview. Ann Surg Oncol. 2008;15:1015–24.
9. van den Esschert JW, de Graaf W, van Lienden KP, et al. Volumetric and functional recovery of the remnant liver after major liver resection with prior portal vein embolization: recovery after PVE and liver resection. J Gastrointest Surg. 2009;13:1464–9.
10. Glazer ES, Curley SA. Technical aspects of hepatic resection. In: Basow DS, editor. UpToDate. Waltham: UpToDate (in press).

Chapter 17
Esophageal Cancer

Linus Ho, Wayne Hofstetter, Ritsuko Komaki, and Steven Hsesheng Lin

Introduction

According to American Cancer Society statistics, 16,470 new cases and 14,530 deaths due to esophageal cancer were expected in 2009. Current estimates of 5-year overall survival in a SEER cohort were approximately 37% for localized disease and only 17% for all stages combined [1]. These statistics reflect a number of contributing factors. First, patients typically present with a history of progressive dysphagia and weight loss often spanning weeks to months, and with such symptoms of locally advanced disease, it is not surprising that most patients present with stage III or IV disease [historically at MD Anderson Cancer Center, fewer than 1% of patients presented with in situ disease, and only one in five presented with local disease (Table 17.1)]. Second, the esophagus lacks a limiting serosal layer that would otherwise tend to restrict the local extension of tumor. Third, the esophagus possesses a rich network of lymphatics spanning its entire length, thereby facilitating longitudinal spread anywhere between the neck and the abdomen. As a result, regional lymph node involvement is found in more than 75% of patients at the time of presentation.

L. Ho
Department of Gastrointestinal Medical Oncology, The University of Texas MD Anderson Cancer Center, 1515 Holcombe Boulevard, Unit 0426, Houston, TX 77030, USA

W. Hofstetter
Department of Thoracic and Cardiovascular Surgery, The University of Texas MD Anderson Cancer Center, 1515 Holcombe Boulevard, Unit 1489, Houston, TX 77030, USA

R. Komaki
Department of Radiation Oncology, The University of Texas MD Anderson Cancer Center, 1515 Holcombe Boulevard, Unit 0097, Houston, TX 77030, USA

S.H. Lin (✉)
Department of Radiation Oncology, The University of Texas MD Anderson Cancer Center, 1515 Holcombe Boulevard, Unit 0097, Houston, TX 77030, USA
e-mail: shlin@mdanderson.org

M.A. Rodriguez et al. (eds.), *60 Years of Survival Outcomes at The University of Texas MD Anderson Cancer Center*, DOI 10.1007/978-1-4614-5197-6_17,

Table 17.1 Initial presentation by stage of patients with esophageal cancer at MD Anderson, 1944–2004

	SEER stage at presentation					
	In situ	Local	Regional	Distant	Unstaged	Total
Decade	[No. (%) of patients]					
1944–1954	0 (0)	8 (18.2)	24 (54.5)	8 (18.2)	4 (9.1)	44 (100.0)
1955–1964	0 (0)	38 (18.4)	98 (47.6)	64 (31.1)	6 (2.9)	206 (100.0)
1965–1974	0 (0)	51 (28.0)	73 (40.1)	55 (30.2)	3 (1.6)	182 (100.0)
1975–1984	0 (0)	86 (31.3)	107 (38.9)	77 (28.0)	5 (1.8)	275 (100.0)
1985–1994	3 (0.5)	121 (21.7)	221 (39.6)	172 (30.8)	41 (7.3)	558 (100.0)
1995–2004	5 (0.5)	184 (19.6)	401 (42.6)	318 (33.8)	33 (3.5)	941 (100.0)
Total	*8 (0.4)*	*488 (22.1)*	*924 (41.9)*	*694 (31.5)*	*92 (4.2)*	*2,206 (100.0)*

SEER Surveillance, Epidemiology, and End Results program

Finally, esophageal cancer is associated with a high incidence of both early invasion to adjacent structures (e.g., cardia of the stomach, pericardium, pleura, trachea, and aorta) and distant metastasis (most commonly to the lungs, liver, and bone).

Epidemiology

Worldwide, 95% of esophageal cancers are of squamous cell origin. In the USA, squamous cell carcinomas and adenocarcinomas represent the majority (>95%) of esophageal malignancies, with neuroendocrine carcinomas, melanomas, lymphomas, and sarcomas making up the remainder. The epidemiology of esophageal cancer in the USA, however, has changed radically over the past few decades. Before 1970, squamous cell carcinomas accounted for >90% of all U.S. esophageal malignancies. Since that time, however, adenocarcinomas have gradually overtaken squamous cell carcinomas as the predominant histology in the USA and the rest of the Western world. The reasons for this are not entirely clear, but there is an association with gastroesophageal reflux disease (GERD) due to obesity and Barrett's esophagus [2].

This shift in histology is important because each histologic type is associated with a distinct epidemiologic profile. Squamous cell carcinomas arise from the normal non-keratinizing squamous mucosa lining the esophagus and tend to arise more proximally along the esophagus (70% arise in the proximal and middle thirds of the esophagus). They are strongly associated with alcohol and tobacco use; in fact, an estimated 90% of squamous cell carcinomas of the esophagus can be attributed to alcohol and/or tobacco exposure. Furthermore, combined alcohol and tobacco use leads to a multiplicative increase in the risk of developing esophageal cancer. Other risk factors for squamous cell carcinomas of the esophagus include prior radiotherapy, caustic injury (e.g., lye ingestion), tylosis, Plummer–Vinson syndrome, esophageal diverticula, achalasia, and human papillomavirus infection. Compared with other demographic groups, African American males are more likely to develop squamous cell carcinomas and demonstrate worse survival rates.

Adenocarcinomas, on the other hand, are most strongly associated with GERD and often arise in the context of Barrett's esophagus; consequently, most adenocarcinomas (75%) arise in the distal third of the esophagus. Obesity is another major risk factor for esophageal adenocarcinomas, probably in large part due to the associated risk for GERD in obese people. However, alcohol and tobacco use is associated with much less risk for adenocarcinomas than it is for squamous cell carcinomas. Curiously, there is an inverse correlation between *Helicobacter pylori* infection and esophageal adenocarcinomas, possibly because of the decreased acid production associated with chronic atrophic gastritis. White middle-aged males, often obese, are the predominant demographic group with adenocarcinomas, although the rate of increase in white females has been almost as great.

Approximately 90% of patients with esophageal cancer present with symptoms of progressive dysphagia, often lasting for several weeks to months before diagnosis. By the time of initial endoscopic examination, the esophageal lumen is typically narrowed by more than 50%. Clearly, patients presenting with new dysphagia should undergo esophagogastroduodenoscopy, and biopsies should be performed if any abnormalities are encountered.

Historical Perspective

Staging

Before 1985, preoperative staging was relatively crude and typically involved a chest X-ray and a barium swallow; thus, the number of understaged cases during this period can only be imagined. However, with the subsequent introduction of and improvements in computed tomography, endoscopic ultrasonography, positron emission tomography, and new surgical techniques, clinical staging has become much more precise. For example, endoscopic ultrasonography has improved our understanding of tumor depth and has allowed for regional nodal sampling. Positron emission tomography has increased the sensitivity for detecting distant metastases, thereby mandating concomitant evolution of the TNM staging system, as evidenced by the most recent (seventh) edition of the *AJCC Cancer Staging Manual* published in 2009. For example, the first edition simplistically defined only three stages, using only tumor size and the presence or absence of extraesophageal spread and/or distant metastases as criteria. This stands in sharp contrast with the seventh edition system, which improved upon the sixth edition by, among other things, subdividing T4 disease into resectable (T4a) and unresectable (T4b) categories (based on improved surgical techniques that now allow resection of previously "unresectable" disease such as pleural involvement), redefining the N classification in terms of the number of involved lymph nodes (N1: 1–2 involved nodes, N2: 3–6 involved nodes, and T3: ≥7 nodes), and simplifying the M classification by eliminating the somewhat ambiguous term "non-regional lymph node." In fact, this latest revised TNM staging system has been shown to demonstrate improved performance characteristics compared with the previous version [3].

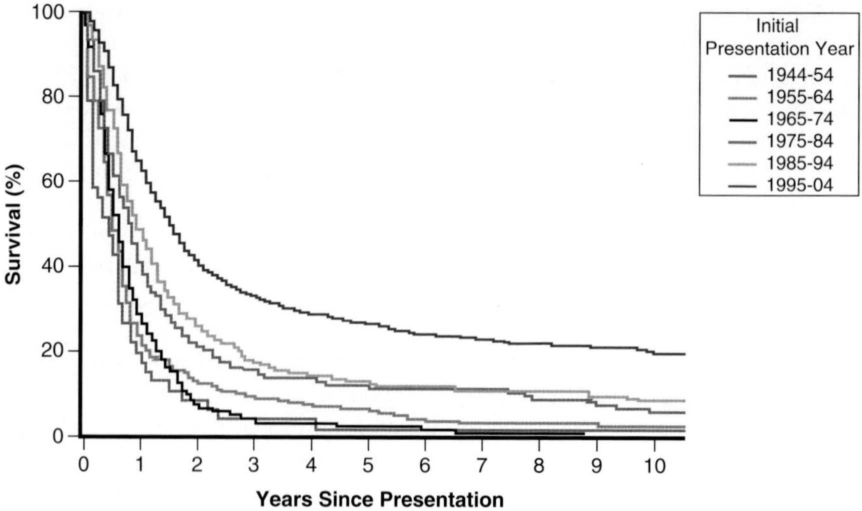

Fig. 17.1 Overall survival rates for patients with esophageal cancer (1944–2004) ($P<0.0001$, log-rank test for trend).

A major caveat in the interpretation of stage-related data from the National Cancer Institute's Surveillance, Epidemiology, and End Results (SEER) database is its simplified staging system, which includes only three stages: localized (disease restricted to the organ of origin), regional (disease that has extended regionally beyond the organ of origin), and distant (disseminated disease) (overall survival rates as well as survival rates for the individual SEER stages of esophageal cancer are shown in Figs. 17.1, 17.2, 17.3, and 17.4). The distinction between regional and distant disease, in particular, is often subjective, making the accuracy and reproducibility of older SEER staging less than optimal. Comparing this staging system with the AJCC staging system (sixth edition; Table 17.2), one can see that localized disease (per SEER) corresponds to AJCC stages I and IIA, distant disease corresponds to stage IV, and regional disease includes everything else (stages IIB and III). The lack of granularity in the SEER system results in oversimplification and is not useful in terms of quoting prognosis or determining treatment for individual patients.

Treatment

As with most solid tumors, surgery has been the mainstay of curative therapy for patients who are medically operable and have localized esophageal cancer. Surgery typically involves resection of the affected portion of the esophagus along with adequate adjoining tissue both above and below the tumor to obtain negative margins and provide for an acceptable functional result. Therefore, this involves removal of a large part of the esophagus (the extensive submucosal lymphatic network is one reason for this) with appropriate reconstruction to establish alimentary continuity.

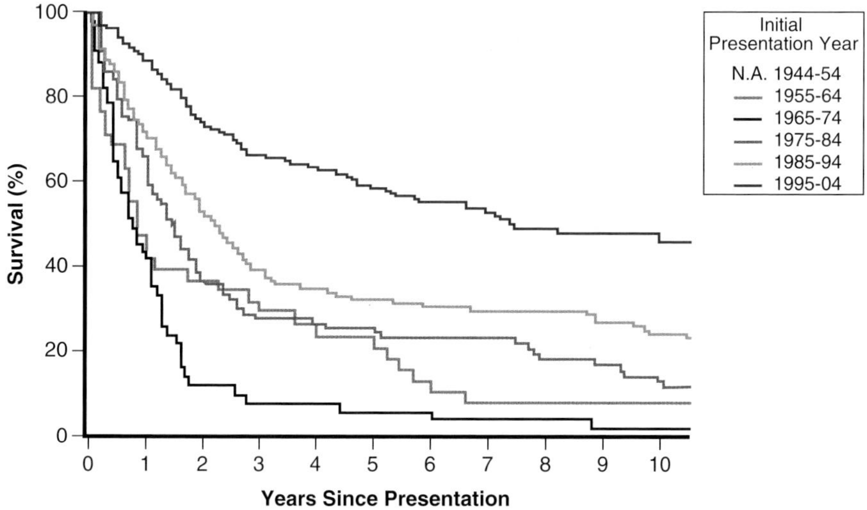

Fig. 17.2 Survival rates for patients with local (SEER stage) esophageal cancer (1944–2004) ($P<0.0001$, log-rank test for trend). Because of the very small number of individuals with local esophageal cancer seen from 1944 to 1954, data from this period were excluded. *N.A.* not applicable.

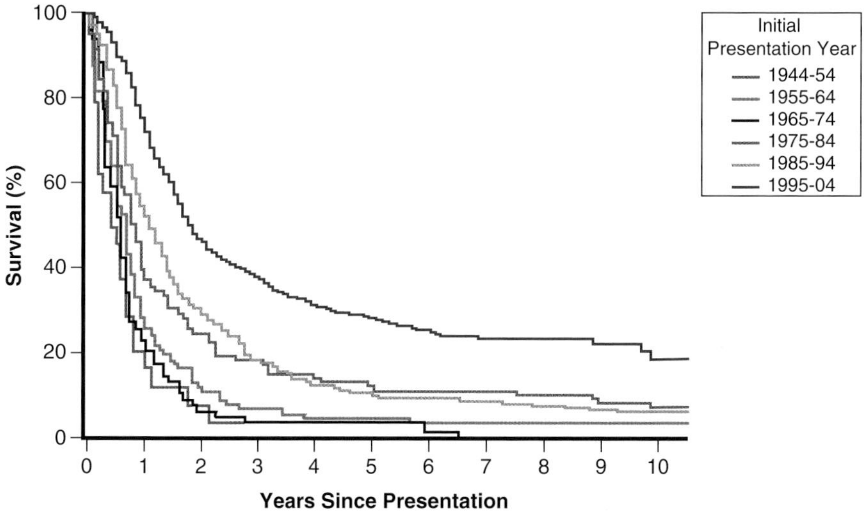

Fig. 17.3 Survival rates for patients with regional (SEER stage) esophageal cancer (1944–2004) ($P<0.0001$, log-rank test for trend).

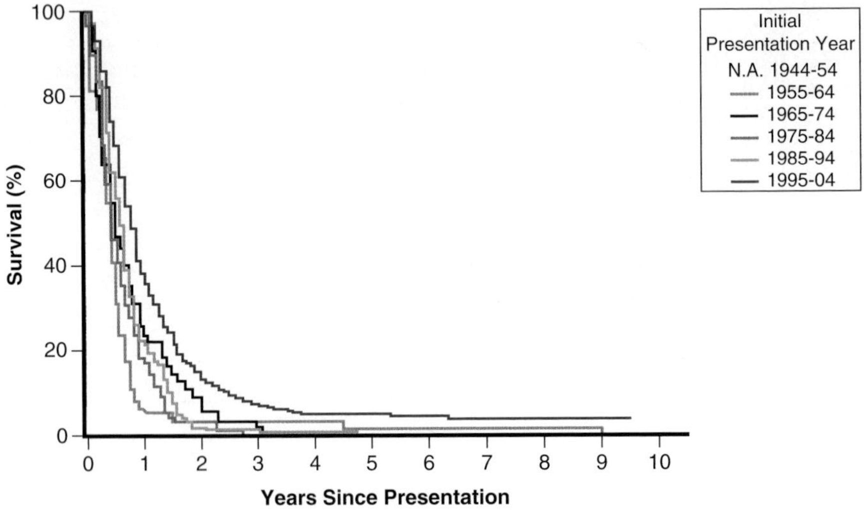

Fig. 17.4 Survival rates for patients with distant (SEER stage) esophageal cancer (1944–2004) ($P<0.0001$, log-rank test for trend). Because of the very small number of individuals with distant esophageal cancer seen from 1944 to 1954, data from this period were excluded. *N.A.* not applicable.

Table 17.2 Esophageal cancer prognosis by stage after surgery

Stage (AJCC, sixth edition)	5-year overall survival
0 (Tis N0 M0)	>95%
I (T2 N0 M0)	50–80%
IIA (T2-3 N0 M0)	30–40%
IIB (T1-2 N1 M0)	10–30%
III (T3 N1 or T4, any N, M0)	10–15%
IVA (Any T, any N, M1a)	<5%
IVB (Any T, any N, M1b)	<1%

In most cases, this involves transposition of the stomach into the chest, but in cases in which a long segment of the esophagus and stomach must be removed, a portion of jejunum or colon may be interposed to serve as a permanent replacement.

Historically, perioperative mortality was a major concern, but this rate has decreased from as high as 30% in the 1970s [4] to between 2% at high-volume centers such as MD Anderson Cancer Center and 21% at lower-volume centers. Numerous studies have concluded that both hospital volume and surgeon experience affect perioperative morbidity and mortality. Not surprisingly, two of the most complicated oncologic operations, namely esophagectomy for esophageal cancer and pancreaticoduodenectomy (Whipple resection) for cancer of the pancreatic head, are instances for which this difference in hospital volume and surgeon experience is most dramatic [5]. The reduction in perioperative complications is due to multiple factors such as improved perioperative care, including better nutritional management and improvement in the delivery of preoperative treatment such as chemotherapy and radiotherapy. Advances in the planning and delivery of radiotherapy, including three-dimensional conformal radiotherapy and intensity-modulated radiotherapy, have contributed to the reduction in toxicity to surrounding normal tissues such as lungs and heart. Also prevention of neutropenic fever or septic death due to preoperative chemotherapy has contributed substantially to improving perioperative complications.

Surgical techniques have evolved considerably over time. In the 1970s, definitive resection was often performed as a two-stage procedure in which esophagectomy and esophageal bypass were performed sequentially in separate operations. More recently, they have been consolidated into a single procedure, approached through either the abdomen and chest or the abdomen and neck.

One of the significant factors in the decrease in surgical mortality has been improved management of leaks that can occur after resection and reconstruction, a potential complication of this surgery. During the 1970s, this complication was considered universally fatal. At our institution, the mortality rate at that time was 43% for patients who developed this complication; today, it is less than 4%. Improved perioperative care, including better nutritional management, has been a contributing factor in reducing overall mortality from this operation [6]. Perioperative mortality at our institution is currently 0–3.4%, depending on the stage of disease and type of treatment.

Although surgery is considered the gold standard for definitive treatment of esophageal cancer, the prognosis after surgery alone remains poor (see Table 17.3). Given the high rates of both local-regional (31%) and distant (50%) recurrence with surgery alone [7] and even worse results with either chemotherapy or radiotherapy alone as definitive treatment, multimodality therapy has become the standard of care in the USA, despite relatively sparse and conflicting phase 3 data. The concurrent use of chemotherapy and radiotherapy has been shown to be superior to radiotherapy alone [8], and combined chemoradiotherapy has therefore been the standard preoperative treatment since 1997.

The advent of three-dimensional conformal radiotherapy, intensity-modulated radiotherapy, and proton beam therapy has enabled safer delivery of higher doses of radiation by better targeting the radiation dose to the tumor while sparing surrounding normal tissues. Before these advances, undesirably high doses of radiation were delivered to adjacent structures—notably the heart, lung, and spine—with concomitant toxicity but inadequate therapeutic doses to the tumor. Also, a four-dimensional radiotherapy plan accounting for respiratory and diaphragmatic motion has enabled more accurate delivery of radiation to the targeted tumor while sparing the surrounding normal tissue from unnecessary high doses of radiation, which is critical when the patient undergoes chemoradiotherapy.

The MD Anderson Cancer Center Experience

The data set used for this discussion was derived from a total of 5,046 patients who presented to MD Anderson Cancer Center with esophageal cancer between 1944 and 2004. Patients with other primary cancers and those who had been treated elsewhere were excluded, resulting in 2,206 patients who received definitive treatment at this institution. Survival was calculated from the time of initial presentation.

Table 17.3 Kaplan–Meier overall survival[a]

Year	Percent survival	
	5 years	10 years
1944–1954	2.3	2.3
1955–1964	7.0	3.5
1965–1974	3.3	0.7
1975–1984	13.1	6.8
1985–1994	13.1	9.4
1995–2004	27.2	20.4

[a]Before 1997, patients with locally advanced esophageal cancers were treated with surgery alone

Presentation

Throughout the observed 60-year period, most patients presented to our institution with locally advanced or metastatic disease, which is consistent with patterns of presentation elsewhere (Table 17.1). However, a radical shift in histology occurred during this time period, reflecting trends seen throughout the USA. Before 1985, more than 70% of patients presented with squamous cell carcinomas, but between 1985 and 1994, that trend reversed, with 68% of patients presenting with adenocarcinoma, and between 1997 and 2001, with 83% of patients presenting with adenocarcinoma. However, using univariate and multivariate analyses, Hofstetter et al. concluded that that no significant survival differences have resulted from this shift in histology [7].

Survival

The overall survival data provided in Fig. 17.1 and Table 17.3 suggest overall improvement in 5-year survival rates, from 2% to 27% over the indicated 60-year time frame, with the most significant increase seen within the most recent decade. Some anomalous results are seen such as those associated with the decade 1955–1964. This temporary shift may be due to a statistical shift rather than a real trend, given the relatively low numbers of patients seen during the first few decades.

The improved survival seen in recent decades is likely due to several factors. First, staging in the earlier era was suboptimal and likely would have resulted in understaging, making survival statistics overly pessimistic. Second, better supportive care has resulted in improved outcomes independent of disease-specific treatment. Such supportive care includes the development of expandable metal stents and other endoscopic techniques to palliate dysphagia as well as the development of readily available feeding tubes and intravenous nutritional support (used during definitive treatment as well as for supportive care). However, a third possible reason for improved outcome in esophageal cancer has been improvement in the various cancer treatment modalities. Advances in surgical and irradiation techniques were mentioned previously, and many new systemic agents have been introduced over the past 10–20 years, including well-tolerated conventional cytotoxic drugs and new molecularly targeted agents. Furthermore, trials of adjuvant therapy (postsurgical medical and/or irradiation treatment) of any type were not commonly reported until the 1980s, with more general acceptance of adjuvant therapy not coming until the 1990s. In this context, one can begin to explain the dramatic improvement in survival in patients with potentially resectable disease (local and regional SEER stages) treated at our institution with multimodality therapy over the past two decades.

Although the overall survival trends are reflected across the board in the SEER stage subgroups, clearly much less progress has been made in patients with metastatic disease. For this subgroup of patients, chemotherapy forms the mainstay of treatment, emphasizing the urgent need for better systemic therapies with acceptable toxicity profiles. Of the drugs currently used to treat esophageal cancer, only 5-fluorouracil and cisplatin were available 20 years ago. Since then, new agents have been introduced, including new fluoropyrimidines (e.g., capecitabine and S-1) and platinum compounds (e.g., carboplatin and oxaliplatin) with improved efficacy and/or toxicity profiles and entirely new classes of compounds (camptothecins such as irinotecan, taxanes such as docetaxel and paclitaxel, and monoclonal antibodies such as bevacizumab and cetuximab). We are incorporating many of these new agents into common clinical practice ahead of generic guidelines.

Current Management Approach

Our current standard of care for patients with stage II/III esophageal cancer treated at our institution involves neoadjuvant chemoradiotherapy followed by surgery, and we believe that the best results are achieved with this approach. We have analyzed our data from sequential phase 2/3 prospective studies conducted at our institution, during which patients were treated with various preoperative therapies involving either chemotherapy alone or chemoradiotherapy [9]. Patients treated with preoperative chemoradiotherapy have had better pathologic complete response rates (28% vs 4%; $P<0.001$) and overall survival rates (3-year: 48% vs 29%; $P=0.04$) than have those treated with preoperative chemotherapy alone. Preoperative chemoradiotherapy was also a significant independent predictor of improved overall survival and disease-free survival in multivariate regression analyses. For patients who are medically or technically inoperable, chemoradiotherapy has been used as definitive therapy. However, recurrence rates remain unacceptably high.

There is a critical need for newer approaches to combat this disease. Future improvements in the treatment of esophageal cancer will depend on continued research in the following areas:

- A better understanding of the molecular and genetic profile of esophageal cancer and the correlation of such profiles with clinical response. In turn, these findings should lead to a better understanding of the subtypes of esophageal cancers and

the determinants of response to therapy, thereby allowing individualization of cancer therapy. For example, current studies indicate the possibility that chemoradiotherapy alone may produce a complete response in at least one molecular subset of esophageal cancer; identification of patients who would respond to this therapy would spare them a potentially morbid procedure and no loss of efficacy.
- Development of more sensitive staging techniques to identify sites of low-volume disease.
- Development of new endoscopic and interventional techniques to address early-stage disease in a definitive manner and to better palliate later stages of disease.
- Continued innovation in surgical techniques, including the use of robotics and minimally invasive approaches to reduce perioperative risk and recovery time.
- Continued refinements in irradiation planning with four-dimensional simulation and delivery by intensity-modulated radiotherapy or proton beam therapy, to minimize the delivery of undesirably high doses of radiation to adjacent normal tissue or organs such as the spinal cord, heart, and lungs. Such refinements are essential to reduce perioperative mortality. Careful conformal planning with use of dose–volume histograms has reduced the number of treatment-related postoperative lung complications [10].
- Identification of novel drugs and drug combinations to improve efficacy and/or treatment-related toxicity. Many of these new agents will be predicated on the improved molecular characterization of esophageal cancers, but even combining currently available drugs in new schedules can improve patient tolerance and hence quality of life without decreasing efficacy. Hence, instead of DCF and ECF (and its variants), a biweekly combination of docetaxel, oxaliplatin, and infusional 5-fluorouracil developed here in the phase 1/2 setting may hold promise as a non-inferior regimen with a superior adverse effect profile.
- Development of new treatment paradigms. For virtually all gastrointestinal malignancies, we have embraced neoadjuvant therapy as a preferable approach to adjuvant therapy, even in diseases in which such an approach is not necessarily the standard of care in the USA (e.g., in patients with adenocarcinomas of the stomach and pancreas). Similarly, in patients with potentially resectable esophageal cancer, we are exploring the role of induction chemotherapy as an adjunct to standard chemoradiotherapy in a randomized phase 2 trial of neoadjuvant chemoradiotherapy preceded or not by induction chemotherapy.

References

1. Altekruse SF, Kosary CL, Krapcho M, et al., editors. SEER cancer statistics review, 1975–2007. National Cancer Institute. http://seer.cancer.gov/csr/1975_2007/, based on November 2009 SEER data submission. Updated 2010. Accessed 23 May 2012.
2. Enzinger PC, Mayer RJ. Esophageal cancer. N Engl J Med. 2003;349(23):2241–52.
3. Hsu PK, Wu YC, Chou TY, et al. Comparison of the 6th and 7th editions of the American Joint Committee on Cancer tumor-node-metastasis staging system in patients with resected esophageal carcinoma. Ann Thorac Surg. 2010;89(4):1024–31.

4. Giuli R, Gignoux M. Treatment of carcinoma of the esophagus: retrospective study of 2,400 patients. Ann Surg. 1980;192:44–52.
5. Birkmeyer JD, Siewers AE, Finlayson E, et al. Hospital volume and surgical mortality in the United States. N Engl J Med. 2002;346(15):1128–37.
6. Martin LW, Swisher SG, Hofstetter W, et al. Intrathoracic leaks following esophagectomy are no longer associated with increased mortality. Ann Surg. 2005;242:392–402.
7. Hofstetter W, Swisher SG, Correa AM, et al. Treatment outcomes of resected esophageal cancer. Ann Surg. 2002;236:376–85.
8. Cooper JS, Guo MD, Herskovic A, et al. Chemoradiotherapy of locally advanced esophageal cancer: long term followup of a prostpective randomized trial (RTOG 85-01). JAMA. 1999;281(17):1623–7.
9. Swisher SG, Hofstetter W, Komaki R, et al. Improved long-term outcome with chemoradiotherapy strategies in esophageal cancer. Ann Thorac Surg. 2010;90(3):892–8 [discussion 898–9].
10. Lee HK, Vaporciyan AA, Cox JD, et al. Postoperative pulmonary complications after preoperative chemoradiation for esophageal carcinoma: correlation with pulmonary dose-volume histogram parameters. Int J Radiat Oncol Biol Phys. 2003;57(5):1317–22.

Chapter 18
Gastric Cancer

Alexandria T. Phan and Paul F. Mansfield

Introduction

Gastric (stomach) cancer, the most frequently occurring cancer and second-leading cause of cancer-related deaths, accounts for 24.2% of cancer deaths worldwide [1–3]. Adenocarcinoma accounts for the vast majority of gastric cancer cases, with the remaining minority consisting of lymphoma, sarcoma, carcinoid tumor, and squamous cell carcinoma; the treatment information in this chapter focuses only on adenocarcinoma, whereas the survival curves include patients with all histologies.

Since the mid-1990s, the most common location of carcinomas in the upper gastrointestinal tract (stomach, gastroesophageal junction, and esophagus) has shifted, resulting in a substantial decline in distal gastric cancers and an increase in proximal gastric/gastroesophageal junction cancers. Distal gastric cancers have become relatively uncommon in North America and in most Northern and Western European countries [4]. In the USA, an estimated 21,000 new cases of gastric cancer were diagnosed and about 10,570 patients died of this disease in 2010 [5]. The causes of the epidemiologic shift from distal to proximal in gastric cancer rates are not completely understood, but environmental factors, chiefly dietary and obesity, are suspected.

Factors associated with higher incidence of gastric cancer include consumption of smoked or salted foods or foods contaminated with aflatoxin, low intake of fruits and vegetables, low socioeconomic status, and possibly a decreased use of refrigeration [6, 7]. Obesity appears to be associated with more proximal cancers within

A.T. Phan (✉)
Department of GI Medical Oncology, The University of Texas MD Anderson Cancer Center, 1400 Holcombe Boulevard, Mailstop 426, Houston, TX 77030, USA
e-mail: ATPhan@mdanderson.org

P.F. Mansfield
Department of Surgical Oncology, The University of Texas MD Anderson Cancer Center, Houston, TX, USA

M.A. Rodriguez et al. (eds.), *60 Years of Survival Outcomes at The University of Texas MD Anderson Cancer Center*, DOI 10.1007/978-1-4614-5197-6_18,

Table 18.1 Surveillance, Epidemiology, and End Results (SEER) staging

Stage	Description
Local	Cancer is still confined to the primary site
Regional	Cancer has spread to regional lymph nodes and/or directly beyond the primary site
Distant	Cancer has spread beyond the primary site into other organs

the stomach. Precursor pathologic conditions include pernicious anemia, achlorhydria atrophic gastritis, gastric ulcers, and adenomatous polyps. Several studies have demonstrated that individuals with *Helicobacter pylori* infection have a three- to six-fold higher risk of gastric cancer than do those without this infection, but the precise role of this bacterium in the etiology of gastric cancer remains unknown [8–10]. However, the increased association of *H. pylori* with gastric cancer seems to be mainly with distal gastric cancers and intestinal-type malignancy. A minority of *H. pylori*-infected individuals develop gastric cancer; however, data do not yet exist on the effect of treatment of *H. pylori* infection on subsequent malignancy.

Germline mutations in the *CDH1* gene, which encodes the E-cadherin protein, have recently been recognized in families with hereditary diffuse gastric adenocarcinoma. Carriers of these mutations have a 70% lifetime risk of developing gastric cancer (which is higher in females than in males). Once these cancers become invasive, survival is rare, thus leading to the use of prophylactic removal of the stomach. Several reports of prophylactic gastrectomy [11–13] have demonstrated the routine presence of microscopic intraepithelial carcinomas in patients having normal endoscopic surveillance that included multiple random biopsies and chromoendoscopy. Early total gastrectomy has been recommended for this small patient population because of the lack of effective early tumor detection by less aggressive techniques.

Presenting symptoms such as pain, dysphagia, early satiety, bleeding, anemia, and weight loss may be more specific to gastric cancers, but they often signify more advanced disease. Diagnosis is made by tissue biopsy, and staging is performed with esophagogastroduodenoscopy along with endoscopic ultrasound and computed tomography (CT). Laparoscopic staging is also done in patients with tumors that invade beyond the mucosa and without radiologic evidence of distant or metastasis. Surveillance, Epidemiology, and End Results (SEER) staging is a classification system used to describe the extent of disease based on the most conclusive information available (Table 18.1). However, the American Joint Committee on Cancer (AJCC) TNM surgical staging system has been used more commonly in recent times (Table 18.2) [14]. Gastric cancers are treated according to their stage at diagnosis. The fact that the gastric staging system is based on surgical pathology further demonstrates that surgery still plays a significant role in the management of this disease.

Table 18.2 American Joint Committee on Cancer TNM system (V7) for surgical staging of gastric cancer

Stage	T	N	M
0	Tis	N0	M0
IA	T1	N0	M0
IB	T2	N0	M0
	T1	N1	M0
IIA	T3	N0	M0
	T2	N1	M0
	T1	N2	M0
IIB	T4a	N0	M0
	T3	N1	M0
	T2	N2	M0
	T1	N3	M0
IIIA	T4a	N1	M0
	T3	N2	M0
	T2	N3	M0
IIIB	T4b	N0	M0
	T4b	N1	M0
	T4a	N2	M0
	T3	N3	M0
IIIC	T4b	N2	M0
	T4b	N3	M0
	T4a	N3	M0
IV	Any T	Any N	M1
Definitions of TNM			
Primary tumor (T)			
TX		Primary tumor cannot be assessed	
T0		No evidence of primary tumor	
Tis		Carcinoma in situ: intraepithelial tumor without invasion of the lamina propria	
T1		Tumor invades lamina propria, muscularis mucosae, or submucosa	
T1a		Tumor invades lamina propria or muscularis mucosae	
T1b		Tumor invades submucosa	
T2		Tumor invades muscularis propria[a]	
T3		Tumor penetrates subserosal connective tissue without invasion of visceral peritoneum or adjacent structures[b,c]	
T4		Tumor invades serosa (visceral peritoneum) or adjacent structures[b,c]	
T4a		Tumor invades serosa (visceral peritoneum)	
T4b		Tumor invades adjacent structures	
Regional lymph nodes (N)			
NX		Regional lymph node(s) cannot be assessed	
N0		No regional lymph node metastasis[d]	
N1		Metastasis in one to two regional lymph nodes	

(continued)

Table 18.2 (continued)

Stage	T	N	M
N2		Metastasis in three to six regional lymph nodes	
N3		Metastasis in seven or more regional lymph nodes	
N3b		Metastasis in 7–15 regional lymph nodes	
N3b		Metastasis in 16 or more regional lymph nodes	
Distant metastasis (M)			
M0		No distant metastasis	
M1		Distant metastasis	

[a]A tumor may penetrate the muscularis propria with extension into the gastrocolic or gastrohepatic ligaments, or into the greater or lesser omentum, without perforation of the visceral peritoneum covering these structures. In this case, the tumor is classified as T3. If there is perforation of the visceral peritoneum covering the gastric ligaments or the omentum, the tumor should be classified as T4.
[b]The adjacent structures of the stomach include the spleen, transverse colon, liver, diaphragm, pancreas, abdominal wall, adrenal gland, kidney, small intestine, and retroperitoneum.
[c]Intramural extension to the duodenum or esophagus is classified by the depth of the greatest invasion in any of these sites, including the stomach.
[d]A designation of pN0 should be used if all examined lymph nodes are negative, regardless of the total number removed and examined.

Historical Perspective

According to the SEER17 (2000–2006) database, only 24% of newly diagnosed gastric cancers are confined to the stomach (localized); in 31% of cases, the disease has already spread beyond the stomach into the regional lymph nodes (regional) and in 32% of cases into other organs (distant) [15]. Median survival duration in advanced gastric cancer is less than 9 months. The 5-year survival rates for gastric cancer according to stage reflect the fact that durable survival is most likely with local disease (Table 18.3). Therefore, surgery remains the cornerstone of therapy for locoregional gastric cancer.

In the 1950s throughout most of the 1980s, because of the lack of effective systemic therapies, patients with newly diagnosed gastric cancer were treated with surgery, either for curative intent or for palliation. Until recently, studies to find effective multimodality therapy to improve outcome in patients with curable disease were unsuccessful. Before the mid-1990s, most gastric cancers in the USA and other Western countries arose from the distal stomach. Surgical publications spanning a decade confirmed that segmental or partial gastrectomy and total gastrectomy had the same survival outcomes [16, 17]. Unfortunately, however, the evidence was inconsistent with regard to the extent of lymph node dissection at the time of curative gastric surgery.

The nodal dissection type is described as D1 when perigastric lymph nodes are excised; D2 when additional lymph nodes along the splenic, hepatic, left gastric, and celiac arteries are removed; and D3 when more lymph nodes in the retroperitoneal or para-aortic regions are dissected. In Japan, gastric cancer is quite common,

Table 18.3 Gastric cancer: 5-year relative survival rates by stages

By TNM stages	
Stage	Five-year survival rate
0	89%
IA	78%
IB	58%
II	34%
IIIA	20%
IIIB	8%
IV	7%
By SEER stages	
Local	63%
Regional	27%
Distant	3%

resulting in a significant public health burden; consequently, screening programs for gastric cancer have been developed in Japan. Japanese surgeons have been able to show a strong correlation between the extent of nodal dissection and overall survival [18]. However, surgeons in Western countries have been unable to duplicate the Japanese results. In fact, in randomized trials comparing D1 to D2 nodal dissection types, survival rates were the same, with D2 resulting in higher morbidity and mortality [19, 20]. The explanation for this divergence of surgical outcomes is not readily transparent, but plausible reasons are as follows: (1) early stages are being diagnosed in Japan as a result of national screening programs; (2) Japanese experience and expertise for gastric surgery and nodal dissection have not been easily translatable across geography; (3) patient populations are very different with different rates of obesity; and (4) stage migration is occurring because of better lymph node removal and evaluation techniques, which explains why stage-for-stage, Japanese patients appear to have earlier disease than their counterparts in Western countries do.

Consistently evident in the historical literature, however, is the finding that although cure is possible only with complete surgical resection, less than half of patients with newly diagnosed gastric cancers present with resectable disease. The survival rate at 5 years after surgery alone is less than 30% [21, 22]. Because of both the low incidence of newly diagnosed resectable gastric cancers and the low 5-year survival rates with surgery alone, the management of gastric cancers relies on multidisciplinary input from surgical, radiation, and medical oncologists.

Many searches for perioperative therapy to improve survival outcome have been fruitless. Furthermore, many randomized trials designed to assess the benefits of postoperative chemotherapy have had conflicting results. Even the results of meta-analyses did not resolve the controversy of adjuvant chemotherapy. Three pivotal studies conducted in the USA, England, and Japan, however, finally provided some answers, although postoperative chemotherapy is now used differently according to the geographically accepted standard of care. For example, based on a Japanese study [23], postoperative chemotherapy after curative gastric surgery became the standard of care in Japan. In the USA, however, based on the Intergroup 116 trial, which showed that postoperative chemotherapy and chemoradiotherapy improved survival outcome over surgery alone [22], the standard of care for patients with resectable gastric cancer included both of these modalities. Resulting from the MAGIC trial in the United Kingdom [21], perioperative chemotherapy became the standard of care in this nation. In other parts of Europe, only preoperative multimodality therapy is used.

There are both risks and benefits associated with giving therapy before vs after curative surgery. For the most part, therapy received after surgery is very difficult to tolerate, and most patients will not be able to complete their postoperative course because of toxicity. On the other hand, starting with preoperative therapy may delay potentially curative surgery; it can be argued, however, that patients whose disease progresses rapidly may not ever benefit from surgery. Currently, there is no worldwide standard of care for patients with potentially curative disease, but clearly additional therapy is necessary. Less than 10% of patients with metastatic gastric cancer survive 24 months after diagnosis [24].

Before the mid-1980s, the foundations of systemic chemotherapy for gastric cancer were mitomycin, carmustine, doxorubicin, and methotrexate. By 1987, a new antimetabolite of the pyrimidine analog was approved for gastrointestinal malignancies. Since that time, the nucleus of systemic therapy for gastric cancer has been 5-fluorouracil (5-FU). For patients with good performance status, retrospective data have suggested that survival improved with 5-FU-based chemotherapy compared with best supportive care [25]. However, progress in the development of therapy for advanced or metastatic gastric cancer has lagged behind all other gastrointestinal cancers. As with perioperative therapy in localized and hence curable disease, there is no accepted worldwide standard of care for frontline therapy in advanced or metastatic gastric cancer. Therefore, reference regimens have differed in various regions, and numerous combinations of chemotherapeutic agents have been compared.

Before the 1990s, very few randomized phase 3 clinical trials in the management of advanced or metastatic gastric cancer had been conducted, resulting in limited advancements [26–30]. At the beginning of the twenty-first century, docetaxel, irinotecan, capecitabine, oxaliplatin, and S-1 were added to the armamentarium of cancer in general. Since that time, more phase 3 clinical trials for gastric cancers have been completed, adding to the research momentum and helping to change the treatment paradigm for this still deadly malignancy [31–38]. Slowly but surely, survival outcome with frontline therapy for metastatic gastric cancer has increased from 5 months [39] with best supportive care to 13.5 months [38] with trastuzumab combined with chemotherapy.

The MD Anderson Cancer Center Experience

The MD Anderson Tumor Registry data set included patients who were diagnosed as having gastric cancer between 1944 and 2004. This total does not include patients with gastroesophageal junction cancer, which had an increasing incidence since the

Table 18.4 Patients with gastric cancer treated at MD Anderson, 1944–2004

	SEER stage at presentation				
	Local	Regional	Distant	Unstaged	Total
Decade	[No. (%) of patients]				
1944–1954	6 (11.8)	28 (54.9)	17 (33.3)	0 (0)	51 (100.0)
1955–1964	32 (12.7)	90 (35.9)	126 (50.2)	3 (1.2)	251 (100.0)
1965–1974	22 (7.3)	101 (33.3)	173 (57.1)	7 (2.3)	303 (100.0)
1975–1984	43 (11.8)	128 (35.3)	186 (51.2)	6 (1.7)	363 (100.0)
1985–1994	77 (16.9)	157 (34.4)	199 (43.6)	23 (5.0)	456 (100.0)
1995–2004	124 (20.2)	174 (28.3)	282 (45.9)	35 (5.7)	615 (100.0)
Total	*304 (14.9)*	*678 (33.3)*	*983 (48.2)*	*74 (3.6)*	*2,039 (100.0)*

SEER Surveillance, Epidemiology, and End Results program

1990s. Furthermore, problems inherent in the historical data sets are the migration of stage over time and the limitations of staging information in the early years. In this data set, stage grouping was based on SEER stages, which were broad. In 1977, the first version of the AJCC TNM staging system was introduced, and in 1997, the staging system for gastric cancer was refined to better reflect surgical pathology. During the earlier years of this data set, stage assignment had been made on the basis of both clinical and limited surgical findings. Clinical findings typically would have been based on physical examination and limited plain film radiographs, without the benefit of current standards of staging such as endoscopic ultrasound, laparoscopic peritoneal evaluation, and CT scans. Consequently, stage assignment across the 60-year course of data recording was not uniform, and a lot of detailed staging data were not available.

A total of 6,215 patients with gastric cancer were seen on or before 31 December 2004. Of this group, 3,819 had received no therapy for their gastric cancer before presenting to MD Anderson Cancer Center. After excluding patients with multiple primary cancers and those treated elsewhere, 2,393 patients received definitive primary treatment at MD Anderson. The distribution of patients presenting by time interval and SEER stage is summarized in Table 18.4. Not surprising, 82% of patients presenting to MD Anderson had advanced (regional and distant) disease. This high percentage of patients with advanced-stage disease reflects the referral pattern of the institution as well as the natural history of the disease, whereby gastric cancer diagnosis is usually made with signs and symptoms of advanced stages [15].

The pattern of treatments administered to patients at MD Anderson is represented in Table 18.5. Over the years, significantly less surgery ($P=0.01241$) and significantly more chemotherapy ($P=0.00001$) was used as primary therapy for gastric cancer patients. This trend reflects an epidemiologic phenomenon as well as advances in both staging and treatment for gastric cancer. As discussed above, the incidence of gastric cancer in the USA is decreasing, but with a greater proportion of gastroesophageal junction cancers being diagnosed. Therefore, the ability of this data set to capture surgery for gastric cancers may be diminished with advancing time intervals. Explanations for the possible inaccurate reflection of the crude

Table 18.5 Pattern of treatment modality for patients with gastric cancer treated at MD Anderson, 1944–2004

	Treatment modality					
	Surgery	Chemo-therapy	Radio-therapy	Multiple[a]	Other	Total
Decade	[No. (%) of patients]					
1944–1954	48 (94.1)	1 (2.0)	1 (2.0)	1 (2.0)	0 (0)	51 (100.0)
1955–1964	147 (58.6)	67 (26.7)	3 (1.2)	29 (11.6)	5 (2.0)	251 (100.0)
1965–1974	89 (29.4)	154 (50.8)	5 (1.7)	51 (16.8)	4 (1.3)	303 (100.0)
1975–1984	157 (43.3)	113 (31.1)	4 (1.1)	64 (17.6)	25 (6.9)	363 (100.0)
1985–1994	130 (28.5)	154 (33.8)	11 (2.4)	91 (19.9)	70 (15.4)	456 (100.0)
1995–2004	128 (20.9)	250 (40.8)	26 (4.2)	77 (12.5)	132 (21.5)	613 (100.0)
Total	*699 (34.3)*	*739 (36.3)*	*50 (2.5)*	*313 (15.3)*	*236 (11.6)*	*2,037 (100.0)*

SEER Surveillance, Epidemiology, and End Results program
[a]Always included surgery

statistics of gastric cancer cases seen and treated at MD Anderson include frequent overlap as to how tumors of the gastroesophageal junction are classified. The distinction of gastric from gastroesophageal junction, from esophageal cancers has been evolving through the decades. Since the start of MD Anderson history until 2010, the classification and staging for gastric cancer was revised at least three times. The AJCC staging has recently updated gastric cancer to no longer include the gastric cardia (Greene FL et al., AJCC Cancer Staging Manual 6th Edition, 2010). The survival outcomes of patients in this dataset do not reflect the change in patient referral to the institution through the years. MD Anderson is seeing more complicated, high-risk, refractory, and advanced gastric cancer cases. Finally, management of locoregional gastric cancers has also advanced through the years. Although surgery still plays a pivotal role in the management of locoregional disease, the integration of surgery with chemotherapy and radiotherapy results in better outcomes. Often, surgery is no longer the first step in patients with local or regional disease. The increasing trend of adding chemotherapy ($P<0.0001$) and radiotherapy ($P<0.005$) to surgery in more recent decades is significant. Eventually, if therapies become effective enough, surgery may become obsolete, although this is still many years in the future. All of these limitations of the dataset generate an inaccurate reflection of gastric cancer through the decades at MD Anderson. Hence, caution must be applied to the interpretation of survival and overall outcomes.

The SEER database encompasses registries of patients from many states and is thus more representative of national averages. The SEER database (1988–2005) indicated that overall survival rates for all stages of gastric cancer were 23.6% at 5 years and 19.5% at 10 years [15]. In addition, 5-year survival rates were 62.5% for localized, 26.6% for regional, and 3.4% for distant disease [15]. For gastric cancer patients treated at MD Anderson at approximately the same time interval (1984–2004), median overall survival rates were 27.4% at 5 years and 21.9% at 10 years; and 5-year survival rates were 70.1% for localized, 34.1% for regional, and 3.8% for distant disease. Comparing SEER results with those of gastric cancer patients treated

Table 18.6 Overall survival rates (at 5 and 10 years) of patients with gastric cancer who were treated at MD Anderson, 1944–2004 (by time interval and SEER stage)

	Overall survival rates (%)							
	All		Local		Regional		Distant	
Decade	5 years	10 years	5 years	10 years	5 years	10 years	5 years	10 years
1944–1954	11.8	5.9	50.0	33.3	10.7	3.6	0.0	0.0
1955–1964	13.5	6.4	65.6	37.5	11.1	4.4	2.4	0.0
1965–1974	7.5	4.6	35.4	20.2	10.9	6.8	2.3	1.5
1975–1984	17.5	12.9	53.8	42.7	25.4	18.8	3.0	1.2
1985–1994	22.6	18.4	65.2	39.4	29.1	20.2	2.6	2.1
1995–2004	32.1	25.3	74.9	63.5	39.0	26.3	4.9	3.0

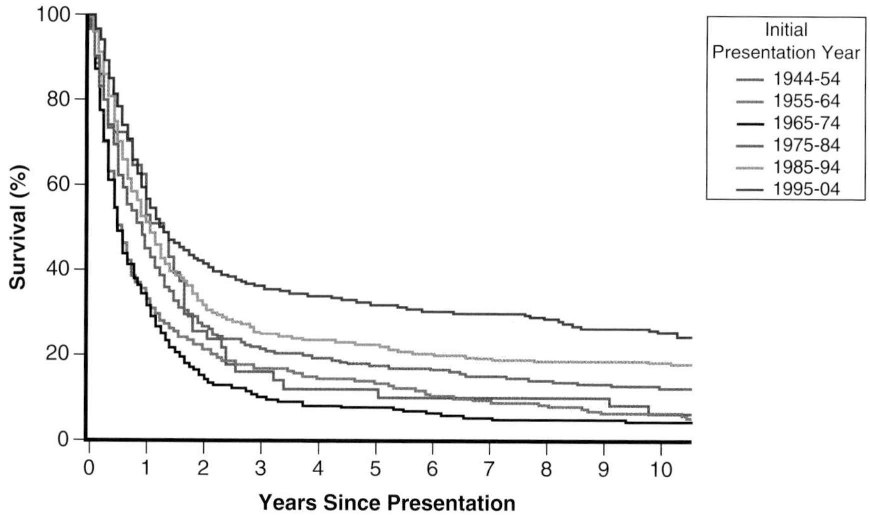

Fig. 18.1 Overall survival rates for patients with gastric cancer (1944–2004) ($P<0.0001$, log-rank test for trend).

at MD Anderson, stage for stage, MD Anderson patients have had the same or better survival outcomes.

Table 18.6 and Fig. 18.1, which show overall survival rates for gastric cancer patients treated at MD Anderson from 1944 to 2004, indicate survival improvement. During this period, among the 2,393 patients treated at MD Anderson, overall survival rates at 5 years improved with time ($P<0.0001$). Overall survival rates at 10 years were also incrementally and significantly better ($P<0.0001$). Figures 18.2, 18.3, and 18.4 depict survival curves based on time period of treatment for gastric cancer patients treated at MD Anderson and according to SEER stage. The 5- and 10-year outcomes significantly improved for local (50% vs 75% and 33% vs 64%;

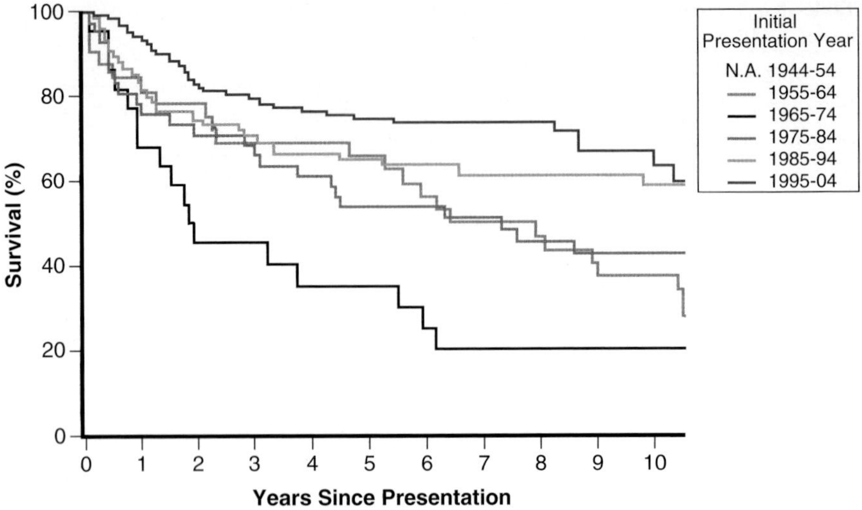

Fig. 18.2 Survival rates for patients with local (SEER stage) gastric cancer (1944–2004) ($P<0.0001$, log-rank test for trend). Because of the very small number of individuals with local gastric cancer seen from 1944 to 1954, data from this period were excluded. *N.A.* not applicable.

$P<0.0001$), regional (11% vs 39% and 4% vs 26%; $P<0.0001$), and even distant (0% vs 5% and 0% vs 3%; $P<0.0001$) disease, respectively, over time.

There are several possible explanations for the improved survival outcome among patients with local or regional disease over this 60-year period. Since 1944, advancements in presurgical staging methods, such as laparoscopic evaluation for low-volume peritoneal metastases, endoscopic ultrasound for more accurate assessment of regional lymph node spread, and certainly high-resolution CT imaging, to name just a few, have allowed for more accurate assessment of stage. Furthermore, better and more aggressive nutritional support, along with advancement in postoperative care, contributed to improved gastric cancer survival at MD Anderson for local and regional diseases.

However, improved survival outcome among patients with local and regional diseases was most likely influenced by (1) surgical experience and expertise and (2) the multidisciplinary approach to all patients with local and regional disease. Observational studies in survival outcome from larger databases of gastric cancer cohorts have confirmed the association between surgical mortality and institutional surgical volume. The Nationwide Inpatient Sample from 1998 to 2003, consisting of 13,354 patients who had undergone gastric resection during their hospitalization, demonstrated an operative mortality rate of 6.0%. One predictive factor of significantly increased in-hospital mortality was low annual hospital surgical volume. Hospitals that performed fewer than 4 gastric resections per year had a higher in-hospital mortality rate than did hospitals that performed more than 11 gastrectomies per year [40]. This concept has been consistently demonstrated in other

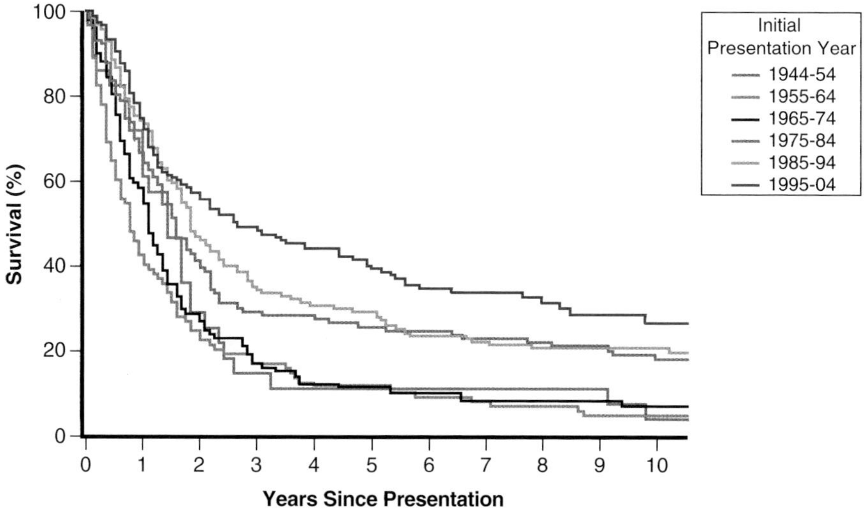

Fig. 18.3 Survival rates for patients with regional (SEER stage) gastric cancer (1944–2004) ($P < 0.0001$, log-rank test for trend).

databases, such as those of SEER, Medicare, and academic institutions [41–44]. In Texas, for example, over a 3-year period, among 214 hospitals that performed 1,864 gastrectomies, the high-volume hospitals (>15 gastrectomies per year) had significantly lower in-hospital mortality rates and perioperative complications than did low-volume hospitals (<3 gastrectomies per year) [44]. A significant factor in this improved survival at high-volume centers was the demonstrated ability to rescue patients who experienced a major complication after gastric resection.

Since the mid-1990s, multimodality care of patients with local or regional gastric cancer has become a foundation of clinical trial development and ultimately clinical decision making. Each patient with newly diagnosed local or regional gastric cancer is examined by a multidisciplinary team consisting of medical, radiation, and surgical oncology specialists, and decisions for each patient's case are made by this multidisciplinary team. In recent pivotal clinical trials, the management of local and regional gastric cancer has become increasingly based on evidence [21–23]. In particular, the Intergroup 116 [22] and MAGIC [21] trials, which were based on different approaches to additional therapy to curative gastric surgery, led to two consistent messages translatable into practice: (1) survival outcome is improved with additional therapy; and (2) postoperative therapy, whether chemoradiotherapy or chemotherapy, is poorly tolerated. At MD Anderson, since the mid-1980s, selected patients with local and regional disease have been treated in clinical trials with preoperative multimodality therapy, which included either chemotherapy and/or chemoradiotherapy. We believe this approach was the major contributor to the improved survival outcome seen on survival curves for regional disease (Fig. 18.3).

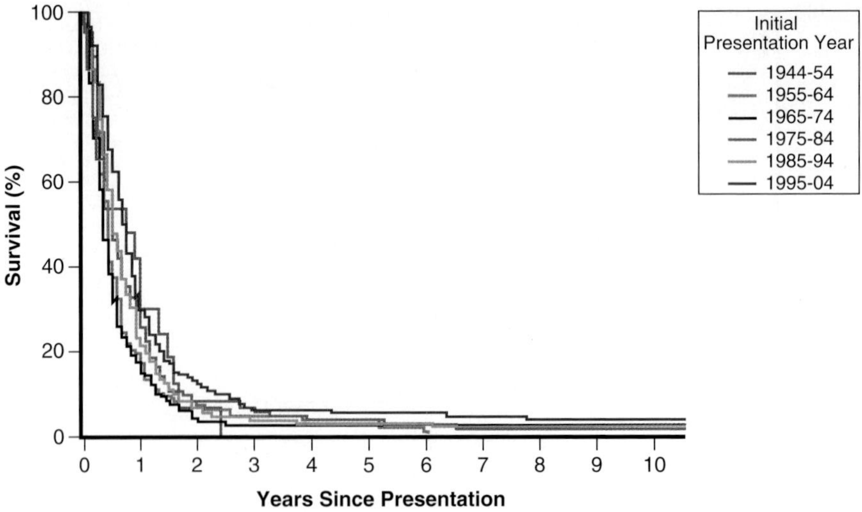

Fig. 18.4 Survival rates for patients with distant (SEER stage) gastric cancer (1944–2004) ($P<0.0001$, log-rank test for trend).

Even within the distant disease group of gastric cancer patients at MD Anderson, survival curves demonstrated incremental but significant improvement in 5- and 10-year outcomes (Fig. 18.4). This modest change is probably explained by the more recent expansion of available cytotoxic agents, such as capecitabine, S-1, docetaxel, and oxaliplatin. Although active, these agents each have a narrow therapeutic index between survival benefit and therapy-related toxicity. Therefore, despite improvements seen in survival rates for patients with distant disease over the past 60 years, these rates have been in the single digits and will remain so until effective durable systemic therapy becomes available.

Current Management Approach

Our approach to patients with gastric cancer is based on TNM staging of the disease. To predict the natural history of disease and determine the direction of disease management, we have all patients undergo extensive disease staging with use of imaging, endoscopy, and laparoscopy, as indicated. Because we support a multidisciplinary approach to cancer management, we provide all patients with multimodality therapy, when appropriate, as well as nutritional and symptom assessment and support. Patients with local or regional disease are almost always seen by a multidisciplinary team of medical, radiation, and surgical oncologists. Many consider the standard of care for local and regional disease to include (1) surgery alone for early disease, (2) postoperative chemoradiotherapy after curative surgery, or (3) perioperative chemotherapy sandwiching curative surgery; in addition, because of our commitment to research, we encourage patients to participate in clinical trials, when appropriate.

Because of the lack of a commonly accepted primary chemotherapy regimen for distant disease, the standard of care for treating advanced gastric cancer consists of several 5-FU-based chemotherapy regimens. Patients with distant gastric cancer typically have poor performance status, especially if they received therapy before coming to MD Anderson. Although enrollment into clinical trials is encouraged, it is often not practical for patients seeking second or third opinions at MD Anderson.

Ongoing and future research will improve our understanding of the molecular pathogenesis of gastric cancer and will enable us to develop molecular biomarkers and targets for drug development. Personalized therapy for gastric cancer patients is the goal of the future. However, to get there, we are working on short-term goals. For example, for patients with local or regional (potentially curable) disease, we must have better models to predict response to therapy and to stratify the risk of recurrence. Furthermore, more effective cytotoxic agents, along with improved targeted therapies, are needed to increase durable responses with less toxicity. Just as in the clinical management of gastric cancer, the combined efforts of all disciplines will be necessary for research, to further improve survival in patients with this disease.

References

1. International Agency for Research on Cancer (IARC). http://www.iarc.fr/. Accessed 23 May 2012.
2. Parkin DM, Bray F, Ferlay J, Pisani P. Global cancer statistics, 2002. CA Cancer J Clin. 2005;55(2):74–108.
3. Shibata A, Parsonnet J. Stomach cancer. 3rd ed. New York: Oxford University Press; 2006.
4. Bosetti C, Malvezzi M, Chatenoud L, Negri E, Levi F, La Vecchia C. Trends in cancer mortality in the Americas, 1970–2000. Ann Oncol. 2005;16(3):489–511.
5. Jemal A, Siegel R, Ward E, Hao Y, Xu J, Thun MJ. Cancer statistics, 2009. CA Cancer J Clin. 2009;59(4):225–49.
6. Howson CP, Hiyama T, Wynder EL. The decline in gastric cancer: epidemiology of an unplanned triumph. Epidemiol Rev. 1986;8:1–27.
7. Coggon D, Barker DJ, Cole RB, Nelson M. Stomach cancer and food storage. J Natl Cancer Inst. 1989;81(15):1178–82.
8. Talley NJ, Zinsmeister AR, Weaver A, et al. Gastric adenocarcinoma and Helicobacter pylori infection. J Natl Cancer Inst. 1991;83(23):1734–9.
9. Parsonnet J, Friedman GD, Vandersteen DP, et al. Helicobacter pylori infection and the risk of gastric carcinoma. N Engl J Med. 1991;325(16):1127–31.
10. Fuchs CS, Mayer RJ. Gastric carcinoma. N Engl J Med. 1995;333(1):32–41.
11. Lewis FR, Mellinger JD, Hayashi A, et al. Prophylactic total gastrectomy for familial gastric cancer. Surgery. 2001;130(4):612–7 [discussion 7–9].
12. Huntsman DG, Carneiro F, Lewis FR, et al. Early gastric cancer in young, asymptomatic carriers of germ-line E-cadherin mutations. N Engl J Med. 2001;344(25):1904–9.
13. Chun YS, Lindor NM, Smyrk TC, et al. Germline E-cadherin gene mutations: is prophylactic total gastrectomy indicated? Cancer. 2001;92(1):181–7.

14. Edge SB, Byrd DR, Compton C, Fritz AG, Greene FL, Trotti A, editors. AJCC cancer staging manual. 7th ed. New York: Springer; 2010.
15. SEER. SEER statistics facts sheet. http://www.seer.cancer.gov/statfacts/html/stomach.html. Accessed 27 Dec 2009.
16. Bozzetti F, Marubini E, Bonfanti G, Miceli R, Piano C, Gennari L. Subtotal versus total gastrectomy for gastric cancer: five-year survival rates in a multicenter randomized Italian trial. Italian Gastrointestinal Tumor Study Group. Ann Surg. 1999;230(2):170–8.
17. Gouzi JL, Huguier M, Fagniez PL, et al. Total versus subtotal gastrectomy for adenocarcinoma of the gastric antrum. A French prospective controlled study. Ann Surg. 1989;209(2):162–6.
18. Maruyama K, Sasako M, Kinoshita T, Sano T, Katai H. Surgical treatment for gastric cancer: the Japanese approach. Semin Oncol. 1996;23(3):360–8.
19. Bonenkamp JJ, Hermans J, Sasako M, et al. Extended lymph-node dissection for gastric cancer. N Engl J Med. 1999;340(12):908–14.
20. Hartgrink HH, van de Velde CJ, Putter H, et al. Extended lymph node dissection for gastric cancer: who may benefit? Final results of the randomized Dutch gastric cancer group trial. J Clin Oncol. 2004;22(11):2069–77.
21. Cunningham D, Allum WH, Stenning SP, et al. Perioperative chemotherapy versus surgery alone for resectable gastroesophageal cancer. N Engl J Med. 2006;355(1):11–20.
22. Macdonald JS, Smalley SR, Benedetti J, et al. Chemoradiotherapy after surgery compared with surgery alone for adenocarcinoma of the stomach or gastroesophageal junction. N Engl J Med. 2001;345(10):725–30.
23. Sakuramoto S, Sasako M, Yamaguchi T, et al. Adjuvant chemotherapy for gastric cancer with S-1, an oral fluoropyrimidine. N Engl J Med. 2007;357(18):1810–20.
24. Ajani JA. Recent developments in cytotoxic therapy for advanced gastric or gastroesophageal carcinoma: the phase III trials. Gastrointest Cancer Res. 2007;1(Suppl):S16–21.
25. Wagner AD, Grothe W, Haerting J, Kleber G, Grothey A, Fleig WE. Chemotherapy in advanced gastric cancer: a systematic review and meta-analysis based on aggregate data. J Clin Oncol. 2006;24(18):2903–9.
26. Moertel CG, Lavin PT. Phase II-III chemotherapy studies in advanced gastric cancer. Eastern Cooperative Oncology Group. Cancer Treat Rep. 1979;63(11–12):1863–9.
27. Schnitzler G, Queisser W, Heim ME, et al. Phase III study of 5-FU and carmustine versus 5-FU, carmustine, and doxorubicin in advanced gastric cancer. Cancer Treat Rep. 1986;70(4):477–9.
28. Klein HO, Wils J, Bleiberg H, Buyse M, Duez N. An EORTC gastrointestinal (GI) group randomized evaluation of the toxicity of sequential high dose methotrexate and 5-fluorouracil combined with adriamycin (FAMTX) vs 5-fluorouracil, adriamycin and mitomycin (FAM) in advanced gastric cancer. Med Oncol Tumor Pharmacother. 1989;6(2):171–4.
29. Barone C, Cassano A, Astone A, et al. Association of epirubicin, etoposide and cisplatin in gastric cancer. A phase II study. Oncology. 1991;48(5):353–5.
30. Kim NK, Park YS, Heo DS, et al. A phase III randomized study of 5-fluorouracil and cisplatin versus 5-fluorouracil, doxorubicin, and mitomycin C versus 5-fluorouracil alone in the treatment of advanced gastric cancer. Cancer. 1993;71(12):3813–8.
31. Roth AD, Maibach R, Martinelli G, et al. Docetaxel (Taxotere)-cisplatin (TC): an effective drug combination in gastric carcinoma. Swiss Group for Clinical Cancer Research (SAKK), and the European Institute of Oncology (EIO). Ann Oncol. 2000;11(3):301–6.
32. Van Cutsem E, Moiseyenko VM, Tjulandin S, et al. Phase III study of docetaxel and cisplatin plus fluorouracil compared with cisplatin and fluorouracil as first-line therapy for advanced gastric cancer: a report of the V325 Study Group. J Clin Oncol. 2006;24(31):4991–7.
33. Roth AD, Fazio N, Stupp R, et al. Docetaxel, cisplatin, and fluorouracil; docetaxel and cisplatin; and epirubicin, cisplatin, and fluorouracil as systemic treatment for advanced gastric carcinoma: a randomized phase II trial of the Swiss Group for Clinical Cancer Research. J Clin Oncol. 2007;25(22):3217–23.

34. Al-Batran SE, Hartmann JT, Probst S, et al. Phase III trial in metastatic gastroesophageal adenocarcinoma with fluorouracil, leucovorin plus either oxaliplatin or cisplatin: a study of the Arbeitsgemeinschaft Internistische Onkologie. J Clin Oncol. 2008;26(9):1435–42.
35. Cunningham D, Starling N, Rao S, et al. Capecitabine and oxaliplatin for advanced esophago-gastric cancer. N Engl J Med. 2008;358(1):36–46.
36. Dank M, Zaluski J, Barone C, et al. Randomized phase III study comparing irinotecan combined with 5-fluorouracil and folinic acid to cisplatin combined with 5-fluorouracil in chemotherapy naive patients with advanced adenocarcinoma of the stomach or esophagogastric junction. Ann Oncol. 2008;19(8):1450–7.
37. Koizumi W, Narahara H, Hara T, et al. S-1 plus cisplatin versus S-1 alone for first-line treatment of advanced gastric cancer (SPIRITS trial): a phase III trial. Lancet Oncol. 2008;9(3):215–21.
38. van Cutsem E, Kang YK, Chung H, et al. Efficacy results from the ToGA trial: a phase III study of trastuzumab added to standard chemotherapy (CT) in first-line human epidermal growth factor receptor 2 (HER2)-positive advanced gastric cancer (GC). J Clin Oncol. 2009;27(18s):LBA4509.
39. Vanhoefer U, Rougier P, Wilke H, et al. Final results of a randomized phase III trial of sequential high-dose methotrexate, fluorouracil, and doxorubicin versus etoposide, leucovorin, and fluorouracil versus infusional fluorouracil and cisplatin in advanced gastric cancer: a trial of the European Organization for Research and Treatment of Cancer Gastrointestinal Tract Cancer Cooperative Group. J Clin Oncol. 2000;18(14):2648–57.
40. Smith JK, McPhee JT, Hill JS, et al. National outcomes after gastric resection for neoplasm. Arch Surg. 2007;142(4):387–93.
41. Brennan MF, Radzyner M, Rubin DM. Outcome—more than just operative mortality. J Surg Oncol. 2009;99(8):470–7.
42. Bare M, Cabrol J, Real J, et al. In-hospital mortality after stomach cancer surgery in Spain and relationship with hospital volume of interventions. BMC Public Health. 2009;9:312.
43. Verhoef C, van de Weyer R, Schaapveld M, Bastiaannet E, Plukker JT. Better survival in patients with esophageal cancer after surgical treatment in university hospitals: a plea for performance by surgical oncologists. Ann Surg Oncol. 2007;14(5):1678–87.
44. Smith DL, Elting LS, Learn PA, Raut CP, Mansfield PF. Factors influencing the volume-outcome relationship in gastrectomies: a population-based study. Ann Surg Oncol. 2007;14(6):1846–52.

Chapter 19
Acute Myeloid Leukemia

Emil J. Freireich

Acute myeloid leukemia (AML) is a systemic disease that is "metastatic" from diagnosis; therefore, the problems typically associated with local and regional control, i.e., those associated with surgery and radiation therapy, do not play a role. Since virtually all patients who die as a result of a malignant disease die of systemic (metastatic) cancer, AML has served as a prototype illness for the development of systemic therapies, and advances in the control of this disease have been rapidly applied to the control of the more common metastatic cancers in man.

The median age at diagnosis for these patients, as for all patients with cancer, is between 50 and 60 years; and like the more common malignancies, the incidence of AML increases progressively with age.

In 1944, when MD Anderson opened, there was no effective or palliative therapy for AML. The disease was uniformly fatal, with a median survival from diagnosis of approximately 8 weeks, and 99% of patients died within 12 months of diagnosis. The first palliative chemotherapy for AML was 6-mercaptopurine, an antitumor agent synthesized by Hitchings and Elion in 1953 and reported to induce temporary remissions of AML in adults. Between 1944 and 1954, only 25 patients with AML were seen at MD Anderson Cancer Center, largely because there was no known therapy for this disease and thus little basis for referral to a major cancer center.

In 1955, I had the opportunity to serve in the United States Public Health Service and to be stationed at the newly opened clinical center of the National Institutes of Health in Bethesda, Maryland. This was an extraordinary facility because of its excellent resources, but more importantly, it was one of the first clinical care institutions devoted entirely to patient-oriented research. The physicians who served in this institution controlled their own practice. There were no service requirements,

E.J. Freireich (✉)
Department of Special Medical Education, Leukemia, The University of Texas MD Anderson Cancer Center, 1515 Holcombe Blvd, Box 55, Houston, TX 77030, USA
e-mail: efreirei@mdanderson.org

M.A. Rodriguez et al. (eds.), *60 Years of Survival Outcomes at The University of Texas MD Anderson Cancer Center*, DOI 10.1007/978-1-4614-5197-6_19,

and patient care was free, including travel for all patients who participated in the clinical research in that institution.

Between 1955 and 1964, the first prospective randomized clinical trials in cancer were conducted and the first cooperative clinical therapy group (Acute Leukemia Group B) formed. Also during that decade, combination chemotherapy and new antibiotics to control infection were developed, new therapeutic agents and adjuvant chemotherapy were discovered, and platelet replacement therapy to control hemorrhage was introduced, all of which demonstrated that the first systemic (metastatic) cancer in man could be "cured" with systemic therapy. That first systemic cancer was childhood acute lymphoblastic leukemia: approximately 40% of children treated with the multi-agent combination chemotherapy vincristine, amethopterin (methotrexate), mercaptopurine (6-mercaptopurine), and prednisone (VAMP) were found to have prolonged survival compatible with cure [1]. This achievement demonstrated that systemic therapy could cure systemic cancers.

Unfortunately, although there were four systemic chemotherapeutic agents active against childhood acute lymphoblastic leukemia, i.e., methotrexate (an antifolic acid compound), prednisone (an adrenal corticosteroid), vincristine (an antitubilin agent), and 6-mercaptopurine (an antipurine nucleoside antagonist), only the 6-mercaptopurine showed any activity against the adult form of AML. Specifically, the use of 6-mercaptopurine resulted in complete hematological remission but in only 9% of patients treated. The median duration of these remissions was approximately 3 months; therefore, by 1965, AML was still essentially an untreatable form of malignancy. During that decade, the number of patients with AML who were treated at MD Anderson (a total of 155) increased, both because the institution had grown and because palliative therapy was now available.

Improvement in therapy for adult AML really began in 1965. Dr. Clark, the President and Director of MD Anderson, after observing the rapid progress in leukemia therapy being made at the National Institutes of Health in Bethesda, recognized that MD Anderson had the potential to become a major therapeutic research center patterned after the developments at the National Cancer Institute in Bethesda. Toward that end, he aggressively recruited Dr. Emil Frei III, Head of the Medicine Program at the National Cancer Institute, who in turn recruited Dr. Emil J. Freireich to join him as head of a new department called Developmental Therapeutics, whose mission was to develop therapy for systemic metastatic cancer.

The following decade, 1965–1974, was one of rapid progress in the management of AML. An important breakthrough was the discovery of the activity of the nucleoside analog arabinosyl cytosine (ARA-C) [2]. Importantly, the unique pharmacology of this drug required that continuous infusion be used to maintain blood levels; once this was discovered, the outlook for patients with AML changed dramatically. The activity of ARA-C was soon recognized to be synergistic with alkylating agents such as cyclophosphamide. The major breakthrough, however, occurred with the discovery of anthracycline antibiotics, specifically daunorubicin, which was found to have major synergistic activity with ARA-C [3]. This increased the frequency of response, but more importantly, it was soon discovered that when therapy was given early in remission, i.e., early intensification and with intermittent reinduction as maintenance, remission could be significantly prolonged [4]. When AML was no longer considered a hopeless diagnosis, the number of patients referred to MD Anderson increased dramatically; in fact, twice as many patients were referred in that decade as in the previous 20 years.

The next decade, 1975–1984, was one of progressive improvements in the use of the drugs discovered in the previous decade, such that for the first time, a significant minority of patients were surviving 5 years or more beyond diagnosis [5]. In fact, one study showed that 20 patients who had been treated for AML at MD Anderson and then monitored after diagnosis were still alive and in remission (free of disease) more than 5 years later; this meant that this single institution had treated more surviving AML patients than had the rest of the world [6].

As a result of this progress, the number of AML patients referred to MD Anderson for treatment continued to increase; specifically, in the 20 years between 1965 and 1984, 980 patients newly diagnosed with AML were referred to MD Anderson, five times more than were referred in the previous 20 years (1944–1964).

In the decade 1985–1994, the advent of cytogenetics used in classifying AML into distinct subgroups was an important development [7]. Patients who had acute promyelocytic leukemia with a translocation between chromosomes 15 and 17, patients with core-binding factor leukemias with a translocation between chromosomes 8 and 21, and those with inversion 16 chromosome abnormality constituted approximately 20% of all patients with AML. This group, which included virtually all of the cured surviving patients (i.e., longer than 5 years), had a high response rate to therapy—more than 80%—and experienced remissions lasting longer than those of any other subgroups. At the other extreme were the patients with a poor prognosis who had more complex cytogenetic characteristics such as the loss of all of chromosome 5, chromosome 7, or trisomy 8; the loss of the long arm of these chromosomes; or other miscellaneous abnormalities. The response rate in this group was extremely low (below 20%), and virtually none of these patients had prolonged survival. This group made up approximately 30% of all patients with AML. The remaining 50% of AML patients were intermediate in outcome.

In the decade 1995–2004, advances in supportive therapy and in intensive combination chemotherapy improved the prognoses for patients with residual disease. During this decade, almost 1,000 new patients were referred to the institution for care because of the prospects for palliation and cure of this disease.

In summary, over a brief period of only 60 years, prognoses and outcomes for patients with AML changed from the hopelessness of 100% mortality within a year to prolonged survival—the equivalent of a cure—in more than a quarter of patients; furthermore, virtually all patients now benefit from treatment [8] (Fig. 19.1). The most important factor predicting outcome of the disease is age at diagnosis. In all cytogenetic and prognostic subgroups, age remains an important prognostic factor. For patients older than 70 years, the prognosis is still poor, and treatment remains highly unsatisfactory. In future decades, more specific and less organ-toxic therapies will almost certainly lead to improved prognoses.

However, the most important result from reviewing this 60-year history at MD Anderson has been discovering the impact that advances in the treatment of this

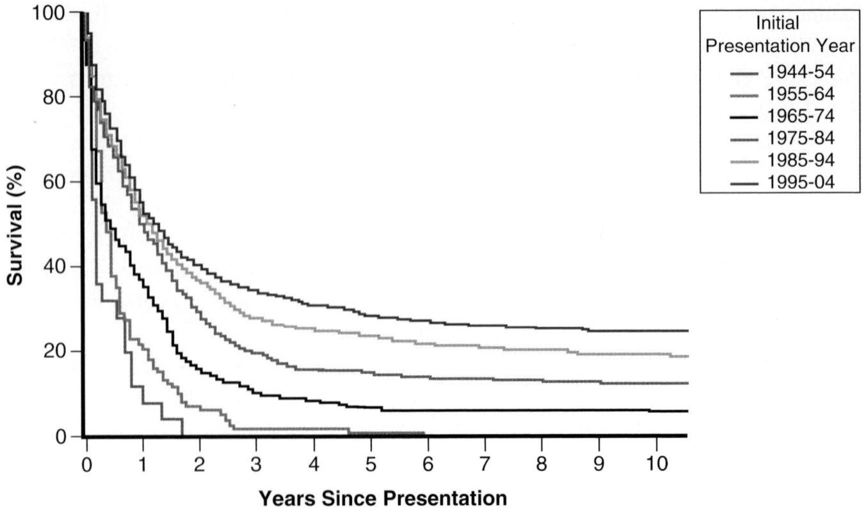

Fig. 19.1 Overall survival rates for patients with acute myeloid leukemia (1944–2004) ($P<0.0001$, log-rank test for trend).

relatively uncommon form of cancer have had on the development of therapy for common malignancies. Principles of remission, induction, combination chemotherapy, adjuvant chemotherapy, intensive maintenance, supportive therapy with platelet transfusions, and control of infections with antibiotics have all been pioneered in AML and have found immediate application to the other common malignancies. The progress made in one short generation at a single institution offers great hope for improving outcome for patients with this diagnosis and other forms of cancer [9].

References

1. Freireich EJ, Frei III E. Recent advances in acute leukemia. In: Moore CV, Brown EB, editors. Progress in hematology. New York: Grune and Stratton; 1964. p. 189–202.
2. Freireich EJ, Bodey GP, Hart JS, Rodriguez V, Whitecar JP, Frei III E. Remission induction in adults with acute myelogenous leukemia. In: Mathe G, editor. Recent results in cancer research, vol. 30. Berlin: Springer; 1970. p. 85–91.
3. Bodey GP, Hewlett JS, Coltman Jr CA, Rodriguez V, Freireich EJ. Therapy of adult acute leukemia with daunorubicin and L-asparaginase. Cancer. 1974;33:626–30.
4. McCredie KB, Bodey GP, Freireich EJ, Gutterman JU, Hester JP, Drewinko B. Adult leukemia. In: Clark RL, Howe CD, editors. Cancer patient care at M.D. Anderson Cancer Center. Chicago: Year Book Medical Publishers; 1976. p. 165–97.
5. Bodey GP, Freireich EJ, McCredie KB, et al. Prolonged remissions in adults with acute leukemia following late intensification chemotherapy and immunotherapy. Cancer. 1981;47: 1937–45.
6. Keating MJ, McCredie KB, Bodey GP, Smith TL, Gehan E, Freireich EJ. Improved prospects for long-term survival in adults with acute myelogenous leukemia. JAMA. 1982;248:2481–6.

7. Keating MJ, Cork A, Broach Y, et al. Toward a clinically relevant cytogenetic classification of acute myelogenous leukemia. Leuk Res. 1987;11:119–33.
8. Freireich EJ. Four decades of therapy for acute myeloblastic leukemia. Leukemia. 1998;12 Suppl 1:S54–6.
9. Kantarjian H, O'Brien S, Cortes J, et al. Therapeutic advances in leukemia and myelodysplastic syndrome over the past 40 years. Cancer. 2008;113(7):1933–52.

Chapter 20
Chronic Lymphocytic Leukemia/Small Lymphocytic Lymphoma

Apostolia-Maria Tsimberidou and Michael J. Keating

Introduction

Chronic lymphocytic leukemia (CLL) and small lymphocytic lymphoma (SLL) are B-cell lymphoproliferative disorders characterized by a proliferation of mature-appearing but functionally incompetent lymphocytes. The result of this proliferation is an accumulation of lymphocytes that progressively infiltrate the lymph nodes, bone marrow, liver, and spleen. CLL and SLL are classified by the World Health Organization as the same disease entity [1]. They are identical histologically and immunophenotypically, but their manifestation is different: CLL manifests primarily in peripheral blood or bone marrow and SLL in the lymph nodes.

The American Cancer Society estimated that among U.S. patients who will be diagnosed as having leukemia in the coming year, about a third will have CLL. In 2011, CLL affected an estimated 14,570 people in the USA, and of the 21,780 deaths expected from leukemias in 2012, about 4,380 will be caused by CLL [2].

CLL/SLL is primarily a disease of older adults, with an average patient age at diagnosis of 72 years [3]. Many patients diagnosed as having CLL/SLL present asymptomatically and are without significant findings on physical examination. Often, the disease is discovered incidentally when blood is evaluated for unrelated or routine reasons.

CLL/SLL is often characterized as an indolent disease. Many patients (about 30%) may have a long and unremarkable course of disease—up to two decades—and do not

A.-M. Tsimberidou (✉)
Department of Investigational Cancer Therapeutics, The University of Texas MD Anderson Cancer Center, 1515 Holcombe Blvd, Unit 455, Houston, TX 77030, USA
e-mail: atsimber@mdanderson.org

M.J. Keating
Department of Leukemia, The University of Texas MD Anderson Cancer Center, Houston, TX, USA

M.A. Rodriguez et al. (eds.), *60 Years of Survival Outcomes at The University of Texas MD Anderson Cancer Center*, DOI 10.1007/978-1-4614-5197-6_20,

require treatment. In recent years, "benign monoclonal B-lymphocytosis" or "smoldering CLL" has been identified as an entity that denotes clonal B-lymphocytes in otherwise healthy individuals [4]. However, another third may have disease progression within the first 5 years, and the remaining third will present with aggressive disease that proves fatal within months.

Approximately 5% of patients with CLL/SLL—independently of disease stage—develop a lymphoma (most commonly a diffuse large B-cell lymphoma) that is more aggressive than the underlying CLL. This disease, known as Richter syndrome (or Richter transformation), is believed to arise through histologic transformation of the original CLL clone, although in several cases it appears to be a new neoplasm. Patients who develop Richter transformation have a poor prognosis, with a median survival of less than 6 months.

On the basis of clinical presentation, therefore, CLL/SLL is characterized as a disease with a highly variable clinical course, with survival ranging from 1 to 20 years. Given the high degree of variability, one of the historical challenges for this disease has been to try to develop clinically informative risk-stratification models to help ascertain which patients among those who present without symptoms, whose disease was perhaps diagnosed incidentally, would benefit from initiating treatment.

In the past two decades, advances in the identification of risk factors used to select optimal therapy and the discovery of new therapeutic agents have significantly improved clinical outcome, including survival, in patients with CLL/SLL. Before these recent developments, only the advent of stem cell transplantation (SCT) was associated with durable responses and cure in selected patients.

Epidemiology and Patient Demographics

CLL/SLL is most often diagnosed in people older than age 60 years. It occurs most commonly in Caucasians. Men are twice as likely as women to be affected, and men generally present with more advanced disease than do women.

Although pesticides and other chemical agents have been targets of suspicion in leukemia development, no specific environmental exposures have been conclusively linked to the development of CLL. However, CLL has been recognized as a service-related illness for military veterans exposed to Agent Orange. Radiation exposure has also been a target of inquiry but has not been shown to cause CLL. In fact, CLL is the only leukemia whose incidence did not increase after radiation exposures in Hiroshima and Chernobyl.

The most specific known risk factor for CLL is inheritance—approximately 10% of patients who are diagnosed as having CLL have a first- or second-degree relative with CLL. It is interesting, however, that a single close relative is more common for this disease than is a family history with multiple affected relatives, as is the case with many other cancers.

Second malignancies are common in patients with CLL. Our own retrospective analysis found a threefold risk for all cancers overall and an eightfold risk for skin cancers [5]. Excluding skin cancers, the risk of developing another cancer was twice as high for CLL patients as for age- and sex-matched controls. Secondary cancers included malignant melanoma, soft tissue sarcomas, and lung cancers. Since these are similar to the secondary cancers that develop in patients who undergo renal transplantation, immunosuppression associated with CLL is a presumed likely cause of second malignancies. However, immunosuppression may lead to the development of both CLL and other cancers. Molecular profiling of patients with secondary cancers will improve the understanding of pathogenesis of other cancers in CLL.

In addition to the role of immunosuppression in secondary cancers, the possible contributing role of chemotherapeutic agents has been another concern, in particular the nucleoside analogs such as fludarabine, used in the treatment of CLL. Our 2009 study, however, determined that there was no difference in secondary cancer development between patients with CLL who had received nucleoside analogs and those who had not [5]. Since patients generally present with CLL/SLL at more advanced ages, other noncancer comorbidities may also pose significant considerations in treatment planning.

The MD Anderson Cancer Center Experience

The data set used for this discussion was derived from 7,422 patients who initially presented to MD Anderson Cancer Center between 1944 and 2005 with a diagnosis of CLL or SLL. Of these 7,422 patients, 4,303 had not received prior treatment elsewhere at the time of presentation to MD Anderson. Of the 4,303 patients, 1,342 had been diagnosed with multiple primary cancers (except for superficial skin cancers) and were excluded from this analysis. The remaining population of 2,961 patients, who were included in this analysis, resulted from merging eligible cases from the Tumor Registry (for those patients initially presenting between 1944 and 1983) and the CLL database from the Department of Leukemia (for those patients initially presenting between 1984 and 2005). Survival was calculated from initial presentation.

Presentation

The distribution of patients presenting to MD Anderson by decade is shown in Table 20.1. Notably, 47% of the total number presented in the final decade (1995–2005). Since the overall incidence of CLL/SLL is not thought to have changed dramatically, it is plausible that this high incidence in the final decade principally reflects an increase in referrals to our institution, particularly of patients in younger

Table 20.1 Patients with CLL/SLL presenting to MD Anderson by decade, 1944–2005

Decade	No. of patients	Percentage	Cumulative percentage
1944–1954	113	3.8	3.8
1955–1964	360	12.2	16.0
1965–1974	333	11.2	27.2
1975–1984	334	11.3	38.5
1985–1994	426	14.4	52.9
1995–2005	1,395	47.1	100.0
Total	*2,961*	*100.0*	

Table 20.2 Median patient age at initial presentation

Decade	Age (years)
1944–1954	63
1955–1964	63
1965–1974	62
1975–1984	61
1985–1994	58
1995–2005	57

Overall median patient age for all decades is 59 years

age groups, to enroll in clinical trials. Table 20.2 shows the median ages of patients who presented to our institution for treatment by decade of presentation. Notably, they trend significantly younger than the general population with this condition at the time of diagnosis.

A major factor contributing to the increasing number of patients presenting for evaluation and treatment at MD Anderson in recent years was the approval of fludarabine by the Food and Drug Administration in 1991, which led to an increased number of effective clinical trials of fludarabine for the treatment of CLL/SLL.

Treatment Patterns

A change in treatment patterns can be seen over the decades. Table 20.3 shows the proportion of patients treated with specific modalities within the first 4 months of their diagnosis. Notably, during the first two decades (1944–1964), treatment with chemotherapy and/or radiation therapy was initiated in the majority of patients. This trend plateaued and then reversed over the following decades, signifying two major changes in the treatment paradigm during that time: (a) radiation therapy ceased to be considered a primary treatment except for locoregional treatment for selected patients with SLL whose disease is confined to a single lymph node group, which remains an accepted standard treatment [6] and (b) timing of the initiation of treatment, depending on stage of the disease and identification of prognostic factors.

Table 20.3 Initial presentation by treatment group within the first 4 months of diagnosis

	MD Anderson treatment group						
	None	Chemo only	XRT only	Chemo + XRT	Chemo + Other	Other	Total
Decade	[No. (%) of patients within initial presentation year]						
1944–1954	18 (15.9)	15 (13.3)	35 (31.0)	43 (38.1)	2 (1.8)	0 (0)	113 (100.0)
1955–1964	82 (22.8)	145 (40.3)	33 (9.2)	86 (23.9)	12 (3.3)	2 (0.6)	360 (100.0)
1965–1974	148 (44.4)	143 (42.9)	5 (1.5)	16 (4.8)	18 (5.4)	3 (0.9)	333 (100.0)
1975–1984	204 (61.1)	64 (19.2)	3 (0.9)	0 (0)	54 (16.2)	9 (2.7)	334 (100.0)
1985–1994	280 (65.7)	55 (12.9)	1 (0.2)	0 (0)	80 (18.8)	10 (2.3)	426 (100.0)
1995–2005	1,071 (76.8)	224 (16.1)	1 (0.1)	1 (0.1)	84 (6.0)	14 (1.0)	1,395 (100.0)
Total	*1,803 (60.9)*	*646 (21.8)*	*78 (2.6)*	*146 (4.9)*	*250 (8.4)*	*38 (1.3)*	*2,961 (100.0)*

Chemo chemotherapy, *XRT* radiation therapy

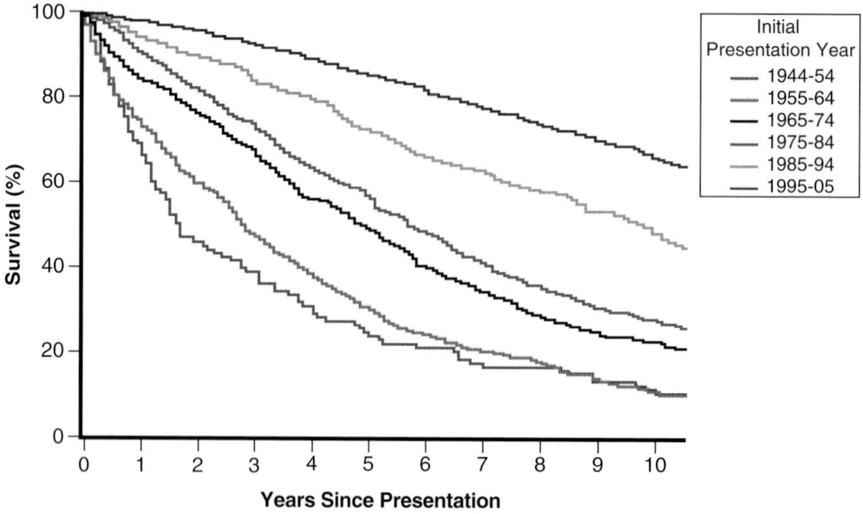

Fig. 20.1 Overall survival rates for patients with chronic lymphocytic leukemia (*CLL*) and small lymphocytic lymphoma (*SLL*) (1944–2005) ($P<0.0001$, log-rank test).

These changes coincided in time with the development of the Rai and Binet staging systems, which were intended to provide prognostic categories to help guide treatment decisions, reflecting a growing recognition that not all patients presenting with CLL/SLL required immediate treatment.

Survival

The overall survival trend reflected in Fig. 20.1 and Table 20.4 indicates a stepwise improvement in survival rates over the 60-year time span. The 5-year survival rates increased from 23.9% (1944–1954) to 85.6% (1995–2005) and the 10-year survival rates from 10.6% (1944–1954) to 65.9% (1995–2005). The most significant increase in survival was seen in the final two decades.

The improved survival rates of patients with CLL/SLL in recent decades are attributed to the following factors:

Advances in the diagnosis and classification of CLL. The wide variation in the natural behavior of this disease became more evident and was standardized by new staging systems in the 1970s and early 1980s. The Rai and Binet staging systems established criteria that enabled physicians to determine prospectively whether, when, and how aggressively they should initiate treatment. The original Rai staging system for CLL, published in 1975, classified the disease into low-, intermediate-, and high-risk groups according to whether lymphocytosis was accompanied by other factors, including lymphadenopathy, splenomegaly, hepatomegaly, anemia, and thrombocytopenia [7]. The Binet system, which followed in 1981, used

Table 20.4 Kaplan–Meier overall survival

	Percent survival		
Decade	5 years	10 years	Median survival (months)
1944–1954	23.9	10.6	20
1955–1964	30.1	11.2	33
1965–1974	48.9	22.9	59
1975–1984	56.2	28.2	68
1985–1994	72.1	48.0	118
1995–2005	85.6	65.9	Not reached

lymphocyte counts and the degree of bone marrow infiltration as correlates of disease progression [8]. Both systems are still in use today. Biologic and genetic information, in addition to the Rai and Binet systems, add critical information for risk stratification of patients with this disease.

Additional efforts to identify useful criteria followed, which included the National Cancer Institute-sponsored Working Group (NCI-WG) guidelines for the diagnosis and treatment of CLL in 1988 and 1996, and the World Health Organization Classification of Lymphoid Neoplasms (2001), which proposed additional criteria to identify patients at higher risk who should be considered for treatment [9].

More recent advances in diagnostic testing such as immunohistochemical and flow cytometric analyses have led to more exacting differential diagnoses, and more sophisticated cytogenetic and molecular analyses have made it possible to identify specific chromosomal translocations occurring in subtypes, for which there are treatment implications.

In our 2007 retrospective analysis of 2,126 patients with CLL/SLL examined at MD Anderson from 1985 to 2005, the median time to treatment was 4.2 years (95% CI, 3.8–4.7 years). Patients with high-risk features, including poor-risk genomic aberrations (particularly 17p or 6q deletions), unmutated IGHV, and ZAP-70 overexpression, required treatment earlier than did patients without these characteristics [10] (Figs. 20.2, 20.3, and 20.4). When combined, these factors can provide more complete predictive information to guide treatment choices than has ever been available before. Identification of these markers was made possible by advances in testing such as flow cytometry and cytogenetic testing such as fluorescence in situ hybridization (FISH).

Advances in first- and second-line chemotherapy. Until the late 1980s, frontline chemotherapy was limited to chlorambucil- and cyclophosphamide-containing regimens. These agents rarely led to complete remission.

The introduction of the purine analogs fludarabine, pentostatin, and cladribine into clinical trials in the 1980s was a major milestone in the treatment of this disease. Studies using fludarabine as first-line therapy demonstrated significant improvements in response rates, complete remission rates, and progression-free survival but not in overall survival [11].

During the 1994–2005 timeframe, the use of these agents in combination began to show promise as well, first with the addition of cyclophosphamide and later

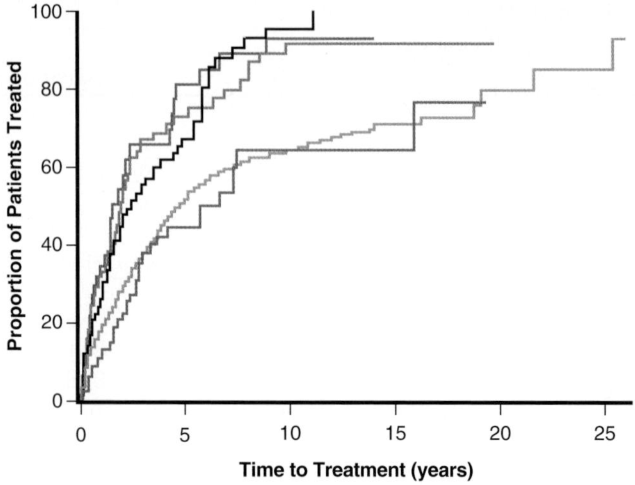

Cyto/FISH Group	N	Treated	Median (years)
17p del +/– other	40	30	1.5
11q del +/– other	85	63	1.9
+12 +/– other	120	76	2.4
13q del +/– other	129	42	6.6
Normal	1,076	547	4.8

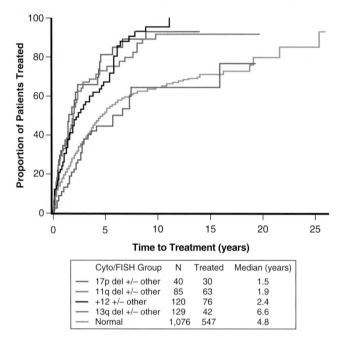

Fig. 20.2 Time to treatment by cytogenetic (*Cyto*)/fluorescence in situ hybridization (*FISH*) group ($P<0.0001$).

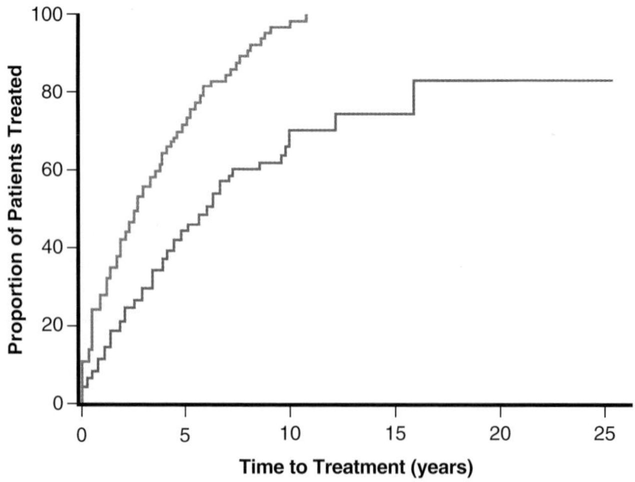

IGHV	N	Treated	Median (years)
Mutated	277	105	6.3
Unmutated	213	143	2.8

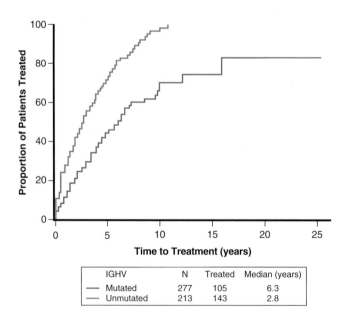

Fig. 20.3 Time to treatment by IGHV mutational status ($P<0.0001$).

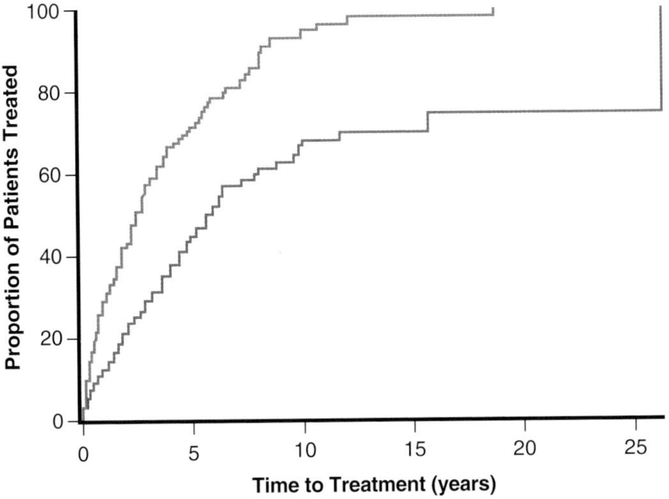

ZAP-70	N	Treated	Median (years)
Negative	294	106	5.8
Positive	185	123	2.5

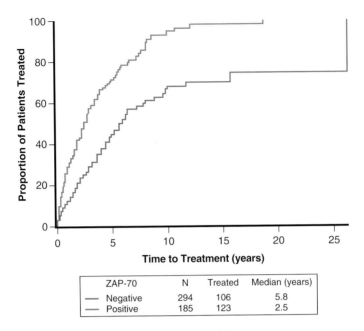

Fig. 20.4 Time to treatment by ZAP-70 status ($P<0.0001$).

with the monoclonal antibody rituximab. The combination of fludarabine and cyclophosphamide proved superior to single-agent therapy, raising complete remission rates from 29% with fludarabine alone to 35% with fludarabine and cyclophosphamide, and the addition of rituximab to the combination resulted in 70% complete remission rates, suggesting not only an additive effect but also a synergistic one [12]. Failure-free survival was also significantly longer in patients treated with the fludarabine, cyclophosphamide, and rituximab combination or with fludarabine and rituximab-containing regimens than in patients who received other therapies ($P<0.0001$, Fig. 20.5).

Advances in treatment for advanced or refractory disease. Improved chemotherapeutic agents and the advent of targeted drug therapies have led to prolonged disease-free survival and improvements in survival. However, many patients invariably experienced relapse, often with resistant or refractory disease.

Stem cell transplantation (SCT) became a viable treatment option in the 1970s and has remained an important tool for treating relapsed or refractory CLL/SLL. Although autologous SCT has not been shown to be effective and is rarely feasible, given the nature of the disease, allogeneic transplantation has resulted in durable remissions. This treatment, however, has been associated with considerable mortality and morbidity, limiting candidacy to younger patients with good performance status.

Progressive refinements in technique over the past two decades have resulted in transplantation approaches that use reduced intensity conditioning (nonmyeloablative or "mini" transplants) and donor lymphocyte infusion to treat or prevent

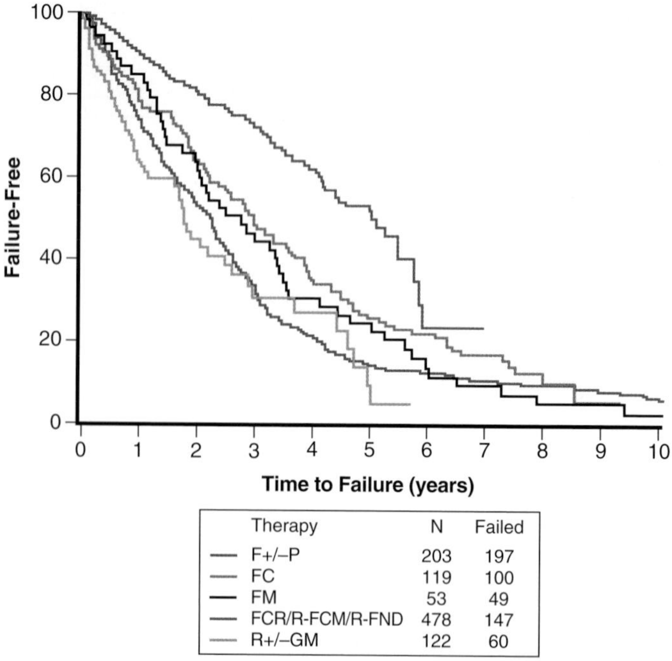

Fig. 20.5 Failure-free survival by therapy. *N*, total number of patients in each subgroup; *Failed*, number of patients for whom treatment failed; *F+/–P*, fludarabine +/– prednisone; *FC*, fludarabine and cyclophosphamide; *FM*, fludarabine and mitoxantrone; *FCR*, fludarabine, cyclophosphamide, and rituximab; *R-FCM*, fludarabine, cyclophosphamide, mitoxantrone, and rituximab; *R-FND*, fludarabine, mitoxantrone, dexamethasone, and rituximab; *R+/–GM*, rituximab +/– granulocyte-macrophage colony stimulating factor ($P<0.0001$).

posttransplant relapse. These treatments were major milestones that grew out of the recognition that the efficacy of transplantation did not come solely from dose-intense preconditioning of chemotherapy, but also from a graft-versus-leukemia effect [13].

The ability to use donor cells harvested from peripheral blood rather than from bone marrow, along with improved donor-matching techniques, wider access to stem cell banks, and better supportive care, has improved availability of SCT to patients with CLL.

The anti-CD52 monoclonal antibody alemtuzumab was approved in 2001 by the U.S. Food and Drug Administration specifically for its activity in relapsed CLL, particularly fludarabine-refractory disease that is limited to blood and bone marrow. Other novel agents have emerged subsequent to the timeframe discussed here and continue to be studied in various combination regimens [14]. Although none have yet replaced allogeneic SCT as a curative option, some show promise and are useful for patients who are not candidates for SCT [15].

Novel agents. A large number of early-phase clinical trials are investigating the role of new agents in the treatment of CLL.

Advances in supportive care. Improved supportive care has reduced the number of immune-compromised patients with CLL who might otherwise succumb to the overwhelming infectious processes and has enabled many to receive therapies that in previous decades would not have been feasible. These improvements include infection prophylaxis with antibiotics and antiviral agents and vaccines, early interventions for autoimmune cytopenias, prevention and proactive management of cytomegalovirus reactivation associated with monoclonal antibodies such as alemtuzumab, and safer blood product support.

Current Management Approach

The National Comprehensive Cancer Network guidelines currently recommend that patients enroll in clinical trials when treatment is indicated by symptoms, including fever without infection, night sweats, weight loss, and severe fatigue, or by disease conditions, including threatened end-organ function, progressive bulky disease evidenced by splenomegaly or lymphadenopathy, disease progression with progressive anemia or thrombocytopenia, and rapid lymphocyte doubling time [6].

The current approach to management of CLL/SLL at our institution begins with a thorough workup that includes immunophenotyping, cytogenetic and/or FISH testing to detect chromosomal deletions, assessment of IGHV mutational status, and determination of CD38 and ZAP-70 expression by flow cytometric and immunohistochemical analyses. The goal of our workup is to identify patients who should initiate treatment and to secure guidance about the best treatment choices based on the patient's disease characteristics and risk factors.

For all patients who require treatment, selection of therapy is individualized on the basis of disease factors, including clinical, laboratory, histologic, and genomic features that represent risk of disease progression, and on patient factors including performance status. In selected patients, clinical trials offer the best treatment option.

Future Directions

Improvements in outcome for CLL/SLL will likely be derived from continued research in the following areas:

- Continued advances in our understanding of the biology and pathogenesis of CLL/SLL, particularly the identification of genetic factors and the role of the B-cell receptor and B-cell receptor signaling, and the continued investigation of intricate cellular and molecular interactions of CLL cells with other immune cells and stromal elements known as the "microenvironment."

- Continued refinement in risk stratification based on molecular and genetic profiles that accurately identify patients who will benefit from specific treatments.
- Continued development of effective, minimally toxic, novel targeted drug therapies for use in frontline and refractory disease.
- Understanding refractoriness to treatment and the development of progression after initial response to treatment.
- Continued development of algorithms and standardization of patient evaluation and selection of therapy, including therapies targeting the biology of the disease.

Our understanding of the molecular and biologic nature of this disease has changed dramatically in recent years. In earlier years, CLL was considered a pathologic but simple accumulation of quiescent leukemic cells that had failed to undergo apoptosis. The identification of pathways involved in CLL pathogenesis and of the interaction of CLL cells with the microenvironment are expected to lead to better treatment and eventually to the cure of CLL.

References

1. Swerdlow SH, Campo E, Harris NL, et al. WHO classification of tumours of haematopoietic and lymphoid tissues. 4th ed. Lyon: IARC Press; 2008.
2. Jemal A, Siegel R, Xu J, et al. Cancer statistics, 2010. CA Cancer J Clin. 2010;60:277–300.
3. Lin TS, Awan FT, Byrd JC. Clinical manifestations, staging, and treatment of indolent non-Hodgkin's lymphoma. In: Hoffman R, Benz EJ, Shattil SJ, et al., editors. Hematology: basic principles and practice. 5th ed. Philadelphia: Elsevier; 2009. p. 1327–47.
4. Amato D, Oscier DG, Davis Z, et al. Cytogenetic aberrations and immunoglobulin VH gene mutations in clinically benign CD5- monoclonal B-cell lymphocytosis. Am J Clin Pathol. 2007;128(2):333–8.
5. Tsimberidou AM, Wen S, McLaughlin P, et al. Other malignancies in chronic lymphocytic leukemia/small lymphocytic lymphoma. J Clin Oncol. 2009;27(6):904–10.
6. NCCN Clinical Practice Guidelines in Oncology: Non-Hodgkin's Lymphoma v4.2011. National Comprehensive Cancer Network. Accessed 23 May 2012.
7. Rai KR, Sawitsky A, Cronkite EP, Chanana AD, Levy RN, Pasternack BS. Clinical staging of chronic lymphocytic leukemia. Blood. 1975;46(2):219–34.
8. Binet JL, Aquier A, Dighiero G, et al. A new prognostic classification of chronic lymphocytic leukemia derived from a multivariate survival analysis. Cancer. 1981;48:198–206.
9. Campo E, Swerdlow SH, Harris N, Pileri S, Stein H, Jaffe ES. The 2008 WHO classification of lymphoid neoplasms and beyond: evolving concepts and practical applications. Blood. 2011;117(19):5019–32.
10. Tsimberidou AM, Wen S, O'Brien S, et al. Assessment of chronic lymphocytic leukemia and small lymphocytic lymphoma by absolute lymphocyte counts in 2,126 patients: 20 years of experience at The University of Texas MD Anderson Cancer Center. J Clin Oncol. 2007;25(29):4648–56.
11. Keating MJ, Kantarjian H, Talpaz M, et al. Fludarabine: a new agent with major activity against chronic lymphocytic leukemia. Blood. 1989;74:19–25.
12. Keating MJ, O'Brien S, Albitar M, et al. Early results of a chemoimmunotherapy regimen of fludarabine, cyclophosphamide, and rituximab as initial therapy for chronic lymphocytic leukemia. J Clin Oncol. 2005;23:4079–88.

13. Khouri IF, Keating M, Korbling M, et al. Transplant-lite: Induction of graft-versus-malignancy using fludarabine-based nonablative chemotherapy and allogeneic blood progenitor-cell transplantation as treatment for lymphoid malignancies. J Clin Oncol. 1998;16(8):2817–24.
14. Tsimberidou AM, Keating MJ. Treatment of patients with fludarabine-refractory chronic lymphocytic leukemia: need for new treatment options. Leuk Lymphoma. 2010;51(7):1188–99.
15. Brown JR. The treatment of relapsed refractory chronic lymphocytic leukemia. Hematology Am Soc Hematol Educ Program. 2011;2011:111–3.

Chapter 21
Hodgkin Lymphoma

Michelle Fanale, Bouthaina Dabaja, Uday Popat, Paolo Anderlini, and Anas Younes

Introduction

An estimated 8,490 Americans were diagnosed as having Hodgkin lymphoma (HL) in 2010 [1]. HL is a B-cell lymphoma that arises from germinal center or post-germinal center B cells. Two types of classic HL (cHL) make up 95% of HL diagnoses; in contrast, nodular lymphocyte predominant Hodgkin lymphoma (NLPHL) is rare and has distinct pathologic features. cHL is unique in that the CD30-positive Reed–Sternberg (RS) cells often make up less than 1% of the tumor and are surrounded by a rich microenvironment, including CD20-positive reactive B cells that are believed to provide survival signals to the RS cells.

There are four distinct subtypes of cHL: nodular sclerosis (NS), mixed cellularity (MC), lymphocyte rich (LR), and lymphocyte depleted (LD). cHL has a bimodal age distribution, first peaking in patients in their 20–30s and then in patients in their 50s. Most patients with cHL present with asymptomatic enlargement of the lymph nodes.

NLPHL is characterized by the presence of CD20-positive lymphocytic and histiocytic (LH) cells. The age at onset for NLPHL is later than that for cHL, occurring in the 30–40s, and has a male predominance. NLPHL patients, similar to cHL

M. Fanale (✉) • A. Younes
Department of Lymphoma and Myeloma, The University of Texas MD Anderson Cancer Center, 1515 Holcombe Boulevard, Unit 429, Houston, TX 77030, USA
e-mail: mfanale@mdanderson.org

B. Dabaja
Department of Radiation Oncology, The University of Texas MD Anderson Cancer Center, Houston, TX, USA

U. Popat • P. Anderlini
Department of Stem Cell Transplantation and Cellular Therapy, The University of Texas MD Anderson Cancer Center, Houston, TX, USA

M.A. Rodriguez et al. (eds.), *60 Years of Survival Outcomes at The University of Texas MD Anderson Cancer Center*, DOI 10.1007/978-1-4614-5197-6_21,

Table 21.1 Ann Arbor staging system with Costwold's modifications for Hodgkin lymphoma[a]

Stage	Description
I	Involvement of a single lymph node region or lymphoid structure such as the thymus, Waldeyer's ring, or spleen
II	Involvement of two or more lymph node regions or lymphoid structures on the same side of the diaphragm
III	Involvement of lymph node regions or lymphoid structures on both sides of the diaphragm
IV	Diffuse or disseminated involvement of one or more extranodal organs or tissue beyond that designated E, with or without associated lymph nodded involvement
	Modifying features
A	Absence of systemic symptoms
B	Presence of systemic symptoms (fever >38 °C, night sweats, or unexplained weight loss >10% of body weight within the preceding 6 months)
E	Involvement of a single extranodal site that is proximal or contiguous to the known nodal site
X	A bulky mediastinal mass with a maximum width that is ≥1/3 the transverse diameter of the thorax or >10 cm in maximum diameter

[a]Data from [2]

patients, tend to present with asymptomatic adenopathy, although the lymph nodes involved are generally more peripheral than central. However, in contrast to patients with cHL, patients with NLPHL rarely present with B symptoms of fever, night sweats, or significant weight loss.

Patients with HL are staged according to the Ann Arbor system with modifications developed at the Costswold Conference in 1989 (Table 21.1) [2]. Stage assignment is used to tailor treatment strategies. Current outcomes for cHL patients are stage-dependent: patients with early-stage disease generally have low 5-year relapse rates of 7–15%, whereas patients with advance-stage disease typically have 5-year relapse rates of 20–40%. Although relapse tends to occur early in patients with cHL, it is not uncommon for relapse to occur 5–10 years after initial treatment in patients with NLPHL. As with cHL, rates of relapse are correlated with stage: patients with early-stage disease have 10-year relapse rates of 10–30%. Although patients with relapsed cHL generally present with aggressive disease and receive intensive treatment, patients with relapsed NLPHL generally present with indolent disease and can be treated more conservatively.

Historical Perspective

Over the past 60 years, significant advances in treatments have led to shifts in paradigms of management, resulting in substantial improvements in patient outcome. Initial treatment approaches were focused on improving overall survival (OS). This was followed by an emphasis on decreasing risk of disease relapse by increasing disease-free survival. Currently, treatments are being tailored toward decreasing the amount of therapy given to low-risk patients and toward integrating biologically targeted therapies for patients with high-risk and relapsed or refractory disease. The treatment of HL is a multidisciplinary effort involving medical and radiation oncologists, which at MD Anderson Cancer Center encompasses the Departments of Lymphoma, Radiation Oncology, and Stem Cell Transplantation. Advances can be subgrouped into changes in frontline management of newly diagnosed disease and of relapsed or refractory disease.

Advances in Frontline Disease Management

The treatment of patients with cHL involved a series of sweeping changes that occurred over half a century. The radical approach of radiation therapy (RT), which was pioneered at Stanford University in the 1960s by Henry Kaplan and Saul Rosenberg, offered patients with HL the first hope for cure. To compensate for the lack of systemic treatment, which became available in the early 1970s, RT used large fields that treated the entire lymphatic system with relatively high doses of radiation. Often the entire heart was included in the radiation field, and the biologic doses were much higher than those delivered in contemporary treatment.

The advent of combination chemotherapy with mechlorethamine, vincristine (Oncovin), procarbazine, and prednisone (MOPP) in the mid-1960s significantly improved responses. In a meta-analysis of 12 trials and 1,666 patients, combined chemotherapy plus RT significantly reduced the risk of relapse by 53% at 10 years [3]. Notably, the reduced relapse rates were similar among trials that used combined chemotherapy plus involved-field RT (IFRT) versus more extensive RT such as extended-field RT, subtotal nodal irradiation (STNI), or total lymphoid irradiation. However, because of the long-term risks of secondary malignancies from alkylating agent exposure in patients treated with MOPP, only borderline improvement was seen in OS.

The Milan group conducted a landmark trial comparing four cycles of doxorubicin (Adriamycin), bleomycin, vinblastine, and dacarbazine (ABVD) followed by IFRT versus STNI [4]. After 10 years of follow-up, ABVD plus IFRT was found to be equivalent to ABVD plus STNI. In addition, outcomes with ABVD therapy compared with historical outcomes with MOPP therapy revealed significantly fewer cases of secondary malignancies. After the Milan trial, IFRT replaced extended-field RT, doses of 36–40 Gy replaced doses of 45–54 Gy, and a dose per fraction of 1.8–2 Gy replaced the 3-Gy dose per fraction. This new approach, which was the dominant practice from the early 1980s until the end of the 1990s, increased patient survival rates in part by decreasing mortality secondary to adverse effects.

In the past decade, there have been further reductions in radiation fields and doses, as well as further stratification of treatment approaches for patients with early-stage disease. The application of computed tomography (CT) to the generation of three-dimensional radiation therapy (3DRT) planning was the single most important development that enabled radiation oncologists to reduce radiation fields without compromising tumor coverage and at the same time spare the surrounding critical organs. Other technological developments currently used at MD Anderson include inverse planning with intensity-modulated radiation therapy (IMRT), cone beam CT for daily tumor tracking, breath-holding techniques that reduce the radiation dose to the lungs and heart, and the mantle board that reduces the dose to the breasts. The application of these techniques further decreased the toxic effects associated with the delivery of RT by better defining the target and by accurately delivering the radiation to the intended sites of disease.

Since the late 1970s, the German Hodgkin Study Group (GHSG) has enrolled more than 15,000 patients in their randomized clinical trials. The GHSG developed criteria to define two distinct prognosis groups in patients with early-stage disease: favorable and unfavorable. Patients are considered to have unfavorable disease if they have a large mediastinal mass, extranodal involvement, elevated erythrocyte sedimentation rate, more than two involved lymph node areas, or B symptoms. This has allowed further tailoring of treatment approaches. The recently published results of the HD10 trial established that for patients with an early-stage favorable prognosis, two cycles of ABVD followed by 20 Gy of IFRT is as efficacious as, and less toxic than, four cycles of ABVD followed by 30 Gy of IFRT [5]. In the paired early-stage unfavorable prognosis GHSG HD11 trial, four cycles of ABVD and 30 Gy of IFRT remained the best treatment strategy; intensification with a regimen of bleomycin, etoposide, doxorubicin (Adriamycin), cyclophosphamide, vincristine (Oncovin), procarbazine, and prednisone (BEACOPP) did not significantly improve outcome in these patients and resulted in more toxicity including infertility [6].

Further improvements beyond ABVD are warranted for patients with advanced-stage cHL since 20% of these patients will not experience complete remission (CR) and among those who do, 33% will ultimately experience relapse. Several philosophies exist on how to decrease relapse rates. The first is based on intensification of the chemotherapy regimen. A series of GHSG trials beginning in the 1990s, HD9, HD12, and HD15, explored BEACOPP-based treatment approaches and showed freedom from disease relapse in the mid-80% range [7–9]. The Intergroup 20012 randomized trial initiated by the European Organization for Research and Treatment of Cancer (EORTC) is currently evaluating whether BEACOPP is superior to ABVD. A second philosophy focuses on combining biologically targeted therapies with standard chemotherapy regimens. Rituximab is an anti-CD20 monoclonal antibody and is a standard treatment for non-Hodgkin lymphoma (NHL). Part of the rationale for incorporating rituximab into cHL therapy is that by targeting the CD20-positive microenvironment B cells that surround the RS cells, one can decrease the survival signals sent to the RS cells. Given the benefit seen in an MD Anderson trial of rituximab treatment in patients with relapsed cHL, a follow-up frontline MD Anderson phase 2 trial evaluating rituximab combined with ABVD (R-ABVD) was conducted. The International Prognostic Score (IPS), which uses seven risk factors to predict outcome in patients with advanced-stage disease, was used to stratify patients [10]. Advanced-stage patients with a high IPS of 3–7 had a predicted 5-year event-free survival (EFS) of 60–42%. A 2009 update with 5 years of follow-up showed 25% improvement in EFS in patients with a high IPS of three or greater who had been treated with R-ABVD compared with historical outcomes after six to eight cycles of ABVD alone [11]. A randomized phase 2 MD Anderson trial evaluating R-ABVD versus ABVD for newly diagnosed cHL in patients with an IPS of three or higher is ongoing.

The introduction of positron emission tomography (PET) scans to assess response has led to multiple studies, beginning in the mid-2000s, to determine the ability of these scans to predict long-term outcome. The benefit of PET scans is encompassed by their ability to distinguish whether residual sites of adenopathy are likely to represent treated versus active cHL, and PET scan response for cHL was incorporated into the 2007 revised response criteria [12]. A recent study explored whether interim PET scan response obtained after two cycles of therapy (PET-2) is stronger than the IPS in predicting outcome. In this study, the 2-year progression-free survival (PFS) for patients with positive PET-2 was only 13% [13]. The use of PET-2 to predict long-term outcome remains controversial; however, the use of PET-2 has enabled a third philosophy of advanced-stage cHL treatment to emerge, focused on using PET-2 to intensify treatment for only those patients with the highest risk of disease relapse. This strategy is incorporated within the Southwest Oncology Group (SWOG) 0816 Intergroup trial in which PET response is assessed after two cycles of ABVD and treatment is intensified to BEACOPP for PET-2-positive patients, whereas PET-2-negative patients complete an additional four cycles of ABVD.

Frontline management of NLPHL has remained relatively stable over the past several decades, in part because of the rarity of this diagnosis. Several publications in the 2000s evaluating patients treated since 1985 established radiation treatment alone as the standard for stage IA and IIA disease [14, 15]. However, recent publications highlight an ongoing rate of relapse, with 10-year PFS rates of 85% and 61% for stage I and II patients, respectively, who were treated with RT; these studies show that unlike cHL patients, NLPHL patients have a 7% risk of transformation to large B-cell NHL at 10 years [16, 17]. Patients with advanced-stage NLPHL are known to have poorer long-term outcome; however, given the lack of prospective trials, no single chemotherapy regimen is preferred, and R-ABVD or a combination of rituximab, cyclophosphamide, hydroxydaunomycin (doxorubicin), Oncovin (vincristine), and prednisone (R-CHOP) is often used. Data from an MD Anderson retrospective study show a trend toward outcome improvement in patients treated with R-CHOP, and a prospective trial with SWOG is being considered to evaluate R-CHOP versus R-ABVD [18].

Advances in Relapsed/Refractory Disease Management

Despite aforementioned advances in chemotherapy and RT, 7–15% of patients with stage I and II disease and 20–40% of patients with advanced disease will have refractory or recurrent cHL. Current standard management of relapsed/refractory cHL includes the use of salvage or second-line chemotherapy followed by high-dose chemotherapy (HDCT) and autologous stem cell transplantation (ASCT). The primary goal of salvage chemotherapy is to achieve CR before ASCT, as this predicts for improved disease-free survival. The development of effective salvage regimens since the 1990s has had a significant impact on outcome for this patient population. Common salvage chemotherapy options include platinum- and gemcitabine-containing regimens, and overall response rates (ORRs) range from 70% to 80% with CR rates of 10–35% [19–22].

At MD Anderson, we are also conducting trials pairing targeted therapies with traditional salvage chemotherapy to assess whether we can further improve CR rates. Activation of the nuclear factor-κβ (NF-κβ) pathway allows for transcription of proteins that drive cell survival and decrease apoptosis. Bortezomib is a proteasome inhibitor that inhibits this pathway. Bortezomib was initially approved for treatment of multiple myeloma and was more recently approved for relapsed mantle cell lymphoma. In cHL cells, bortezomib has been shown to decrease apoptosis. Although single-agent responses in cHL patients were low, solid tumor trials suggested that bortezomib can overcome chemotherapy resistance. Thus, at MD Anderson, we recently conducted a phase 1 trial that combined standard salvage chemotherapy consisting of ifosfamide, carboplatin, and etoposide (ICE) with bortezomib. This combination was well tolerated and showed a good CR rate of 25% in a poor risk factor patient group; a randomized phase 2 trial has recently completed enrollment at MD Anderson [23].

Autologous or "self" stem cell transplantation for cHL was developed in the late 1970s and the first ASCT for cHL was performed at MD Anderson in 1978; by the 1990s, this procedure was commonly used. Several discoveries were important for this development. First, E. Donnall Thomas showed feasibility and success of allogeneic or "donor" bone marrow transplantation in patients with refractory leukemias. Specifically, he showed that stem cells in donor's marrow are able to repopulate and replenish the recipient's hematopoietic system after myeloablative chemoradiotherapy. Second, techniques for cryopreservation and storage of hematopoietic cells were developed, and the ability to use stored cells to reconstitute the hematopoietic system was established. Third, a dose-dependent increase in tumor kill from chemotherapy was shown in in vitro studies. However, this dose escalation was limited by myelotoxicity, which can be overcome by infusion of previously cryopreserved autologous hematopoietic stem cells. On the basis of this belief, ASCT was studied in patients with relapsed or refractory HL at transplant centers worldwide, including MD Anderson Cancer Center.

Early studies in the 1980s focused on patients in whom multiple prior regimens had failed. In these studies, 5-year PFS rates of 30–60% were observed. Recent update of long-term outcome in 184 consecutive patients treated with cyclophosphamide, BCNU, and etoposide (CBV) and ASCT at MD Anderson between 1978 and 1994 showed OS and PFS rates at 10 years of 34% and 29%, respectively, suggesting durability of these results [24]. To determine whether results obtained with high-dose chemotherapy and ASCT were superior to results obtained with salvage chemotherapy without ASCT, two randomized trials were conducted in patients with chemosensitive (CR or partial remission with standard salvage therapy) cHL. Both showed significant improvement in PFS. A British study of HDCT compared with standard-dose chemotherapy had to be closed early after enrolling only 40 patients because patients declined randomization to the standard dose arm [25]. A larger German study, which enrolled 61 patients to the high-dose BCNU, etoposide, ara-C (cytarabine), and melphalan (BEAM) and ASCT arm and 56 patients to the conventional-dose arm, showed a significantly superior PFS of 55% in the HDCT plus ASCT group compared with 34% in the standard chemotherapy group [26]. These two trials, published in 1993 and 2002, respectively, changed the management of disease by defining HDCT with BEAM plus ASCT as the standard treatment for relapsed or refractory cHL.

Since the 1990s, better transplantation outcome has been achieved by choosing patients with chemosensitive disease for ASCT, using a peripheral blood stem cell graft instead of bone marrow, using filgrastim, and improving supportive care. At MD Anderson, our treatment-related mortality rate decreased 15% in the 1980s to 1.6% between 1996 and 2007 (in 246 patients). In patients treated with the BEAM conditioning regimen, the 48-month overall and PFS rates were 72% and 57%, respectively. The cumulative incidence of secondary myelodysplastic syndrome or acute myelogenous leukemia was 8%, which remains a major long-term adverse effect of extensive prior treatment with HDCT. Similar results have been reported by others. Consolidation with RT will also be considered after ASCT for patients who did not previously receive RT, particularly if they presented with a bulky mediastinal mass.

Other prognostic factors predicting poor outcome after ASCT include primary refractory disease, remission duration of less than 12 months, B symptoms at the time of relapse, extranodal disease, and the number of prior chemotherapy regimens. Patients with one or more of these adverse factors have poor outcomes and alternative strategies are needed. One such strategy is the development of novel HDCT regimens. An ongoing phase 1 trial at MD Anderson combines gemcitabine with busulfan and melphalan, and a phase 2 trial is planned.

Survival of cHL patients who experience relapse after ASCT is highly predicted by their time to relapse. This has been shown through a review of MD Anderson patients as part of an international multicenter retrospective study published in 2008 [27]. Striking similarity of outcome was seen in patients treated in various cancer centers. The data demonstrated that patients whose disease relapses within 6–12 months after ASCT have a median OS of 2.4 years, whereas patients whose disease relapses within 3 months of ASCT have a very short median OS of only 8 months. Thus, this study emphasized the crucial need for additional treatment options.

Advances in our understanding of cHL pathology and biology over the past decade have led to the development of targeted agents that are currently undergoing clinical trials in the hope of obtaining approval for new drugs for treating cHL. CD30 expression is highly restricted and is densely seen on RS cells in cHL. Initial trials evaluated unconjugated anti-CD30 antibodies and showed overall low response rates. To increase efficacy, a conjugated or linked anti-CD30 antibody was developed. Brentuximab vedotin is an anti-CD30 antibody that is conjugated to a microtubule inhibitor—monomethyl auristatin E (MMAE)—that acts similar to vinblastine and is termed an antibody drug conjugate (ADC). Brentuximab vedotin has been evaluated in patients with relapsed cHL in several multicenter clinical trials at MD Anderson. The ORR for both phase I trials was in the mid-50–60%, and CR was seen in 25–30% of cHL patients; the overall median duration of responses was 10 months [28, 29]. Given the promising level of clinical activity, a pivotal trial for cHL patients was conducted and enrolled 102 patients with relapsed disease after prior ASCT. Patients were treated with brentuximab vedotin every 3 weeks and dramatic responses were seen with an ORR of 75%, a CR rate of 34%, and a median duration of CRs lasting 20.5 months. The data from this pivotal trial led to Food and Drug Administration (FDA) approval of this therapy in August 2011 for the third-line management of cHL. This approval represents a landmark advance in therapeutic options for cHL patients and is the first ADC to be approved for the treatment of lymphoma [30]. Currently, brentuximab is being evaluated in a randomized phase 3 trial at MD Anderson as a maintenance therapy after ASCT for cHL patients who have a high risk of disease relapse.

Another method of targeting cHL is with use of histone deacetylases (HDAC), since gene transcription is in part regulated by posttranscriptional histone modification. Several HDAC inhibitors (HDACi's) have shown efficacy. MGCD0103 is a pill HDACi which in a phase 2 cHL trial demonstrated an ORR in the mid-30% range, and correlative studies supported down-regulation of proteins expressed by the RS cells [31]. Another oral HDACi, panobinostat, has shown similar efficacy in a phase 2 cHL trial; it is being evaluated as a pre-ASCT salvage therapy in combination with ICE [32].

In addition to targeted therapies for patients with relapsed cHL after ASCT, patients whose disease enters remission can also be considered for allogeneic stem cell transplantation (allo-SCT). Historically, the role of allo-SCT in the management of relapsed and refractory HL has been controversial. Published data in the 1980s and 1990s remain largely limited to registry series and retrospective historical data from large transplantation centers, including MD Anderson [33]. The vast majority of these patients were young and received transplants from related donors. The consistent pattern that emerged from these reports painted a rather disappointing picture of high transplant-related mortality and relapse rates. This poor outcome was likely a reflection of the nature and poor prognosis of the patients undergoing transplantation, with the vast majority having been extensively pretreated and many having chemoresistant or refractory disease. Still, a minority of patients, 15–20%, did indeed achieve long-term remission.

To improve and expand on these results, the major new development in the allo-SCT area from 2000 on has been the introduction in the field of allo-transplantation of reduced-intensity conditioning (RIC) regimens, made possible by fludarabine. Fludarabine, pioneered here at MD Anderson, is a purine analog with significant immunosuppressive activity but little systemic or organ toxicity. Fludarabine has been incorporated into the conditioning regimen for patients with relapsed/refractory HL and is usually coupled with an alkylating agent (e.g., melphalan). In other studies, fludarabine was used with low-dose total body irradiation. Although not entirely accurate, the term "mini transplant" has also been used to designate this new development. Over the past decade, many published reports have confirmed the feasibility of this approach [34, 35], resulting in substantial decreases in early-transplant-related mortality and in hospitalization duration. In addition, patient outcome may be improved. This mini-transplant allows older HL patients with comorbidities such as hypertension, diabetes, and poor cardiac or pulmonary function, as well as patients whose disease relapses after ASCT, to undergo the procedure. Moreover, the rapid evolution of human leukocyte antigen typing techniques is allowing the identification of suitably matched unrelated donors for many patients lacking a sibling donor.

Due to marked improvement in supportive care, as well as in the prevention and treatment of graft-versus-host disease, RIC transplant results in these patients are closely approaching the results achieved with related donors. Indeed, investigators are now trying to identify high-risk refractory patients who are unlikely to benefit from high-dose chemotherapy and ASCT for upfront treatment with allo-SCT. Alternative donor transplants, using umbilical cord blood units as well as haploidentical donors (i.e., partially matched related donors), have also shown promising results in pilot trials [34].

Although these improvements have been encouraging, it should be acknowledged that many hurdles remain. A prospective, randomized comparison between conventional myeloablative and RIC regimens has not been carried out and is unlikely to be finalized. Disease relapse remains a fairly common occurrence, despite the use of allo-SCT, particularly if the patient is not in remission at the time of transplantation. Although better controlled, graft-versus-host disease and infection continue to contribute significantly to the risk and toxicity of the procedure. Results in older patients continue to leave significant room for improvement. The optimal RIC regimen is still not well defined, and the addition of new and different agents active in HL such as gemcitabine is being contemplated. More patients being treated, better patient selection, longer follow-up, and more detailed analyses of the data will ultimately better define the role of RIC allo-SCT in cHL.

Whereas patients with relapsed cHL receive intensive treatment, patients with relapsed NLPHL often present with indolent disease at relapse and can receive more conservative management approaches. The anti-CD20 antibody rituximab has been evaluated for the treatment of relapsed NLPHL. Two studies presented in 2007–2008 demonstrated a 100% ORR and CR of 40–60% [36, 37]. In addition, patients who received maintenance or extended rituximab had a higher CR of 88%; at 2.5 years of follow-up, only 12% of patients treated with maintenance rituximab had experienced further progression of their NLPHL compared with 48% of patients treated with a limited number of cycles of rituximab [37]. Transformation to diffuse large B-cell lymphoma or T-cell–rich B-cell lymphoma also occurred at a rate of 14% after 6.5 years [17]. These patients are generally treated according to diffuse large B-cell lymphoma and T-cell–rich B-cell lymphoma guidelines and can be considered for HDCT and ASCT. Overall, the rarity of the disease makes it difficult to prospectively evaluate the role of ASCT for patients with relapsed or refractory NLPHL. A 2009 review of MD Anderson patients described the outcomes of 26 patients who underwent HDCT plus ASCT, and after 4 years of follow-up, 69% remain in remission [38].

The MD Anderson Cancer Center Experience

The MD Anderson data set for HL was derived from the 6,513 patients who were seen at MD Anderson between 1944 and 2004 (Table 21.2). Of this total group, 3,326 patients (51%) had received no prior treatment and were newly diagnosed at the time of referral to MD Anderson. A total of 2,723 (81%) of the newly diagnosed patients received definitive primary front-line treatment at MD Anderson.

The number of HL patients presenting by time interval (Table 21.3) is greatest beginning in 1965, with only about 13% of the total patients being seen from 1944 to 1964. The histologic features of patients with HL seen (Table 21.4) mirror those

Table 21.2 Hodgkin lymphoma (HL) patients referred to MD Anderson, 1944–2004

Description	No. of patients
Patients with HL initially presenting to MD Anderson on or before 12/31/04	6,513
Newly diagnosed without prior treatment	3,326
Definitive primary MD Anderson treatment	2,723
No other primary malignancies except for superficial skin cancers	2,445

Table 21.3 Initial presentation year of Hodgkin lymphoma patients at MD Anderson (N=2,445)

Decade	No. (%) of patients
1944–1954	54 (2.2)
1955–1964	261 (10.7)
1965–1974	517 (21.1)
1975–1984	578 (23.6)
1985–1994	578 (23.6)
1995–2004	457 (18.7)

Table 21.4 Histologic features of Hodgkin lymphoma patients referred to MD Anderson, 1944–2004[a]

Histologic feature	% of patients
Classic Hodgkin lymphoma (cHL)	91.2
Nodular sclerosis (NS)	58.5
Mixed cellularity (MC)	30.3
Lymphocyte depleted (LD)	2.4
Nodular lymphocyte predominant Hodgkin's lymphoma (NLPHL)	5.4

[a]Diagnosis was unable to be further classified in 3.5% of patients

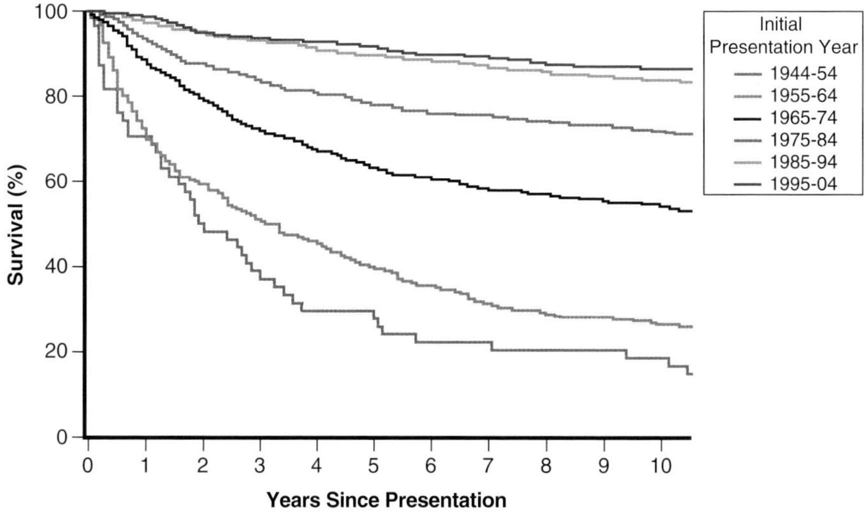

Fig. 21.1 Overall survival rates for patients with Hodgkin lymphoma (1944–2004) ($P<0.0001$, log-rank test for trend).

Table 21.5 Survival of Hodgkin lymphoma patients treated at MD Anderson, 1944–2004

Decade	Percent survival	
	5 years	10 years
1944–1954	27.8	18.5
1955–1964	39.8	26.6
1965–1974	63.3	54.2
1975–1984	78.2	71.9
1985–1994	89.7	83.8
1995–2004	91.7	86.5

of the general population in that the overwhelming majority of patients had cHL, whereas only about 5% had pathologically confirmed diagnoses of the rarer NLPHL. Within the cHL group, as anticipated, the most common subtype was NS, followed by MC, with LD being diagnosed in only a small fraction of patients. In 3.5% of patients, the diagnosis could not be further classified because of overlapping morphologic or immunohistochemical findings between diagnoses of HL and NHL. Since staging definitions have changed over the past several decades, detailed information about patients' stage of disease is not fully available from the MD Anderson database. However, most patients with newly diagnosed disease who present to MD Anderson have early-stage disease as similar to the general population.

The survival curves for patients with HL demonstrate significantly improved 5- and 10-year outcomes for patients treated during the most recent decades compared with those treated earlier (Fig. 21.1; Table 21.5). For instance, patients treated from 1995 to 2004 had very high 5- and 10-year survival rates of 91.7% and 86.5%, respectively, which showed a respective 64% and 68% improvement when compared with patients treated from 1944 to 1954.

The dramatic impact of the development and advancement of frontline chemotherapy for cHL can be seen by the clear improvements in OS. Outcomes from 1944 to 1954 reflect a period when cHL was managed with surgery alone, and thus prognosis was dismal. The addition of radiation treatment in the 1960s is reflected by an increase in survival rates; however, approximately 75% of patients treated in this decade still died within 10 years. This high mortality rate is a result of high relapse rates after radiation treatment alone and the lack of further treatment options at that time for relapsed disease beyond repeat irradiation. In addition, patients treated during this period received very large irradiation fields that often encompassed nearly the whole body, resulting in high rates of secondary cancers, coronary artery disease, and other complications that also affected survival.

Patients treated from 1975 to 1984 had a clear stepwise improvement in survival compared with patients treated during the earlier two decades. The introduction of the MOPP chemotherapy regimen for systemic management of cHL in the mid- to late-1960s was a turning point. Long-term adverse effects from this regimen, however, included the risks of developing myelodysplastic syndrome and acute myelogenous leukemia. The Milan group both introduced ABVD and demonstrated that smaller radiation fields through IFRT could have similar benefits as STNI with fewer adverse effects. Positive data on ABVD, first published in 1975, supported findings that ABVD was more effective and less toxic than MOPP. The incorporation of ABVD into standard management was reflected by significant improvement in survival rates for patients treated from 1975 to 1984 when compared with both the immediately preceding and early decades. A further stepwise enhancement in outcome was seen between 1985 and 2004, as this is the period over which salvage chemotherapy treatments were developed and expanded. Also during this time, high-dose chemotherapy with ASCT became a standard treatment for patients with relapsed disease. Beginning in 2000, additional treatments became available at MD Anderson for patients with relapsed cHL disease after ASCT, including an increased number of targeted treatment approaches on clinical protocols and the option for allogeneic stem cell transplantation.

Current Management Approach

Our current management approach for newly diagnosed HL is tailored to the stage of disease, and the assessment of risk factors is used to further stratify treatment options for patients with cHL. Patients are assessed for protocol treatment options when available. Patients with relapsed or refractory cHL are treated with additional salvage chemotherapy, and those entering remission proceed with high-dose chemotherapy and ASCT. Patients who do not experience remission with salvage chemotherapy or those whose disease relapses after ASCT are evaluated for treatment options that include the recently approved brentuximab vedotin treatment as well as targeted therapies on protocol; if they subsequently experience remission, they can be further considered for allogeneic stem cell transplantation. Patients with relapsed NLPHL have in general a more indolent disease course and are treated less intensively. However, patients with relapsed NLPHL with transformation to diffuse large B-cell lymphoma or T-cell–rich large B-cell lymphoma who previously received R-CHOP are often treated with HDCT and ASCT.

Future improvements in survival outcomes are anticipated and will result from evolving strategies in patient care. One such improvement includes the ability to improve methods of risk assessment to better select the level of treatment needed, thereby intensifying treatment for patients with predicted poorer outcomes and de-escalating therapy for patients with favorable risk profiles. The GHSG HD 10 trial is an example of treatment de-escalation for cHL patients with favorable risk. The SWOG 0816 is an example of intensification of therapy for patients with high risk of developing refractory or relapsed cHL. The process of determining risk will come from both clinical and tumor biology factors. A second evolving strategy in patient care is the incorporation of novel targeted treatments into the frontline and second-line setting, first with chemotherapy and eventually potentially paired with each other. The rituximab-ABVD, brentuximab-ABVD, bortezomib-ICE, and panobinostat-ICE MD Anderson trials are examples of this. A third future improvement is the further use of tumor biology to develop rationally combined and eventually personalized combinations of targeted therapies such as combinations of the anti-CD30 treatment brentuximab vedotin with drugs that target other pathways in active in cHL. Fourth will be the further potential reduction of the radiation field size through involved nodal rather than field radiation. Fifth is the refinement of HDCT through the introduction of new regimens beyond standard BEAM; MD Anderson's evaluation of gemcitabine, busulfan, and melphan is an example of this. Finally, although not in the near future, is the ultimate development of management strategies tailored to target tumor biology, which could result in patients with newly diagnosed relapsed cHL being treated in a less intensive fashion, using approaches not based on chemotherapy or irradiation. Although not all strategies for future management are obviously known, what is clear is the belief that the treatment of HL will continue to advance as it has over the past 60 years.

References

1. Jemal A, Siegel R, Xu J, Ward E. Cancer statistics, 2010. CA Cancer J Clin. 2010;60: 277–300.
2. Lister T, Crowther D, Sutcliffe S, et al. Report of a committee convened to discuss the evaluation and staging of patients with Hodgkin's disease: Cotswolds meeting. J Clin Oncol. 1989;7:1630–6 [published erratum appears in J Clin Oncol. 1990;8(9):1602].
3. Specht L, Gray RG, Clarke MJ, Peto R. Influence of more extensive radiotherapy and adjuvant chemotherapy on long-term outcome of early-stage Hodgkin's disease: a meta-analysis of 23 randomized trials involving 3,888 patients. International Hodgkin's Disease Collaborative Group. J Clin Oncol. 1998;16:830–43.

4. Bonadonna G, Bonfante V, Viviani S, Di Russo A, Villani F, Valagussa P. ABVD plus subtotal nodal versus involved-field radiotherapy in early-stage Hodgkin's disease: long-term results. J Clin Oncol. 2004;22:2835–41.
5. Engert A, Plutschow A, Eich HT, et al. Reduced treatment intensity in patients with early-stage Hodgkin's lymphoma. N Engl J Med. 2010;363:640–52.
6. Eich HT, Diehl V, Gorgen H, et al. Intensified chemotherapy and dose-reduced involved-field radiotherapy in patients with early unfavorable Hodgkin's lymphoma: final analysis of the German Hodgkin Study Group HD11 trial. J Clin Oncol. 2010;28:4199–206.
7. Diehl V, Franklin J, Pfreundschuh M, et al. Standard and increased-dose BEACOPP chemotherapy compared with COPP-ABVD for advanced Hodgkin's disease. N Engl J Med. 2003;348:2386–95.
8. Engert A, Franklin J, Mueller R-P, et al. HD12 randomised trial comparing 8 dose-escalated cycles of BEACOPP with 4 escalated and 4 baseline cycles in patients with advanced stage Hodgkin lymphoma (HL): an analysis of the German Hodgkin Lymphoma Study Group (GHSG), University of Cologne, D-50924 Cologne, Germany. ASH annual meeting abstracts. Blood. 2006;108:99.
9. Kobe C, Dietlein M, Franklin J, et al. Positron emission tomography has a high negative predictive value for progression or early relapse for patients with residual disease after first-line chemotherapy in advanced-stage Hodgkin lymphoma. Blood. 2008;112:3989–94.
10. Hasenclever D, Diehl V. A prognostic score for advanced Hodgkin's disease. International prognostic factors project on advanced Hodgkin's disease. N Engl J Med. 1998;339:1506–14.
11. Copeland AR, Cao Y, Fanale M, et al. Final report of a phase-II study of rituximab plus ABVD for patients with newly diagnosed advanced stage classical Hodgkin lymphoma: results of long follow up and comparison to institutional historical data. ASH annual meeting abstracts. Blood. 2009;114:1680.
12. Cheson BD, Pfistner B, Juweid ME, et al. Revised response criteria for malignant lymphoma. J Clin Oncol. 2007;25:579–86.
13. Gallamini A, Hutchings M, Rigacci L, et al. Early interim 2-[18 F]fluoro-2-deoxy-D-glucose positron emission tomography is prognostically superior to international prognostic score in advanced-stage Hodgkin's lymphoma: a report from a joint Italian-Danish study. J Clin Oncol. 2007;25:3746–52.
14. Wirth A, Yuen K, Barton M, et al. Long-term outcome after radiotherapy alone for lymphocyte-predominant Hodgkin lymphoma: a retrospective multicenter study of the Australasian Radiation Oncology Lymphoma Group. Cancer. 2005;104:1221–9.
15. Nogova L, Reineke T, Eich HT, et al. Extended field radiotherapy, combined modality treatment or involved field radiotherapy for patients with stage IA lymphocyte-predominant Hodgkin's lymphoma: a retrospective analysis from the German Hodgkin Study Group (GHSG). Ann Oncol. 2005;16:1683–7. doi:10.1093/annonc/mdi323.
16. Chen RC, Chin MS, Ng AK, et al. Early-stage, lymphocyte-predominant Hodgkin's lymphoma: patient outcomes from a large, single-institution series with long follow-up. J Clin Oncol. 2010;28:136–41.
17. Al-Mansour M, Connors JM, Gascoyne RD, Skinnider B, Savage KJ. Transformation to aggressive lymphoma in nodular lymphocyte-predominant Hodgkin's lymphoma. J Clin Oncol. 2010;28:793–9.
18. Fanale MA, Fayad L, Romaguera J, et al. Experience with R-CHOP in patients with lymphocyte predominant Hogdkin lymphoma (LPHL). Haematologica. 2007;92(s5):57.
19. Aparicio J, Segura A, Garcera S, et al. ESHAP is an active regimen for relapsing Hodgkin's disease. Ann Oncol. 1999;10:593–5.
20. Santoro A, Magagnoli M, Spina M, et al. Ifosfamide, gemcitabine, and vinorelbine: a new induction regimen for refractory and relapsed Hodgkin's lymphoma. Haematologica. 2007;92:35–41.
21. Moskowitz CH, Nimer SD, Zelenetz AD, et al. A 2-step comprehensive high-dose chemoradiotherapy second-line program for relapsed and refractory Hodgkin disease: analysis by intent to treat and development of a prognostic model. Blood. 2001;97:616–23.

22. Bartlett NL, Niedzwiecki D, Johnson JL, et al. Gemcitabine, vinorelbine, and pegylated liposomal doxorubicin (GVD), a salvage regimen in relapsed Hodgkin's lymphoma: CALGB 59804. Ann Oncol. 2007;18:1071–9.
23. Fanale MA, Fayad LE, Pro B, et al. A phase I study of bortezomib in combination with ICE (BICE) in patients with relapsed/refractory classical Hodgkin lymphoma. ASH annual meeting abstracts. Blood. 2008;112:3048.
24. Popat U, Hosing C, Saliba RM, et al. Prognostic factors for disease progression after high-dose chemotherapy and autologous hematopoietic stem cell transplantation for recurrent or refractory Hodgkin's lymphoma. Bone Marrow Transplant. 2004;33:1015–23.
25. Linch DC, Winfield D, Goldstone AH, et al. Dose intensification with autologous bone-marrow transplantation in relapsed and resistant Hodgkin's disease: results of a BNLI randomised trial. Lancet. 1993;341:1051–4.
26. Schmitz N, Pfistner B, Sextro M, et al. Aggressive conventional chemotherapy compared with high-dose chemotherapy with autologous haemopoietic stem-cell transplantation for relapsed chemosensitive Hodgkin's disease: a randomised trial. Lancet. 2002;359:2065–71.
27. Horning S, Fanale M, deVos S, et al. Defining a population of Hodgkin lymphoma patients for novel therapeutics: an international effort. 10th international conference on malignant lymphoma (10-ICML) [abstract 118]. Ann Oncol. 2008;19:iv120.
28. Younes A, Forero-Torres A, Bartlett NL, et al. Multiple complete responses in a phase 1 dose-escalation study of the antibody-drug conjugate SGN-35 in patients with relapsed or refractory CD30-positive lymphomas. ASH annual meeting abstracts. Blood. 2008;112:1006.
29. Fanale M, Bartlett NL, Forero-Torres A, et al. The antibody-drug conjugate brentuximab vedotin (SGN-35) induced multiple objective responses in patients with relapsed or refractory CD30-positive lymphomas in a phase 1 weekly dosing study. ASH annual meeting abstracts. Blood. 2009;114:2731.
30. Younes A, Gopal AK, Smith SE, et al. Results of a pivotal phase II study of brentuximab vedotin for patients with relapsed or refractory Hodgkin's lymphoma. J Clin Oncol. 2012;30:1–7.
31. Younes A, Pro B, Fanale M, et al. Isotype-selective HDAC inhibitor MGCD0103 decreases serum TARC concentrations and produces clinical responses in heavily pretreated patients with relapsed classical Hodgkin lymphoma (HL). ASH annual meeting abstracts. Blood. 2007;110:2566.
32. Younes A, Ong T-C, Ribrag V, et al. Efficacy of panobinostat in phase II study in patients with relapsed/refractory Hodgkin lymphoma (HL) after high-dose chemotherapy with autologous stem cell transplant. ASH annual meeting abstracts. Blood. 2009;114:923.
33. Anderlini P, Champlin RE. Reduced intensity conditioning for allogeneic stem cell transplantation in relapsed and refractory Hodgkin lymphoma: where do we stand? Biol Blood Marrow Transplant. 2006;12:599–602.
34. Peggs KS, Anderlini P, Sureda A. Allogeneic transplantation for Hodgkin lymphoma. Br J Haematol. 2008;143:468–80.
35. Anderlini P, Saliba R, Acholonu S, et al. Fludarabine-melphalan as a preparative regimen for reduced-intensity conditioning allogeneic stem cell transplantation in relapsed and refractory Hodgkin's lymphoma: the updated MD Anderson Cancer Center experience. Haematologica. 2008;93:257–64.
36. Schulz H, Rehwald U, Morschhauser F, et al. Rituximab in relapsed lymphocyte-predominant Hodgkin lymphoma: long-term results of a phase 2 trial by the German Hodgkin Lymphoma Study Group (GHSG). Blood. 2008;111:109–11.
37. Horning SJ, Bartlett NL, Breslin S, et al. Results of a prospective phase II trial of limited and extended rituximab treatment in Nodular Lymphocyte Predominant Hodgkin's Disease (NLPHD). ASH annual meeting abstracts. Blood. 2007;110:644.
38. Popat U, Hosing C, Fanale M, et al. Autologous transplantation for Nodular Lymphocyte-Predominant Hodgkin Lymphoma (NLPHL). ASH annual meeting abstracts. Blood. 2009;114:2310.

Chapter 22
Non-Hodgkin Indolent B-Cell Lymphoma

Sattva S. Neelapu

Introduction

Non-Hodgkin lymphomas (NHLs) are a diverse group of lymphoproliferative neoplasms arising from lymphocytes that differ in terms of their morphology, natural history, response to therapy, and prognosis. As a group, NHLs are the sixth most common cancer in the USA, with an estimated 65,540 new cases diagnosed in 2010. They are also the sixth most common cause of cancer death in the USA, with an estimated 20,210 deaths in 2010. Approximately 85% of NHLs are of B-cell origin, and the remaining are T-cell malignancies. On the basis of their clinical features and natural history, NHLs of B-cell origin may be broadly categorized as either indolent or aggressive. Follicular lymphoma, the most common indolent B-cell lymphoma, accounts for 22.1% of all NHL cases worldwide [1]. Other indolent B-cell lymphomas include small lymphocytic lymphoma or chronic lymphocytic lymphoma (6.7% of all NHLs); marginal zone lymphomas, consisting of extranodal marginal zone lymphoma (also called mucosa-associated lymphoid tissue [MALT] lymphoma [7.6% of all NHLs]), nodal marginal zone lymphoma (1.8% of all NHLs), and splenic marginal zone lymphoma (<1% of all NHLs); and lymphoplasmacytic lymphoma/Waldenstrom macroglobulinemia (1.2% of all NHLs) [1]. This chapter focuses primarily on follicular lymphoma; the other indolent B-cell lymphomas will be described briefly.

Follicular lymphoma is derived from germinal center B cells; histologically, they are composed of a mixture of centrocytes (small cleaved cells) and centroblasts (large noncleaved cells). Depending on the number of centroblasts per high-power field (hpf), follicular lymphoma is graded in the current World Health Organization

S.S. Neelapu (✉)
Department of Lymphoma and Myeloma, The University of Texas MD Anderson Cancer Center, 1515 Holcombe Blvd, Unit 903, Houston, TX 77030, USA
e-mail: SNeelapu@mdanderson.org

M.A. Rodriguez et al. (eds.), *60 Years of Survival Outcomes at The University of Texas MD Anderson Cancer Center*, DOI 10.1007/978-1-4614-5197-6_22,

(WHO) classification [2] for NHL into grade 1 (0–5 centroblasts/hpf), grade 2 (6–15 centroblasts/hpf), and grade 3 (>15 centroblasts/hpf). Grade 3 follicular lymphoma is further categorized into grade 3A (>15 centroblasts/hpf but with some centrocytes) and grade 3B (sheets of centroblasts without any centrocytes). Grades 1 and 2 follicular lymphoma are considered low-grade and are generally treated as indolent lymphomas. In contrast, grade 3 follicular lymphoma is more aggressive, especially grade 3B, and will not be discussed in this chapter.

The median age at diagnosis for follicular lymphoma is 60 years. Follicular lymphoma is characterized by painless lymphadenopathy, relatively slow progression, and a median survival of 8–10 years. Approximately 15% of patients with follicular lymphoma present with stage I or II disease and may be potentially cured with radiation therapy. However, most follicular lymphoma patients have advanced stage III or IV disease at initial diagnosis and are considered incurable. Although some patients have waxing and waning asymptomatic disease for several years without the need for therapy, others present with more disseminated, rapidly growing disease and require treatment to alleviate symptoms. Although highly responsive to chemotherapy, radiation therapy, and biologic therapy, advanced-stage follicular lymphoma is characterized by repeated patterns of remissions and relapses, and most patients eventually die of their lymphoma, despite its usually indolent course. Follicular lymphoma may also transform into a higher-grade histologic subtype such as diffuse large B-cell lymphoma; this occurs in 3% of patients each year. Transformation may be characterized by a sudden increase in one lymph node mass, elevated lactate dehydrogenase level, pain, or B symptoms and may portend a poor prognosis.

The clinical features and natural history of other indolent B-cell lymphomas are similar to those of follicular lymphoma and are characterized by asymptomatic onset followed by slow progression to symptomatic disease, good response to therapy, and repeated patterns of remissions and relapses. Extranodal marginal zone lymphoma is more commonly localized at initial diagnosis and therefore may be potentially cured with radiation therapy or other therapeutic strategies. In contrast, nodal marginal zone lymphoma, splenic marginal zone lymphoma, lymphoplasmacytic lymphoma, and small lymphocytic lymphoma usually have disseminated disease at diagnosis and are considered incurable. However, as with follicular lymphoma, because of the indolent nature of these diseases, patients have a long median survival.

Historical Perspective

The classification and terminology for NHLs continued to evolve since the 1940s as more was learned about the biology and natural history of these malignancies. Over the past seven decades, several classification systems have been proposed by various groups (Table 22.1) [2–4]. The early classification systems were based on morphology, cell lineage, and/or clinical features of the lymphomas. In 1994, the

Table 22.1 Major lymphoma classifications proposed since the 1940s

Classification	Year	Features used for classification
Gall and Mallory	1942	Morphology
Rappaport	1956	Morphology and pattern
Lukes and Collins	1974	Cell of origin
Kiel	1974	Morphology, cell of origin, and clinical
Working formulation	1982	Clinical prognosis and morphology
REAL [3]	1994	Morphology, immunophenotype, genetic, and clinical
WHO [4]	2001	Morphology, immunophenotype, genetic, and clinical
WHO update [2]	2008	Morphology, immunophenotype, genetic, and clinical

REAL Revised European-American Lymphoma, *WHO* World Health Organization

Revised European-American Lymphoma (REAL) classification system was proposed, which was based on all available information about lymphomas, including their immunophenotypic, genetic, morphologic, and clinical features [3]. The current WHO classification, initially published in 2001 [4] and updated in 2008 [2], was based on the foundations of the REAL classification and represents a consensus on lymphoma classification that was developed from input from pathologists, clinical hematologists, and oncologists from all over the world (Table 22.2) [2].

Historically, staging studies in NHL included a complete physical examination, complete blood count, chemistry survey including renal and liver function tests, chest radiography, bilateral iliac crest bone marrow aspirations and biopsy, and imaging studies. Before computed tomography (CT) scans became available, lymphadenopathy in the abdomen and pelvis was assessed by lymphangiography. From the 1980s until the start of the 2000s, peripheral and central lymphadenopathy was assessed by CT scans of the neck, chest, abdomen, and pelvis. Since the 2000s, positron emission tomography (PET) scans have been used in patients with indolent lymphoma if there is clinical suspicion of transformation to aggressive histology.

The Ann Arbor staging system [5], which was originally proposed for Hodgkin lymphoma in 1971, has also been used to determine the clinical stage for NHL (Table 22.3) [5]. However, despite the Ann Arbor staging system's prognostic value in Hodgkin lymphoma, likely due to the disease's contiguous lymphatic spread, this staging system has had limited usefulness in predicting prognosis in NHL, probably because of the hematogenous spread seen in this disease. Therefore, other prognostic indices have been developed to assess prognosis in NHL. In 1993, the International Prognostic Index (IPI) was proposed to assess prognosis in diffuse large B-cell lymphoma [6]. The IPI was also used to assess prognosis in indolent lymphomas for a number of years. However, the IPI categorized most follicular lymphoma patients into low-risk or low-intermediate-risk groups, with only a small fraction of patients identified as high-risk. Furthermore, other clinical features that had been found to have prognostic value in follicular lymphoma were not included in the IPI. Therefore, in 2004, the Follicular Lymphoma International Prognostic Index (FLIPI) was proposed to assess prognosis in follicular lymphoma. This index divided patients into three risk groups according to the number of adverse prognostic factors associated

Table 22.2 WHO 2008 classification of mature B-cell non-Hodgkin lymphomas [2]

Chronic lymphocytic leukemia/small lymphocytic lymphoma
B-cell prolymphocytic leukemia
Splenic marginal zone lymphoma
Hairy cell leukemia
Splenic lymphoma/leukemia, unclassifiable
Splenic diffuse red pulp small B-cell lymphoma
Hairy cell leukemia-variant
Lymphoplasmacytic lymphoma/Waldenstrom macroglobulinemia
Heavy chain diseases
Alpha heavy chain disease
Gamma heavy chain disease
Mu heavy chain disease
Plasma cell myeloma
Solitary plasmacytoma of bone
Extraosseous plasmacytoma
Extranodal marginal zone B-cell lymphoma of mucosa-associated lymphoid tissue (MALT) type
Nodal marginal zone lymphoma (MZL)
Pediatric type nodal MZL
Follicular lymphoma (grades 1, 2, 3A, and 3B)
Pediatric type follicular lymphoma
Primary cutaneous follicular center lymphoma
Mantle cell lymphoma
Diffuse large B-cell lymphoma (DLBCL), not otherwise specified
T-cell/histiocyte-rich DLBCL
Epstein–Barr virus (EBV)$^+$ DLBCL of the elderly
DLBCL associated with chronic inflammation
Lymphomatoid granulomatosis
Primary mediastinal (thymic) large B-cell lymphoma
Intravascular large B-cell lymphoma
Primary cutaneous DLBCL, leg type
ALK$^+$ large B-cell lymphoma
Plasmablastic lymphoma
Large B-cell lymphoma arising in HHV8-associated multicentric Castleman disease
Primary effusion lymphoma
Burkitt lymphoma
B-cell lymphoma, unclassifiable, with features intermediate between DLBCL and Burkitt lymphoma
B-cell lymphoma, unclassifiable, with features intermediate between DLBCL and Hodgkin lymphoma

with each patient (Table 22.4) [7]. The five adverse prognostic factors in FLIPI include age ≥60 years, Ann Arbor stage III or IV, hemoglobin level <12 g/dL, elevated serum lactate dehydrogenase level, and involvement of ≥5 nodal sites.

Indolent B-cell lymphomas were found to be highly sensitive to radiation therapy in the 1930s. Indeed, involved-field radiation therapy has been the treatment of choice for stage I and II follicular lymphoma and is probably curative in 40–50% of

Table 22.3 Ann Arbor staging system [5]

Stage	Definition
I	Involvement of a single lymph node region or a single extranodal organ or site
II	Involvement of two or more lymph node regions on the same side of the diaphragm, or localized involvement of an extranodal organ or site and one or more lymph node regions on the same side of the diaphragm
III	Involvement of lymph node regions on both sides of the diaphragm with or without localized involvement of an extranodal organ or site or spleen or both
IV	Diffuse or disseminated involvement of one or more distant extranodal organs with or without involvement of lymph nodes

Definition of B symptoms: Fever >38°C, drenching night sweats, and/or weight loss >10% of body weight in the preceding 6 months

Table 22.4 Survival according to risk group by Follicular Lymphoma International Prognostic Index [7]

Risk group	No. of factors	Overall survival rate (5 years)	Overall survival rate (10 years)
Low	0–1	90.6	70.7
Intermediate	2	77.6	50.9
High	≥3	52.5	35.5

these patients [8, 9]. Advanced-stage follicular lymphoma is considered incurable and has traditionally been observed without therapy if the patient is asymptomatic. Symptomatic advanced disease was primarily treated with radiation therapy in the 1930s and 1940s. Subsequently, with the demonstrated clinical efficacy of alkylating agents such as chlorambucil [10] in the 1950s and of cyclophosphamide [11] in the 1960s, chemotherapy became the treatment of choice for advanced-stage indolent B-cell lymphomas. In the 1970s, combination chemotherapy with or without anthracyclines [12, 13] was found to be more effective in inducing clinical remissions than was single-agent chemotherapy and eventually became the first-choice therapy for most patients. Biologic therapies such as interferon and monoclonal antibodies were introduced either as single agents or in combination with chemotherapy in the 1980s and 1990s. Other treatment modalities that became available in the 1990s or later include radioimmunotherapy and stem cell transplantation.

The MD Anderson Cancer Center Experience

Of the 8,199 patients who presented to the MD Anderson Cancer Center between 1944 and 2004 with a diagnosis of indolent B-cell lymphoma, 4,533 were previously untreated; of this group, 2,549 received definitive treatment at MD Anderson. Of these 2,549 patients, 1,962 had indolent B-cell lymphoma as the only site of malignancy

Table 22.5 Patients with indolent B-cell lymphoma treated at MD Anderson between 1944 and 2004

Decade	No. (%) of patients
1944–1954	58 (3.0)
1955–1964	217 (11.1)
1965–1974	317 (16.2)
1975–1984	410 (20.9)
1985–1994	433 (22.1)
1995–2004	527 (26.9)
Total	*1,962 (100.0)*

Table 22.6 Distribution by histologic features of 1,962 patients with indolent B-cell lymphoma who were treated at MD Anderson between 1944 and 2004

Histologic feature	No. (%) of patients
Follicular lymphoma, unspecified	521 (26.6)
Follicular lymphoma, small cleaved	533 (27.2)
Follicular lymphoma, mixed small and large cleaved	295 (15.0)
Small lymphocytic lymphoma	448 (22.8)
Diffuse well-differentiated lymphoma	94 (4.8)
Marginal zone lymphoma	42 (2.1)
MALT lymphoma	19 (1.0)
Splenic B-cell lymphoma	7 (0.4)
Monocytoid B-cell lymphoma	3 (0.2)

MALT mucosa-associated lymphoid tissue

except for superficial skin cancers and were considered for survival analysis. The total number of patients who presented to MD Anderson by decade is shown in Table 22.5, and the distribution of these patients by histologic feature is shown in Table 22.6. The patients were grouped into histological categories that were commonly used in NHL classifications in the 1970s and 1980s. Therefore, some of the patients may not have been grouped in the indolent lymphoma category per the current WHO classification [2]. For example, diffuse lymphomas probably consisted of several histologic features including those currently referred to as follicular, small lymphocytic, lymphoplasmacytic, and mantle cell lymphoma according to WHO classification. Furthermore, mantle cell lymphoma, a relatively aggressive B-cell NHL, was not recognized as a distinct entity until the 1990s and was probably included in follicular, small lymphocytic, or diffuse lymphoma groups before this period.

Survival rates were computed for all 1,962 patients with indolent B-cell lymphomas definitively treated at MD Anderson between 1944 and 2004 (Fig. 22.1). Patients were not stratified by stage or histology. However, most of the patients had follicular lymphoma (Table 22.6) and would have likely had advanced-stage disease at initial presentation because of the nature of these lymphomas. The overall survival rates improved steadily over the past six decades, with 5-year survival rates

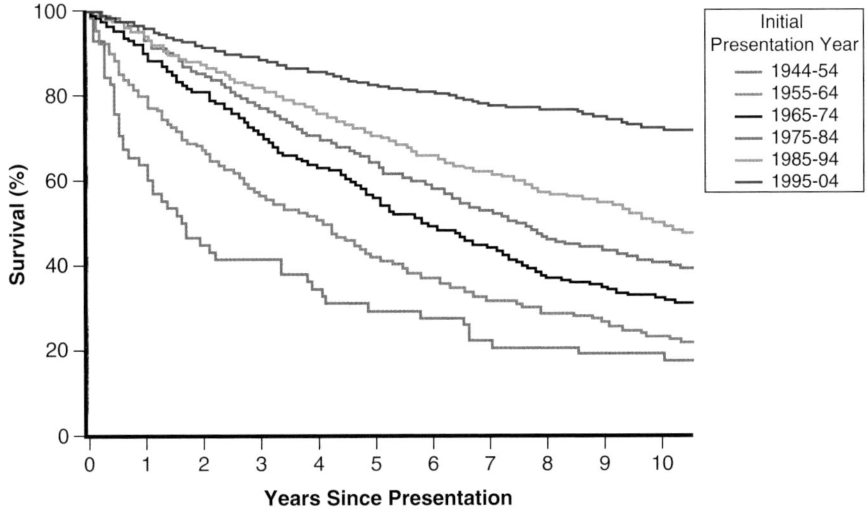

Fig. 22.1 Overall survival rates for patients with non-Hodgkin indolent B-cell lymphoma who were treated at MD Anderson between 1944 and 2004 ($P<0.0001$, log-rank test for trend).

Table 22.7 Five-year and ten-year survival rates for patients with indolent B-cell lymphoma who were treated at MD Anderson between 1944 and 2004

Decade	Overall survival rate (5 years)	Overall survival rate (10 years)
1944–1954	29.3	17.2
1955–1964	41.5	23.2
1965–1974	54.1	31.9
1975–1984	63.5	41
1985–1994	70.6	49.6
1995–2004	82.7	72.3

increasing from 29% to 83% and 10-year survival rates increasing from 17% to 72% between 1944 and 2004 (Table 22.7). With the use of single-agent chemotherapies in the 1950s and 1960s and of multiagent chemotherapy regimens including alkylating agents and anthracyclines in the 1970s for treatment of advanced disease, survival rates almost doubled compared with 1940s rates, when radiation therapy would have been the primary treatment modality for patients with both localized and advanced disease. Interferon was used in multiple clinical trials at MD Anderson in the 1980s as consolidation after standard combination chemotherapy and may have provided further benefit [14]. The introduction of fludarabine, a highly active drug in most indolent B-cell lymphomas in the early 1990s, offered additional options for controlling these tumors when alkylating agents and anthracyclines failed [15]. The significant improvement in survival observed in the late 1990s and 2000s was most likely due to the use of rituximab [16, 17]. Other therapeutic strategies that may have contributed include radioimmunotherapy, autologous and non-myeloablative allogeneic stem cell transplantation [18], and improvements in supportive care.

In addition, it is very likely that factors not associated with therapy may have played a role in improving survival duration in the late 1990s. For example, mantle cell lymphoma, a B-cell lymphoma associated with a median survival of only 3 years in the 1990s, was defined as a distinct entity in the REAL classification in 1994 [3] and was excluded from the indolent B-cell lymphoma category after 1994. Another factor that may have improved survival duration in the late 1990s was increased awareness of the symptoms and signs of lymphoma; by this time, patients may have started seeking medical attention sooner, leading to diagnoses being made at earlier stages of the natural history of these indolent lymphomas, giving a lead-time effect. The increased use of imaging studies for various medical conditions and biopsies of incidental lymphadenopathy detected in the abdomen and pelvis, which otherwise would not have caused symptoms for several years, may also have led to diagnoses at earlier stages of the natural history of these indolent lymphomas in some patients. Although these non-therapy-related factors may have contributed to improvement in survival in the past two decades, the major reason was likely the use of rituximab. In randomized studies, rituximab administered in combination with chemotherapy was shown to improve overall and complete response rates, molecular remission rates, progression-free survival, and overall survival, compared with use of chemotherapy alone [19, 20].

In summary, the development of multiple chemotherapeutic and biologic therapeutic agents over the past six decades has markedly expanded the therapeutic armamentarium available to treat patients with indolent B-cell lymphomas. Until the 1990s, most patients with follicular lymphoma received an average of three systemic therapies during the course of their disease. With the availability of a larger therapeutic armamentarium and because of improvements in supportive care, patients with indolent B-cell lymphomas now have the option of receiving ten or more effective systemic therapies that can induce durable remissions even after multiple relapses. This has translated into a survival benefit, with the current median survival for patients treated at MD Anderson much longer than 10 years (Table 22.7).

Current Management Approach

Currently, our initial staging evaluations for patients with a diagnosis of indolent B-cell lymphoma include a complete physical examination, complete blood count with differential, chemical survey including renal and liver function tests, lactate dehydrogenase, beta-2-microglobulin, CT scans of the neck, chest, abdomen, and pelvis, and bilateral bone marrow biopsies and unilateral aspirate. A PET scan is performed in patients with suspected transformation to guide in choosing a biopsy site. Participation in a clinical trial is encouraged at all stages of disease at initial presentation and at the time of relapse. Outside of a clinical trial, patients presenting with stages I or II follicular lymphoma, grade 1 or 2, are treated with involved-field radiation therapy with or without rituximab-based chemotherapy. Stage III and IV patients with low-volume disease and who are asymptomatic may be observed without therapy or treated with single-agent rituximab therapy. Patients with bulky and/or symptomatic advanced disease are usually treated with rituximab-based chemotherapy. However, elderly patients or patients with multiple comorbid illnesses may be treated with single-agent rituximab therapy. Myelotoxic agents such as fludarabine that may impair the collection of stem cells are avoided if the patient is a potential candidate for autologous stem cell transplantation in the future.

All relapses are confirmed by a biopsy. Treatment decision for relapsed disease is individualized and is based on age, nature of prior therapy, number of prior therapies, duration of remission after prior therapy, comorbid illnesses, tumor bulk, and symptoms. Late relapses, asymptomatic relapses, or relapses with low-tumor volume may be observed or treated with single-agent rituximab therapy. Younger patients whose disease relapses early after prior therapy or patients with multiple prior therapies are considered for salvage therapy followed by consolidation with stem cell transplantation. If a matched donor is available, non-myeloablative allogeneic stem cell transplantation is recommended. If there is no matched donor, patients are considered for consolidation with high-dose chemotherapy with autologous stem cell transplantation. Maintenance rituximab therapy is usually recommended after induction therapy, both at initial presentation and at the time of relapse.

In conclusion, complete remission can be induced in most patients with follicular lymphoma with use of current therapies at initial presentation and at relapse. However, most patients experience recurrent relapses and eventually die of their disease. Rituximab-based therapies improve complete remission rates, progression-free survival, and overall survival in follicular lymphoma, but they do not appear to be curative [19, 20]. Therefore, novel therapeutic strategies that eradicate minimal residual disease are needed to further improve clinical outcome in these patients. Ideally, strategies used to eradicate minimal residual disease should have a different mechanism of action and target different molecules than do agents used in induction therapy since the residual tumor cells are likely to be resistant to the induction therapy agents.

Ongoing research over the past decade has led to a better understanding of the biology of these tumors and has identified targets for development of novel therapies such as monoclonal antibodies, vaccines, immunomodulatory drugs, and small-molecule inhibitors against vital signaling pathways in the tumor. In the future, these therapeutic agents may provide novel options to eradicate minimal residual disease and to control these lymphomas at relapse. It is possible that the combined use of these novel agents with current therapies may lead to a cure for lymphomas or alternatively, convert these diseases into chronic illnesses so that patients can live with a reasonably good quality of life, even if they cannot be cured of their lymphoma.

References

1. A clinical evaluation of the International Lymphoma Study Group classification of non-Hodgkin's lymphoma. The Non-Hodgkin's Lymphoma Classification Project. Blood. 1997;89(11):3909–18.
2. Swerdlow SH, Campo E, Harris NL, et al. WHO classification of tumours of haematopoietic and lymphoid tissues. 4th ed. Lyon: IARC Press; 2008.
3. Harris NL, Jaffe ES, Stein H, et al. A revised European-American classification of lymphoid neoplasms: a proposal from the International Lymphoma Study Group. Blood. 1994;84(5):1361–92.
4. Jaffe ES, Harris NL, Stein H, Vardiman JW. Pathology and genetics of tumours of haematopoietic and lymphoid tissues. WHO classification of tumours, vol. 3. Lyon: IARC Press; 2001.
5. Carbone PP, Kaplan HS, Musshoff K, Smithers DW, Tubiana M. Report of the Committee on Hodgkin's Disease Staging Classification. Cancer Res. 1971;31(11):1860–1.
6. A predictive model for aggressive non-Hodgkin's lymphoma. The International Non-Hodgkin's Lymphoma Prognostic Factors Project. N Engl J Med. 1993;329(14):987–94.
7. Solal-Celigny P, Roy P, Colombat P, et al. Follicular lymphoma international prognostic index. Blood. 2004;104(5):1258–65.
8. Mac Manus MP, Hoppe RT. Is radiotherapy curative for stage I and II low-grade follicular lymphoma? Results of a long-term follow-up study of patients treated at Stanford University. J Clin Oncol. 1996;14(4):1282–90.
9. Wilder RB, Jones D, Tucker SL, et al. Long-term results with radiotherapy for Stage I-II follicular lymphomas. Int J Radiat Oncol Biol Phys. 2001;51(5):1219–27.
10. Galton DA, Israels LG, Nabarro JD, Till M. Clinical trials of p-(di-2-chloroethylamino)-phenylbutyric acid (CB 1348) in malignant lymphoma. Br Med J. 1955;2(4949):1172–6.
11. Gross R, Lambers K. First experience in treating malignant tumors with a new nitrogen mustard-phosphamidester. Dtsch Med Wochenschr. 1958;83(12):458–62.
12. Hoogstraten B, Owens AH, Lenhard RE, et al. Combination chemotherapy in lymphosarcoma and reticulum cell sarcoma. Blood. 1969;33(2):370–8.
13. McKelvey EM, Gottlieb JA, Wilson HE, et al. Hydroxyldaunomycin (Adriamycin) combination chemotherapy in malignant lymphoma. Cancer. 1976;38(4):1484–93.
14. Rohatiner AZ, Gregory WM, Peterson B, et al. Meta-analysis to evaluate the role of interferon in follicular lymphoma. J Clin Oncol. 2005;23(10):2215–23.
15. Redman JR, Cabanillas F, Velasquez WS, et al. Phase II trial of fludarabine phosphate in lymphoma: an effective new agent in low-grade lymphoma. J Clin Oncol. 1992;10(5):790–4.
16. Fisher RI, LeBlanc M, Press OW, Maloney DG, Unger JM, Miller TP. New treatment options have changed the survival of patients with follicular lymphoma. J Clin Oncol. 2005;23(33):8447–52.
17. Liu Q, Fayad L, Cabanillas F, et al. Improvement of overall and failure-free survival in stage IV follicular lymphoma: 25 years of treatment experience at The University of Texas M.D. Anderson Cancer Center. J Clin Oncol. 2006;24(10):1582–9.
18. Khouri IF, McLaughlin P, Saliba RM, et al. Eight-year experience with allogeneic stem cell transplantation for relapsed follicular lymphoma after nonmyeloablative conditioning with fludarabine, cyclophosphamide, and rituximab. Blood. 2008;111(12):5530–6.
19. Marcus R, Imrie K, Belch A, et al. CVP chemotherapy plus rituximab compared with CVP as first-line treatment for advanced follicular lymphoma. Blood. 2005;105(4):1417–23.
20. Hiddemann W, Kneba M, Dreyling M, et al. Frontline therapy with rituximab added to the combination of cyclophosphamide, doxorubicin, vincristine, and prednisone (CHOP) significantly improves the outcome for patients with advanced-stage follicular lymphoma compared with therapy with CHOP alone: results of a prospective randomized study of the German Low-Grade Lymphoma Study Group. Blood. 2005;106(12):3725–32.

Chapter 23
Non-Hodgkin Aggressive B-Cell Lymphoma

M. Alma Rodriguez

Introduction

Advances in biology during the twentieth century have led us to a better understanding of the nature of lymphomas. We now recognize that what was called "lymphosarcoma" 100 years ago is not a sarcoma, but a complex group of malignancies of lymphoid cells that arise at various stages of cell differentiation. Our immune system includes lymphoid cells and the lymphatic network. Lymphomas thus are cancers of our immune system that arise as a result of unique genetic events that lead to various subtypes of lymphomas that can manifest with very different clinical behaviors and outcomes.

Historically, the lymphomas have been stratified into two broad categories: non-Hodgkin lymphomas (NHLs) and Hodgkin lymphomas (HLs). The NHLs were differentiated from HLs at the turn of the twentieth century with recognition of the unique cells (Reed–Sternberg cells) that characterize the latter. Over the past few decades, medical advances and research have led to enhanced diagnostic capabilities and treatments for patients with NHLs, as well as antitumor drug therapies and combination chemotherapies that have been responsible for significant and steady improvements in survival for these patients. In this chapter, we will review the salient clinical innovations made at MD Anderson Cancer Center that contributed to these advances.

M.A. Rodriguez (✉)
Department of Lymphoma and Myeloma, The University of Texas MD Anderson Cancer Center, 1515 Holcombe Blvd, Unit 1485, Houston, TX 77030, USA
e-mail: marodriguez@mdanderson.org

M.A. Rodriguez et al. (eds.), *60 Years of Survival Outcomes at The University of Texas MD Anderson Cancer Center*, DOI 10.1007/978-1-4614-5197-6_23,

Epidemiology and Patient Demographics

Lymphomas are cancers that present most commonly in adults. There is a moderate predominance of males over females in the incidence of NHL, about 1.5:1 in most studies, which has persisted for many years. In the USA, there is a higher incidence among Caucasians than among other racial subgroups. The overall incidence of NHL is increasing steadily, although the underlying cause for this trend is not clear. Significant increases in incidence occurred between 1970 and 1995, some of which may have been attributable to the emergence of HIV/AIDS-related lymphomas. These increases in NHL incidence have abated since the late 1990s, yet the overall lymphoma incidence continues to climb. Thus, NHL remains a significant and growing cause of morbidity and mortality. The American Cancer Society estimated that 65,540 new cases of NHL would be diagnosed in 2010 and that 20,210 people would die of this disease [1]. About 55–60% of NHL cases are categorized as "aggressive" lymphomas, and 85–90% of these are of B-cell origin [2].

Advances in Diagnosis and Classification of Lymphomas

Knowledge about the histology, genetics, and behavior of NHL variants has arisen in the past few decades, as have attempts to classify them. Both of these facts make analysis and discussion of NHL necessarily complex. Once thought to be a single disease, we now know that NHL is a heterogeneous group of malignancies with multiple known subtypes. Although the World Health Organization (WHO) classification system currently recognizes more than 30 distinct subtypes of NHL [3], attempts to classify the subtypes of this disease have been ongoing since the 1940s. In the 1950s and 1960s, Rappaport and Rye categorized the few known subtypes pathologically by cell morphology and lymph node histology. The classification systems of the 1970s recognized new variants, which correlated with a new understanding of the immune system and recognition of cell origins (Lukes and Collins classification). In the 1980s, a classification system was developed that attempted to acknowledge patterns with clinical, rather than just pathologic, relevance. Three broad categories emerged from this system: low-, intermediate-, and high-grade disease. These became the backbone of the 1982 International Working Formulation (IWF), an NCI initiative that attempted to synthesize classifications from various systems [4].

Since the advent of the IWF, there have been more refinements in how we view lymphomas, due in large measure to a growing knowledge of the complexity of the lymphatic system and of the ways in which cell lineages within B and T cells interact to maintain immunity. Furthermore, it became evident that unique molecular and genetic events correlate with categories of lymphoma. These newly appreciated complexities led to increasingly sophisticated (and complex) classifications, most notably the REAL and WHO classification systems, which acknowledged

Table 23.1 Ann Arbor staging system

Stage	Definition
I	Involvement of a single lymph node region or a single extranodal organ or site
II	Involvement of two or more lymph node regions on the same side of the diaphragm, or localized involvement of an extranodal organ or site and one or more lymph node regions on the same side of the diaphragm
III	Involvement of lymph node regions on both sides of the diaphragm with or without localized involvement of an extranodal organ or site or spleen or both
IV	Diffuse or disseminated involvement of one or more distant extranodal organs with or without involvement of lymph nodes

Definition of B symptoms: Fever >38 °C, drenching night sweats, and/or weight loss >10% of body weight in the preceding 6 months

immunophenotypic, genetic, molecular, and some clinical characteristics [3, 5]. Dr. Sattva Neelapu summarizes the classification systems in Tables 22.1 and 22.2 of Chap. 22, "Non-Hodgkin Indolent B-Cell Lymphoma."

"Aggressive" NHL Defined

Clinically, a useful way to look at NHL includes its natural history:

- *Indolent:* Indolent lymphomas are slow-growing and are usually not imminently life-threatening; their clinical course may be stable and not require immediate treatment. Paradoxically, these are less amenable to cure than are more aggressive variants. The indolent lymphomas are discussed by Dr. Sattva Neelapu in Chap. 22.
- *Aggressive:* Aggressive lymphomas require treatment within a short period after presentation; if the illness is not treated, the clinical course will progress and will be fatal. A significant proportion of NHL cases can be cured, but survival outcome can be influenced by a number of critical biological and clinical factors [2]. The first clinical characteristic known to be of significance was the stage of the disease [6] (Table 23.1). A later model of risk, called the International Prognostic Index, included the lymphoma stage and added four other factors: age; whether multiple extranodal sites of involvement are present; the overall performance status of the individual; and the lactic dehydrogenase serum level [7] (Table 23.2).

MD Anderson Cancer Center Experience

Because of the evolving nature of classification in lymphoma diagnostic categories across a span of 60 years, it is difficult to absolutely stratify identical categories as aggressive. However, we mapped the historically described correlation of clinical behavior to categories of lymphomas in each of the major periods of pathologic

Table 23.2 Survival % at 5 years by International Prognostic Index (IPI) score

Each of the following risk factors constitutes 1 IPI score point	
Age	>60 years
Serum LDH	> Upper normal limit
Performance status	≥2 (by ECOG criteria)
Extranodal disease	>1 site
Ann Arbor stage	III or IV
Survival % at 5 years by IPI score	
IPI score	5-year survival (%)
0–1	73
2	51
3	43
4–5	26

ECOG Eastern Cooperative Oncology Group, *LDH* lactic dehydrogenase

classification. Thus, we included the large cell histologies from the older classification systems. From the IWF, we included all of the subtypes in the intermediate- and high-grade categories, but excluded lymphoblastic lymphoma. From the REAL and WHO classification systems, we included the mantle cell subtypes, all large B-cell subtypes, follicular lymphoma grade 3B, Burkitt-like lymphomas, and high-grade B-cell lymphomas otherwise not classified. Because the most common subtype of aggressive lymphoma (diffuse large cell) is predominantly of B-cell origin and the next most common subtype (mantle cell) is always of B-cell origin, we described our analysis as most relevant to aggressive B-cell disorders. However, we acknowledge that before 1980 there was no consistent classification that addressed the immunohistologic identity of the T-cell or NK-cell lymphomas. Retrospectively, however, we know that the percentage of lymphomas that are not of B-cell origin constitute at most 15% of the total and so were included among the other lymphomas in the decades before standardized immunohistology.

Our data set was derived from a population of 10,003 patients who presented with the above-noted histologies at our institution between 1944 and 2004 (Table 23.3). Adding to the complexity of any analysis of NHL outcome is the fact that a certain percentage of patients present with a history of prior malignancy. For this discussion, we excluded patients who had received previous treatment, those treated elsewhere, and those who had additional primary cancers, resulting in 3,271 patients who were treated at MD Anderson for these lymphomas. Of these, most had diffuse large cell lymphoma (73%), followed by mantle cell lymphoma (13%) (consisting of the histology categories of mantle cell + diffuse small and intermediate cleaved cell), follicular large cell (6%) and high-grade lymphomas (high-grade B-cell lymphomas + diffuse small non-cleaved cell (6%), and other histologies (2%) (Table 23.4).

Table 23.3 Patients with aggressive non-Hodgkin lymphoma presenting at MD Anderson Cancer Center between 1944 and 2004

Patient characteristics	No. of patients
Total number	10,003
No previous treatment	5,151
Definitive MD Anderson treatment	3,969
No other primaries except superficial skin cancers	3,271

Table 23.4 Aggressive lymphoma histologies in Tumor Registry, 1944–2004

Histologies	Number (%)
Diffuse large cell	2,380 (73)
Follicular large cell/follicular grade 3b	194 (6)
Mantle cell/diffuse small and intermediate cleaved cell	425 (13)
High-grade B-cell/diffuse small non-cleaved cell	190 (6)
Diffuse mixed cell lymphoma/other histologies	82 (2)
Total	*3,271 (100)*

Survival Trends of Patients with Aggressive Lymphomas

The increase in overall survival for patients with aggressive lymphomas is notable not only for its continuous positive trend over the 60-year time frame (Fig. 23.1), but also for the dramatic survival improvements seen during certain time frames, in particular between 1965 and 1985 and again between 1995 and 2004 (Table 23.5). The overall trend can be attributed to the continuous advances and refinements in the use of chemotherapy and the development of new therapeutic agents. The more dramatic jumps can be attributed to a number of significant breakthroughs and milestones, including the advent of combination chemotherapies, bone marrow stem cell transplantation, second-line combinations for salvage in relapsed disease, and specific cell surface antigens that have led to targeted treatments. The application and innovation of these advances at MD Anderson Cancer Center are discussed in the following sections.

Advances in Frontline Chemotherapy

Combination Chemotherapy

The idea of using a chemotherapeutic approach in the treatment of cancers has a long history. William Osler's 1894 *Textbook of Medicine* referred to Fowler's Solution (an arsenic compound) for the treatment of lymphosarcomas. But it was not until after World War II that research gave us nitrogen mustard, a compound that

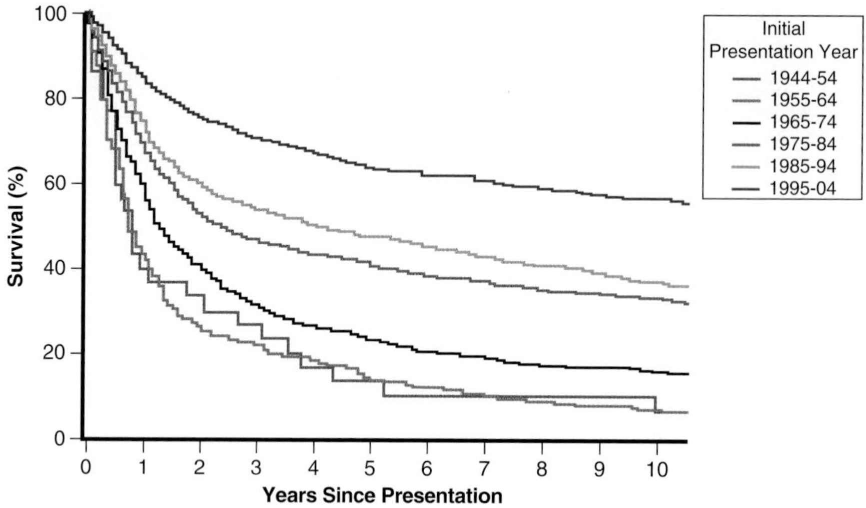

Fig. 23.1 Overall survival rates for patients with non-Hodgkin aggressive B-cell lymphoma who were treated at MD Anderson between 1944 and 2004 ($P<0.0001$, log-rank test for trend). The salient developments that influenced survival outcomes of aggressive lymphomas were as follows: 1960s–1970s: Introduction of doxorubicin, etoposide, and other novel chemotherapy agents into frontline combination regimens for advanced-stage disease, and combined-modality therapy (chemoradiation) for early-stage disease. 1980s: Development of second-line salvage regimens for recurrent disease, introduction of autologous stem cell transplants, and biologic identification of subtypes of lymphomas. 1990s: Hematopoietic growth factor support agents that allowed more intense dose chemotherapy in frontline treatment as well as autologous stem cell transplantation as consolidation for salvage treatments. Late 1990s–2000: Rituximab, a targeted immunotherapeutic agent against B cells, was combined with chemotherapy.

Table 23.5 Percent survival by decade

Decade	Percent survival	
	5 years	10 years
1944–1954	13.3	6.7
1955–1964	13.9	6.7
1965–1974	23.4	16.2
1975–1984	41.0	33.0
1985–1994	47.9	37.0
1995–2004	63.8	57.5

was proven effective in Hodgkin lymphoma. Other effective agents soon followed, including other alkylating agents and vinca alkaloids, antitumor antibiotics such as doxorubicin, epipodophyllotoxins such as etoposide, and multiple regimens for combination therapies. Thus, cancer chemotherapy was established in the latter part of the twentieth century, and the specialty of medical oncology was born.

The first chemotherapy combination to prove effective in treating aggressive lymphomas was CHOP (cyclophosphamide, 750 mg/m^2 intravenously [IV] on day 1; hydroxydaunomycin [doxorubicin], 50 mg/m^2 IV on day 1; vincristine [Oncovin], 1.4 mg/m^2 IV on day 1, not to exceed 2 mg total; and prednisone, 100 mg by mouth daily on days 1–5). Clinical studies by Jeffrey A. Gottlieb at MD Anderson and his colleagues were a significant milestone in the introduction of the then novel drug doxorubicin in the treatment of aggressive lymphomas [8, 9]. The initial phase II protocol of the CHOP regimen designed by Dr. Gottlieb resulted in complete remissions of large cell lymphomas, even in advanced Ann Arbor stage III–IV disease (Table 23.1). From that point forward, the design of all future frontline regimens for aggressive lymphomas included doxorubicin. A subsequent trial by the Southwest Oncology Group (SWOG) confirmed a significant long-term survival benefit for this regimen in the treatment of advanced-stage large cell lymphomas. Thus, the CHOP regimen became the international gold standard in the frontline treatment of large cell lymphomas and has remained so until the early part of the present century, despite the interim development of numerous other regimens, none of which proved superior to CHOP in randomized trials [10].

Synergy of Immunotherapy and Chemotherapy

The next major advance in the frontline treatment of large cell lymphoma did not arrive until more than 20 years after the design of CHOP and was due to more specific knowledge of the biologic characteristics of B-cell lymphomas. The recognition of unique cell surface complex molecules on B cells, such as the CD-20 antigen, led to the development of agents that could specifically target those molecular antigens with the intent of activating the body's own immune response against the lymphoma. The most notable agent in this category of treatments has been rituximab, a monoclonal antibody that targets the CD-20 B-cell surface antigen complex. It was initially tested in indolent NHL, in a large clinical multi-institutional phase II trial led by Peter McLaughlin, a colleague at our institution. This trial led to FDA approval of this immunotherapeutic agent in 1997 for use in indolent relapsed B-cell lymphomas, but it was promptly integrated into therapy for aggressive B-cell lymphomas in multiple trials. A randomized trial was conducted in Europe by the French cooperative GELA group, in which the addition of rituximab to CHOP (RCHOP) was compared with CHOP. The results demonstrated a statistically superior response and overall survival for the patients with large B-cell lymphoma who were treated with RCHOP compared with those who received CHOP [11]. These results were evident across low- and high-risk International Prognostic Index categories (Table 23.2) and have been confirmed by other trials. Thus, RCHOP has become the new international standard for the treatment of large B-cell lymphomas.

Radiation Therapy and Its Role in Large Cell Lymphoma

Before the development of effective chemotherapy regimens, early-stage (localized) aggressive NHL (stages I and II) was historically treated with radiation therapy (RT) alone. Although many studies were undertaken to improve on results by adjusting radiation dosages and field coverage, it was the addition of combination chemotherapy to RT regimens that improved outcome most dramatically. CHOP was integrated with RT in collaborative trials at MD Anderson for limited-stage large cell lymphoma, with favorable and sustained long-term remissions [12].

To date, four randomized trials have been conducted in early-stage aggressive NHL, all before anti-CD-20 rituximab therapy was incorporated into CHOP chemotherapy. The most well known in the USA is the SWOG study in which eight cycles of CHOP were compared with three cycles of CHOP followed by involved-field RT (40–55 Gy) in limited-stage (I/II) diffuse large B-cell lymphoma. The combined-modality arm, versus the CHOP-only arm, achieved superior overall survival [13]. Thus, combined-modality therapy (chemotherapy plus radiation) remains the standard approach for localized-stage large cell lymphoma. A retrospective case-controlled analysis conducted in patients treated with RCHOP plus RT at our institution, compared with control patients who received RCHOP but not RT, suggested that RT combined with RCHOP is beneficial [14]. However, randomized trials comparing RCHOP with and without RT should be conducted to address the two most pressing unresolved issues—the benefit of RT when patients are in complete remission after RCHOP chemotherapy, and the optimal number of chemotherapy cycles when RCHOP is combined with RT.

Intensified-Dose Chemotherapy

Another significant development in the treatment of aggressive lymphomas at MD Anderson Cancer Center was seen when intensified-dose chemotherapy regimens were used to treat adult lymphomas. The increased sophistication of pathologic diagnoses that included immunohistochemical analyses, as well as cytogenetic and molecular genetic studies, led to the recognition of a new entity called mantle cell lymphoma in the 1980s. Mantle cell lymphoma is aggressive, and survival rates have been poor with CHOP treatment. An intense-dose combination regimen known as HyperCVAD had been developed by Sharon Murphy and her colleagues at another institution to treat childhood lymphoblastic leukemias. Hagop Kantarjian and colleagues at our institution pioneered the application of the HyperCVAD regimen to treat adult lymphoblastic and Burkitt lymphomas, with results in adults as favorable as those in children [15]. Using the same HyperCVAD regimen as front-line treatment, followed by consolidation with autologous stem cell transplantation, Issa Khouri, Jorge Romaguera, and their colleagues at our institution demonstrated long-term survival benefits in young patients with mantle cell lymphomas who received this intensive treatment approach [16].

With the reported benefit of combining rituximab with CHOP in large cell lymphomas, the HyperCVAD regimen for mantle cell lymphoma was similarly combined with rituximab (RHCVAD), showing similar synergy of chemotherapy and immunotherapy as that observed in large cell lymphoma. The treatment of mantle cell lymphoma continues to evolve today, with the development and approval of a new class of targeted drugs, the proteosome inhibitors, to treat this disease. The most well studied of the drugs in this class is bortezomib, which in combination with RHCVAD is currently being evaluated in frontline trials.

Advances in Salvage Treatment

Alternative Combinations After CHOP

A series of lymphoma trials in the 1980s and 1990s at MD Anderson Cancer Center, led by Fernando Cabanillas, William Velasquez, and colleagues, confirmed that using different categories of drugs in second-line therapy after CHOP could lead to response and salvage in recurrent large cell lymphoma. The concept behind these trials was that although the malignant cells might have become resistant to the chemotherapy drugs in the frontline regimen, second-line exposure to drugs of different classes could lead to non-cross-resistant tumor response. Before the development of salvage regimens, a recurrence of large cell lymphoma or a refractory (not responsive) case of large cell lymphoma treated with CHOP meant certain death. Today, there are a number of salvage (second-line) regimens in use that were derived from the seminal work of these pioneers, including cytarabine and cisplatinum combinations (DHAP, ESHAP, and ASHAP) and ifosfamide and etoposide combinations (IE, MINE, and MIME) [17, 18]. These trials were very critical to the further development of the present-day treatment strategies for recurrent/refractory disease (such as the regimen ICE).

Autologous Stem Cell Transplant Consolidation

In the 1980s, another critical new treatment concept was born with the introduction of autologous stem cell transplantation to overcome the limitations of high-dose chemotherapy. The use of autologous stem cell transplants in lymphomas was introduced at MD Anderson by Karel Dicke and Gary Spitzer. Phase II studies showed that this method (high-dose chemotherapy consolidation with stem cell rescue post-salvage treatment for relapse) could lead to durable remissions and survival in patients with relapsed large cell lymphoma [19]. These seminal phase II studies were followed by a large international collaborative randomized trial, the PARMA study. The results of this trial demonstrated that patients with large cell lymphoma who responded to second-line chemotherapy had improved survival when this response was consolidated with autologous stem cell transplantation [20]. Thus, autologous stem cell transplant consolidation after response to second-line salvage became the standard of care for aggressive lymphomas.

Advances in Supportive Care

Improvements in supportive care have contributed in a significant way to cancer therapy outcomes by reducing the adverse effects of treatment. The supportive management of neutropenia with hematopoietic growth factors to stimulate recovery of neutrophils is critical to the treatment of lymphomas, in particular for patients receiving more intense chemotherapy regimens as well as salvage regimens and stem cell transplants. These agents decrease early mortality due to infections in patients undergoing chemotherapy [21]. Also important is the consultative expertise of infectious disease specialists who focus on cancer-related infectious complications and the appropriate antibiotic management for febrile neutropenia, since infections are the most significant life-threatening complication for patients undergoing autologous stem cell transplantation and receiving intensified-dose chemotherapy regimens. The patients' quality of life is significantly affected as well by appropriate medical management of pain, nausea, and fatigue. Multidisciplinary care, along with specialized nursing care and access to other allied health professionals who specialize in the care of cancer patients, is in no small part responsible for improved outcomes for patients receiving care in comprehensive cancer centers and is particularly important when patients are undergoing intensive therapies.

Future Directions

Continued improvements—durable remissions and increased survival—for aggressive lymphomas are likely to come from building on the trends that have brought us thus far:

- Continued advances in understanding the molecular and genetic profiles of lymphomas
- Development of additional novel targeted therapies that potentiate or replace traditional chemotherapies and thereby reduce the toxicity of treatment
- Continued development of second-line therapies for refractory or relapsed disease

The challenge remains to refine our knowledge about the unique molecular mechanisms that distinguish the various subtypes of NHL and to develop targeted treatments that are more suited to the illness and better tolerated by patients. The latter would expand the number of patients eligible to receive definitive therapy and hopefully minimize downstream toxicities. The continued refinement in our knowledge of the biologic and molecular genetic nature of NHL is also the key, we hope, to one day being able to prevent them.

References

1. Jemal A, Siegel R, Xu J, et al. Cancer Statistics, 2010. CA Cancer J Clin. 2010;60:277–300.
2. Armitage J, Weisenberger D. New approach to classifying non-Hodgkin's lymphoma: clinical features of the major histologic subtypes. J Clin Oncol. 1998;16:2780–95.
3. Jaffe ES, Harris NL, Stein H, et al. World Health Organization classification of tumours. Pathology and genetics of tumours of haematopoietic and lymphoid tissues. Lyon: IARC Press; 2001. p. 121–253.
4. The Non-Hodgkin's Lymphoma Pathologic Classification Project. National Cancer Institute sponsored study of classifications of non-Hodgkin's lymphomas: summary and description of a working formulation for clinical usage. Cancer. 1982;49:2112–35.
5. The Non-Hodgkin's Lymphoma Classification Project: A clinical evaluation of the International Lymphoma Study Group classification of non-Hodgkin's lymphoma. Blood. 1997;89: 3909–18.
6. Carbone PP, Kaplan HS, Musshoff K, et al. Report on the Committee on Hodgkin's Disease Staging Classification. Cancer Res. 1971;31:1860–1.
7. A predictive model for aggressive non-Hodgkin's lymphoma. The International Non-Hodgkin's Lymphoma Prognostic Factors Project. N Engl J Med. 1993;329:987–94.
8. Gottlieb JA, Gutterman JU, McCredie KB, et al. Chemotherapy of malignant lymphoma with adriamycin. Cancer Res. 1973;33:3024–8.
9. McKelvey EM, Gottlieb JA, Wilson HE, et al. Hydroxyldaunomycin (Adriamycin) combination chemotherapy in malignant lymphoma. Cancer. 1976;38:1484–93.
10. Fisher RI, Gaynor ER, Dahlberg S, et al. Comparison of a standard regimen (CHOP) with three intensive chemotherapy regimens for advanced non-Hodgkin's lymphoma. N Engl J Med. 1993;328:1002–6.
11. Coiffier B, Lepage E, Briere J, et al. CHOP chemotherapy plus rituximab compared with CHOP alone in elderly patients with diffuse large B-cell lymphoma. N Engl J Med. 2002;346:235–42.
12. Velasquez WS, Fuller LM, Jagannath S, et al. Stages I and II diffuse large cell lymphomas: prognostic factors and long-term results with CHOP-Bleo and radiotherapy. Blood. 1991;77:942–7.
13. Miller TP, Dahlberg S, Cassady JR, et al. Chemotherapy alone compared with chemotherapy plus radiation for localized intermediate- and high-grade non-Hodgkin's lymphoma. N Engl J Med. 1998;339:21–6.
14. Phan J, Mazloom A, Medeiros LJ, et al. Benefit of consolidative radiation therapy in patients with diffuse large B-Cell lymphoma treated with R-CHOP chemotherapy. J Clin Oncol. 2010;27:3441–8.
15. Kantarjian H, O'Brien S, Smith TL, et al. Results of treatment with hyper-CVAD, a dose-intensive regimen, in adults with acute lymphocytic leukemia. J Clin Oncol. 2000;18:547–61.
16. Khouri IF, Romaguera JE, et al. Hyper-CVAD and high-dose methotrexate/cytarabine followed by stem-cell transplantation: an active regimen for aggressive mantle-cell lymphoma. J Clin Oncol. 1998;16:3803–9.

17. Velasquez WS, Cabanillas F, Salvador P, et al. Effective salvage therapy for lymphoma with cisplatin in combination with high-dose Ara-C and dexamethasone (DHAP). Blood. 1988;71:117–22.
18. Rodriguez MA, Cabanillas FC, Velasquez W, et al. Results of a salvage treatment program for relapsing lymphoma: MINE consolidated with ESHAP. J Clin Oncol. 1995;13:1734–41.
19. Armitage JO, Jagannath S, Spitzer G, et al. High dose therapy and autologous marrow transplantation as salvage treatment for patients with diffuse large cell lymphoma. Eur J Cancer Clin Oncol. 1986;22:871–7.
20. Philip T, Guglielmi C, Hagenbeek A, et al. Autologous bone marrow transplantation as compared with salvage chemotherapy in relapses of chemotherapy-sensitive non-Hodgkin's lymphoma. N Engl J Med. 1995;333:1540–5.
21. Kuderer NM, Dale DC, Crawford J, Lyman GH. Impact of primary prophylaxis with granulocyte colony stimulating factor on febrile neutropenia and mortality in adult cancer patients receiving chemotherapy: a systematic review. J Clin Oncol. 2007;25:3158–67.

Chapter 24
Multiple Myeloma

Donna Weber and Raymond Alexanian

Introduction

Multiple myeloma is diagnosed in approximately 20,500 people in the USA annually [1] and its incidence has been rising. The frequency is approximately twice as high in blacks as in whites and higher in men than in women. The disease develops as a malignant proliferation of plasma cells that usually results in the production of a monoclonal protein in the serum and/or urine. Although the disease is systemic at diagnosis and must be differentiated from its less advanced counterparts (e.g., monoclonal gammopathy of unknown significance and solitary plasmacytoma of bone), approximately 20% of patients with multiple myeloma are asymptomatic at diagnosis. For these patients with no evidence of symptomatic disease at diagnosis, there has been no clearly demonstrated survival advantage for early treatment, justifying the delay of therapy until progression to symptomatic disease. Survival in this group of patients is usually longer than in their counterparts considered symptomatic at diagnosis. For symptomatic patients, the presence of more advanced stage has been predictive of shorter survival, and the presence of certain chromosomal abnormalities (i.e., deletion of chromosome 13 or 17p, chromosome 1 abnormalities, and IgH translocations involving chromosome 4, 16, or 20) has indicated a more aggressive course and shorter survival [2].

D. Weber (✉) • R. Alexanian
Department of Lymphoma and Myeloma, The University of Texas MD Anderson Cancer Center, 1515 Holcombe Blvd, Box 429, Houston, TX 77030, USA
e-mail: dmweber@mdanderson.org; ralexani@mdanderson.org

M.A. Rodriguez et al. (eds.), *60 Years of Survival Outcomes at The University of Texas MD Anderson Cancer Center*, DOI 10.1007/978-1-4614-5197-6_24,

Historical Perspective

Although radiotherapy or surgery can by curative in approximately 35–65% of patients who present with solitary plasmacytoma (bone or extramedullary, respectively), multiple myeloma is a systemic malignancy at diagnosis, making chemotherapy the mainstay of treatment for symptomatic patients. In 1947, the use of urethane provided the first documented response to treatment and became the standard of care for this disorder for nearly two decades until a randomized trial showed no benefit for this agent [3, 4]. Subsequently, in the late 1950s and early 1960s, the alkylating agent L-phenylalanine mustard (melphalan) was reported to be active in 50% of a small number of patients by Blokhin et al. [5] and then in a larger group of patients in a Southwest Oncology Group (SWOG) trial led by Bergsagel et al. [6] at this center. Although many alkylating agent combinations have been introduced, none have proved superior to melphalan and prednisone (MP), making this regimen the standard of care for the next several decades [7].

Although the introduction of vincristine, doxorubicin (Adriamycin), and dexamethasone (VAD) by Barlogie, Smith, and Alexanian [8] from this center in 1984 provided an effective salvage regimen that improved survival in myeloma, there was no clear advantage to using this regimen for induction compared with MP. In addition, although partial remissions (PRs) in the 1980s were achievable in more than half of myeloma patients, complete remissions (CRs) were seen in less than 10% of patients; cure appeared unattainable. In an attempt to prevent drug resistance, McElwain et al. [9] successfully introduced the concept of myeloablative therapy and autologous stem cell transplantation for myeloma in the 1980s, after which more than 50% of a small number of patients achieved CR. With continued improvements in induction regimens, supportive care, and conditioning regimens, this therapy improved quality of life and subsequent survival compared with continued standard chemotherapy [10, 11]. Despite these improvements, it became apparent that some patients, particularly those with deletion of chromosome 13, had a more aggressive course with shortened survival.

The introduction of thalidomide to therapy in 1998 began a new era of therapeutic advances for myeloma. Although this agent would not be FDA-approved until 2006, when it was combined with dexamethasone, it provided the impetus for investigations of multiple targets within the plasma cell and marrow microenvironment [12, 13]. Subsequently, the proteasome inhibitor, bortezomib, was introduced and is now approved for use alone or in combination with pegylated liposomal doxorubicin in relapsing and/or refractory myeloma, and with MP for previously untreated myeloma [14–16]. In an effort to reduce troublesome adverse effects, such as neuropathy and thromboses, lenalidomide was developed and demonstrated a different efficacy and adverse effect profile from the parent drug, thalidomide, particularly when combined with dexamethasone, resulting in FDA approval in 2006 [17, 18]. The introduction of these agents alone or in combination with other novel or conventional agents, together with intensive therapy supported by autologous stem cells, has extended the median survival rate for patients with myeloma.

The MD Anderson Cancer Center Experience

The MD Anderson myeloma data set includes 4,426 patients who were seen during the 60-year period between 1944 and 2004. Among those considered were 1,983 patients with symptomatic disease who had not previously received treatment for myeloma; the data set was then limited to 1,202 patients who did not have multiple primary cancers, with the exception of superficial skin cancers, and those who received primary treatment at MD Anderson. The number of patients seen by decade is summarized in Table 24.1. Staging for myeloma changed in the past decade; although the previous Dune-Salmon staging system was more dependent on levels of monoclonal protein, calcium, hemoglobin, and creatinine as well as the number of lytic bone lesions, the new International Staging System (ISS) reflects the power of beta-2-microglobulin and albumin as determinants of tumor burden [19]. Perhaps more importantly, during the past several decades, the impact of poor-risk cytogenetics, such as deletions of chromosome 13 or 17p, chromosome 1 abnormalities, and IgH translocations involving chromosome 4, 16, or 20, has predicted a more aggressive course and shorter survival for patients with myeloma [2]. In addition, although staging was used to determine treatment decisions at various times during the 60-year period, at other times it did not affect treatment choices. Due to the lack of uniformity in staging and prognostic factors in the determination of treatment since 1944, it was decided not to report results of the tumor registry based on these factors, but rather to present the results as a whole, as depicted in Table 24.1.

The survival curves (Fig. 24.1) and data (Table 24.2; Fig. 24.2) reflect improvements in 5- and 10-year survival, particularly during the 1955–1964, 1975–1984, and 1995–2004 time periods. Although superior outcomes could be attributed to earlier diagnosis and improved supportive care, particular improvements during these periods were more likely due to therapeutic trials with novel agents, available at our center, often resulting in changes in the standard of care.

The 5-year survival rates nearly doubled during each of these decades, demonstrating the impact of MP during the early 1960s, VAD and myeloablative therapy with autologous stem cell transplantation during the early 1980s and 1990s, and the novel agents thalidomide, bortezomib, and lenalidomide during the most recent

Table 24.1 Previously untreated patients with multiple myeloma treated at MD Anderson, 1944–2004

Years	No. of patients	Percent	Cumulative percent
1944–1954	16	1.3	1.3
1955–1964	95	7.9	9.2
1965–1974	245	20.4	29.6
1975–1984	236	19.6	49.3
1985–1994	284	23.6	72.9
1995–2004	326	27.1	100.0
Total	*1,202*	*100.0*	

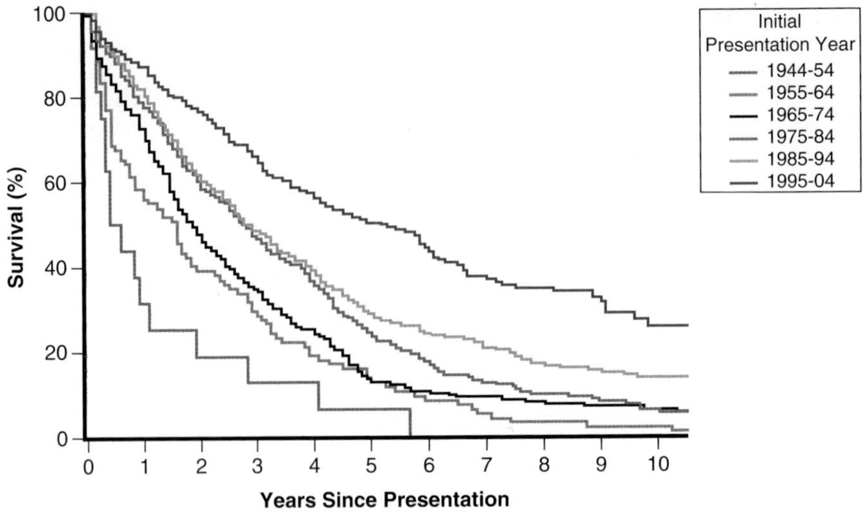

Fig. 24.1 Overall survival rates for patients with multiple myeloma (1944–2004) ($P<0.0001$, log-rank test for trend).

Table 24.2 Kaplan–Meier 5- and 10- year survival (%) for myeloma patients

	Percent survival	
Years	5 years	10 years
1944–1954	6.3	0
1955–1964	12.6	2.1
1965–1974	12.7	6.5
1975–1984	23.7	5.9
1985–1994	28.5	14.2
1995–2004	50.4	25.4

decade. These changes probably began even earlier than reflected in the survival curves since this center led or participated in many of the definitive trials leading to changes in standard therapy, by providing our patients with early access to new and effective drugs, and drug combinations, for this disease. Both bortezomib and lenalidomide-dexamethasone have improved response rates, progression-free survival, and overall survival in patients with relapsed and/or refractory disease in phase III trials that were led by or included strong participation from our center. The 10-year survival rate nearly doubled between 1985 and 1994 (14%) compared with previous decades, when it was less than 7%, and nearly doubled again between 1995 and 2004 (25%). The introduction of and refinements in myeloablative therapy with stem cell support, and the addition of agents with novel mechanisms of action to available treatments, explain these major improvements in survival.

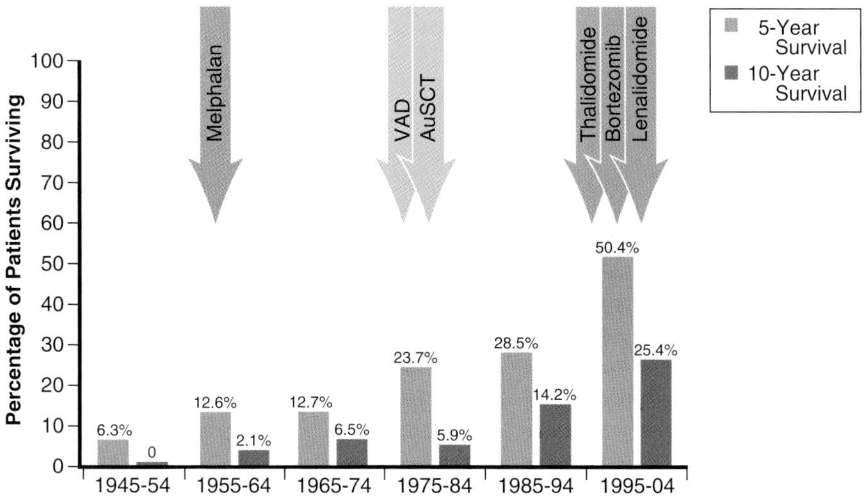

Fig. 24.2 Impact of the introduction of new therapies on 5- and 10-year overall survival of patients with newly diagnosed multiple myeloma treated at MD Anderson Cancer Center. *AuSCT* autologous stem cell transplantation, *VAD* vincristine, doxorubicin (Adriamycin), and dexamethasone.

The most marked changes in overall survival occurred between 1995 and 2004 and may be attributed to the availability of superior regimens; these regimens produced more frequent and marked responses as evidenced by CR rates increasing from approximately 5–10% with regimens such as MP or VAD to as high as 40–50% with more recent regimens. These improved survival rates may also reflect the development of more sensitive tests such as the free light chain assay to define CR and guide treatment decisions, such as the initiation of maintenance therapy. Treatment with bortezomib, and perhaps lenalidomide, also appears to overcome the poor prognostic significance of chromosomal abnormalities such as deletion of chromosome 13 or t(4;14), providing survival benefits for the first time for many patients with high-risk disease. With these improvements in treatment, long-term stability of CR is now possible, raising the question of cure in a small fraction of patients [16, 20, 21].

Current Management Approach

Our current approach to treatment incorporates a novel agent-based induction regimen until at least PR is achieved. This is followed by early intensive therapy (usually with melphalan) with autologous stem cell support in eligible patients. Eligibility for transplantation at our center is not based on a certain age cutoff, but rather on adequate cardiopulmonary and performance status and lack of significant comorbidity.

For patients who do not achieve very good partial remission or better, maintenance therapy should be considered. The optimum number of courses of primary therapy is not clear. Although 3- and 4-drug regimens may provide a greater depth of response, it remains unclear whether it is best to use more drugs for induction or reserve some agents for treatment at relapse. Bortezomib-based therapy, and in preliminary data, possibly lenalidomide-based therapy, may overcome the poor prognosis associated with the deletion of chromosome 13 or 1gH translocations, and bortezomib is included in our frontline approach for most patients. For patients with deletion of chromosome17p, investigational approaches may be best, since no therapy has demonstrated a significant survival benefit for these patients.

Stem cell collection should be considered early for all eligible patients, particularly for those who received lenalidomide-based therapy, which may impair collection. Cyclophosphamide-based chemomobilization therapy may be necessary for some patients who received prolonged therapy with lenalidomide before stem cell harvest. Radiotherapy is generally used sparingly for severe pain to preserve the availability of stem cells for harvesting. For patients with painful compression fractures, vertebroplasty or kyphoplasty usually provides pain relief and allows the preservation of stem cells.

Despite the many recent advances for treatment of multiple myeloma, the disease relapses in nearly all patients. Thus, novel approaches for therapy, including new drug development, and better methods for detection of residual disease remain important for future improvements in survival.

References

1. Jemal A, Siegel R, Ward E, Hao Y, Xu J, Thun MJ. Cancer statistics, 2009. CA Cancer J Clin. 2009;59:225–49.
2. Kapoor P, Rajkumar SV. Update on risk stratification and treatment of newly diagnosed myeloma. Int J Hematol 2011;94:310–320.
3. Alwall N. Urethane and stilbamidine in multiple myeloma: a report on two cases. Lancet. 1947;2:388–9.
4. Holland JR, Hosley H, Scharlau C, et al. A controlled trial of urethane treatment in multiple myeloma. Blood. 1966;27:328–42.
5. Blokhin N, Larionov L, Perevodchikova N, Chebotareva L, Merkulova N. Clinical experiences with sarcolysin in neoplastic diseases. Ann N Y Acad Sci. 1958;68:1128–32.
6. Bergsagel DE, Sprague CC, Austin C, Griffith KM. Evaluation of new chemotherapeutic agents in the treatment of multiple myeloma. IV. L-Phenylalanine mustard (NSC-8806). Cancer Chemother Rep. 1962;21:87–99.
7. Alexanian R, Haut A, Khan AU, et al. Treatment for multiple myeloma: combination chemotherapy with different melphalan dose regimens. JAMA. 1969;208:1680–5.
8. Barlogie B, Smith L, Alexanian R. Effective treatment of advanced multiple myeloma refractory to alkylating agents. N Engl J Med. 1984;310:1353–6.
9. McElwain TJ, Selby PJ, Gore ME, et al. High-dose chemotherapy and autologous bone marrow transplantation for myeloma. Eur J Haematol Suppl. 1989;51:152–6.
10. Attal M, Harousseau J-L, Stoppa A-M, et al. A prospective, randomized trial of autologous bone marrow transplantation and chemotherapy in multiple myeloma. N Engl J Med. 1996;335:91–7.

11. Fermand JP, Ravaud P, Chevret S, et al. High-dose therapy and autologous peripheral blood stem cell transplantation in multiple myeloma: up-front or rescue treatment? Results of a multicenter sequential randomized clinical trial. Blood. 1998;92:3131–6.
12. Singhal S, Mehta J, Desikan R, et al. Antitumor activity of thalidomide in refractory multiple myeloma. N Engl J Med. 1999;341:1565–71.
13. Weber D, Rankin K, Gavino M, et al. Thalidomide alone or with dexamethasone for previously untreated multiple myeloma. J Clin Oncol. 2003;21:16–19.
14. Richardson PG, Sonneveld P, Schuster MW, et al. Bortezomib or high-dose dexamethasone for relapsed multiple myeloma [see comment]. N Engl J Med. 2005;352:2487–98.
15. Orlowski RZ, Nagler A, Sonneveld P, et al. Randomized phase III study of pegylated liposomal doxorubicin plus bortezomib compared with bortezomib alone in relapsed or refractory multiple myeloma: combination therapy improves time to progression. J Clin Oncol. 2007;25:3892–901.
16. San Miguel JF, Schlag R, Khuageva NK, et al. Bortezomib plus melphalan and prednisone for initial treatment of multiple myeloma. N Engl J Med. 2008;359:906–17.
17. Weber DM, Chen C, Niesvizky R, et al. Lenalidomide plus dexamethasone for relapsed multiple myeloma in North America [see comment]. N Engl J Med. 2007;357:2133–42.
18. Dimopoulos M, Spencer A, Attal M, et al. Lenalidomide plus dexamethasone for relapsed or refractory multiple myeloma [see comment]. N Engl J Med. 2007;357:2123–32.
19. Greipp PR, Miguel JS, Durie BGM, et al. International staging system for multiple myeloma. J Clin Oncol. 2005;23:3412–20.
20. Reece D, Song KW, Fu T, et al. Influence of cytogenetics in patients with relapsed or refractory multiple myeloma treated with lenalidomide plus dexamethasone: adverse effect of deletion 17p13. Blood. 2009;114:522–5.
21. Alexanion R, Delasalle K, Wang M, Thomas S, Weber D. Curability of multiple myeloma. Bone Marrow Res. 2012 (Article 10916479).

Chapter 25
Head and Neck Cancer

Ehab Hanna, Bonnie Glisson, Kian Ang, and Randal Weber

Introduction

Head and neck cancer (HNC) is a devastating disease that affects some of the most basic daily functions such as breathing, speaking, and swallowing. Because of its visible nature, HNC is also associated with significant disfigurement. The combined effect of disability and disfigurement and the added toxicity of treatment greatly increase symptom burden and reduce physical, emotional, and social functioning. Since its inception, the Head and Neck Oncology Program at MD Anderson Cancer Center has pioneered multidisciplinary care with the main goal of improving survival and reducing suffering in patients with HNC. Over the past 60 years, significant advances have been made in the treatment and rehabilitation of patients with HNC, resulting in improved disease control, survival, and organ preservation. The purpose of this chapter is to highlight some of the advances in treatment and improvements in outcome of patients with HNC treated in the Head and Neck Multidisciplinary Care Center at MD Anderson.

E. Hanna (✉) • R. Weber
Department of Head and Neck Surgery, The University of Texas MD Anderson Cancer Center, 1515 Holcombe Blvd, Houston, TX 77025, USA
e-mail: EYHanna@mdanderson.org

B. Glisson
Department of Thoracic Head and Neck Oncology, The University of Texas MD Anderson Cancer Center, Houston, TX, USA

K. Ang
Department of Radiation Oncology, The University of Texas MD Anderson Cancer Center, Houston, TX, USA

M.A. Rodriguez et al. (eds.), *60 Years of Survival Outcomes at The University of Texas MD Anderson Cancer Center*, DOI 10.1007/978-1-4614-5197-6_25,

Epidemiology

Cancer of the head and neck is a broad term that comprises malignant tumors, mostly squamous cell carcinoma, originating from the upper aerodigestive tract, namely the lip and oral cavity, nasopharynx, oropharynx, hypopharynx, larynx and nasal cavity, and paranasal sinuses. HNC is the sixth most common cancer worldwide, with approximately 650,000 new cases diagnosed annually and 350,000 deaths each year. In the USA, HNC accounted for approximately 52,140 new cancer cases and 11,460 deaths in 2011 [1]. It is estimated that approximately $3.2 billion is spent in the USA each year on treatment of HNC [2].

Changes in Etiology and Patient Demographics

The Emerging Role of the Human Papilloma Virus

For many decades, the majority of patients presenting with HNC were in their fifth or sixth decade of life, had a long history of tobacco and alcohol use, were of lower socioeconomic class, and experienced substantial comorbidity. In the past decade, however, a "new" demographic profile emerged for patients with HNC: presentation at a younger age and with no prior history of tobacco use. The role of human papilloma virus (HPV) as an etiologic factor in HNC, particularly cancer of the oropharynx, is becoming more evident. The presence of high-risk HPV 16 or 18, or p16 overexpression, or both can usually be detected in tumors of patients with cancer of the oropharynx who have no prior smoking history. There is growing evidence that HPV infection of the oropharynx is sexually transmitted, that HPV-related cancers respond better to therapy, and that HPV-related cancers are associated with improved survival compared with tobacco-related cancers of the head and neck [3]. Another area of ongoing research in MD Anderson's Head and Neck Program is determining the feasibility of both therapy "de-intensification" in patients with HPV cancer to reduce toxicity and the escalation of treatment in patients with tobacco-related cancers to improve efficacy. In addition, the role of vaccination against HPV in HNC remains to be explored [4].

Survival Trends of Patients with HNC Treated at MD Anderson Cancer Center

Figures 25.1, 25.2, 25.3, and 25.4 demonstrate the gradual, although significant, improvements in survival outcome for patients with HNC in the major sites who were treated at MD Anderson over the past six decades. The study population

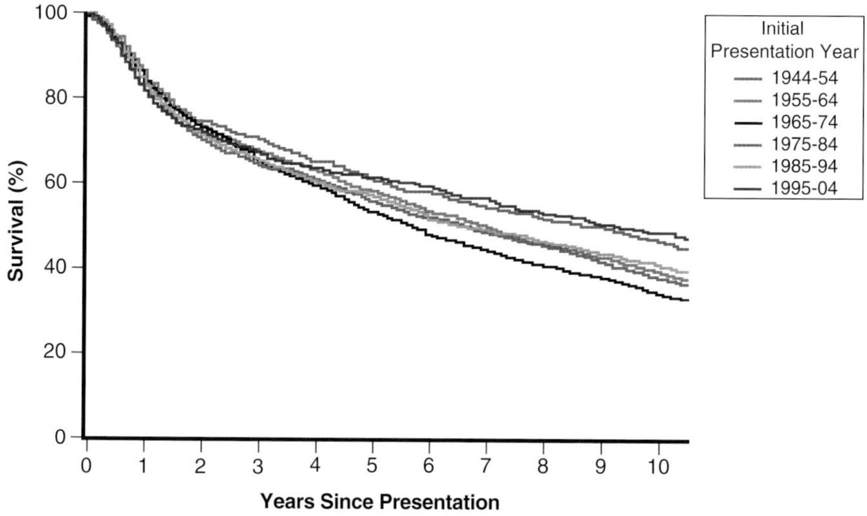

Fig. 25.1 Overall survival rates for patients with cancer of the head and neck with oral cavity primary sites (1944–2004) ($P = 0.014$, log-rank test for trend). See the appendix at the end of this chapter for graphs of local, regional, and distant stages at these primary sites (Figs. 25.8, 25.9, and 25.10).

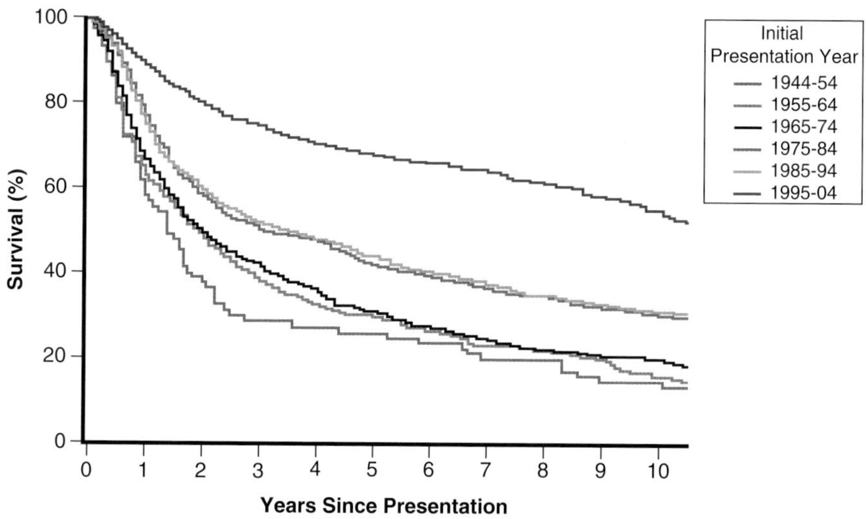

Fig. 25.2 Overall survival rates for patients with cancer of the head and neck with oropharyngeal primary sites (1944–2004) ($P < 0.0001$, log-rank test for trend). See the appendix at the end of this chapter for graphs of local, regional, and distant stages at these primary sites (Figs. 25.11, 25.12, and 25.13).

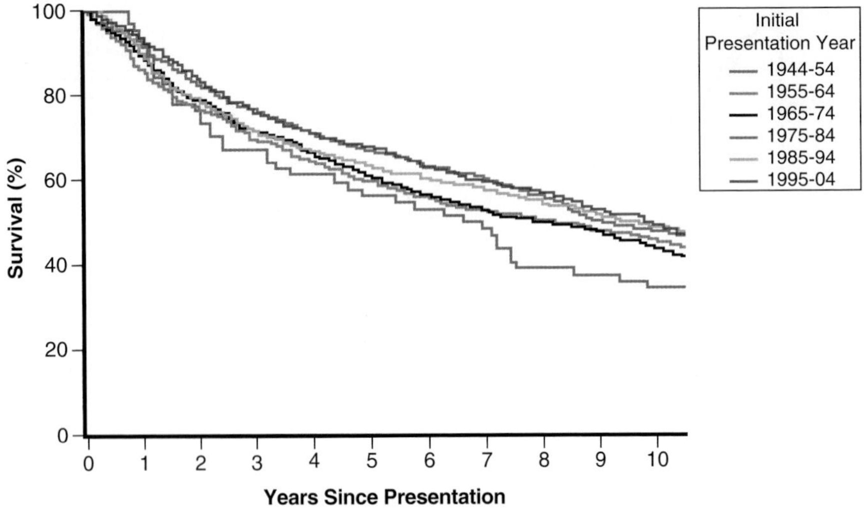

Fig. 25.3 Overall survival rates for patients with cancer of the head and neck with laryngeal primary sites (1944–2004) ($P=0.004$, log-rank test for trend). See the appendix at the end of this chapter for graphs of local, regional, and distant stages at these primary sites (Figs. 25.14, 25.15, and 25.16).

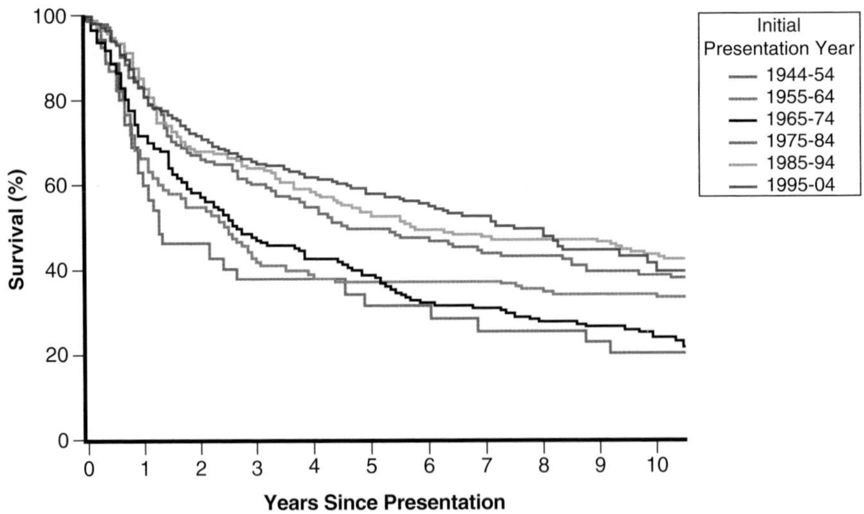

Fig. 25.4 Overall survival rates for patients with cancer of the head and neck with paranasal sinus and nasal cavity primary sites (1944–2004) ($P<0.0001$, log-rank test for trend). See the appendix at the end of this chapter for graphs of local, regional, and distant stages at these primary sites (Figs. 25.17, 25.18, and 25.19).

includes patients with previously untreated cancers of the oral cavity, oropharynx, larynx, and paranasal sinuses who received definitive treatment at MD Anderson from 1944 through 2004. Survival curves are shown for each of these sites by decade of initial presentation to MD Anderson.

Advances in Treatment and Rehabilitation of Patients with HNC at MD Anderson Cancer Center

During the past 60 years, significant improvements have been made in the treatment of HNC, and MD Anderson has led the way in designing and implementing key clinical and translational research that has contributed significantly to improvements in patient outcome. These advances shaped what is now being adopted as the standard of care in head and neck oncology. Key advances in surgery, radiotherapy, chemotherapy, targeted molecular therapy, rehabilitation, and outcome measurement are highlighted. Continued advances in the field of HNC treatment will focus on personalized cancer therapy that will be guided by the molecular profile of the patient's tumor.

Advances in Surgery

The goal of surgery is complete extirpation of cancer. In the 1940s, this meant radical and often mutilating surgery for patients with HNC. Radical neck dissections were routinely practiced and resulted in significant disability of the neck and shoulder. In 1972, Lindberg [5] published a landmark study that established the clinical rationale for selective neck dissection as an effective oncologic procedure that spared patients the morbidity of radical neck dissection. In this study, the records of 2,044 patients with HNC were reviewed at The University of Texas at Houston MD Anderson Hospital and Tumor Institute, the former name of our institution, to identify distribution patterns for cervical metastases clinically apparent at presentation. This study revealed that lymphatic spread of cancers from subsites within the head and neck follow predictable patterns to specific lymph node levels within the neck.

Building on this observation, head and neck surgeons at MD Anderson Cancer Center adopted the practice of less radical neck surgery, and in 1985, Dr. Byers reported the outcomes of 967 patients treated with modified and selective neck dissections. His landmark study demonstrated that for a primary tumor in the oral cavity or oropharynx, a supraomohyoid neck dissection was adequate treatment for the neck that was both clinically staged as N_0 or N_1 and pathologically staged as N_1 without evidence of extracapsular extension. For primary tumors in the larynx and hypopharynx, bilateral selective neck dissection (levels II–IV) is considered proper treatment if the nodes are not multiple or if connective tissue disease is not present. Dr. Byers also demonstrated that the selective use of postoperative radiotherapy can more effectively decrease the incidence of neck recurrence compared with surgery alone in patients with a node more than 3 cm in size, multiple positive nodes, or nodes with extracapsular invasion. Many of the principles of these studies form the basis of modern HNC surgery practiced worldwide.

Another major breakthrough in the surgical management of HNC has been in the area of surgical reconstruction. Before the 1980s, reconstructive head and neck surgery was limited and consisted of local or regional flaps that accomplished little more than wound closure and did not in most cases restore form and function. The introduction of microvascular free flaps at MD Anderson in the 1980s revolutionized head and neck oncologic surgery and permitted for the first time aggressive resections of the laryngopharynx, mandible, and skull base that could effectively and reliably be reconstructed in a single stage. This type of surgical reconstruction also improved patients' posttreatment function, including speech and swallowing, and improved cosmesis. Major bone defects in the mandible and maxilla can now be effectively reconstructed using the fibula, scapula, or iliac crest free flap [6]. These vascularized bone flaps can receive primary or secondary osteo-integrated implants for dental restoration. Soft tissue defects in the oral cavity and pharynx can be meticulously reconstructed with a variety of soft tissue flaps including the radial forearm, rectus abdominus, or latissimus dorsi flaps. The anterior lateral thigh flap is becoming the most popular choice for reconstruction of oral and oropharyngeal defects, as well as circumferential defects of the pharynx, larynx, and trachea [7].

Until the early 1960s, tumors of the paranasal sinuses that invaded the base of the skull were considered inoperable because this area was considered surgically inaccessible. The development of the anterior craniofacial resection, a two-team surgical procedure involving an intracranial approach by neurosurgery and extracranial approach by head and neck surgery, allowed adequate access for safe and effective resection of skull base tumors. The adoption and refinement of these techniques is probably behind the dramatic improvement in survival of these patients, as shown in the survival curves for paranasal sinus and nasal cavity tumors (Fig. 25.4).

More recently, the skull base team at MD Anderson has been leading the development of minimally invasive techniques for resection of malignant tumors of the base of the skull. These techniques avoid the morbidity associated with the traditional open surgical approaches and allow patients a shorter hospital stay and faster recovery. In 2009, Dr. Ehab Hanna and colleagues [8] reported the largest U.S. series to date of patients with malignant tumors of the sinonasal tract treated with endoscopic resection. Their results suggested that, in well-selected patients and with appropriate use of adjuvant therapy, endoscopic resection of sinonasal and skull base cancer results in excellent oncologic outcome.

Advances in minimally invasive surgery have also been made in transoral resection of early laryngeal and pharyngeal tumors with preservation of speech and swallowing [9]. For more advanced tumors of the larynx and pharynx, organ-sparing laryngeal and pharyngeal surgery may be a viable treatment option for carefully selected patients [10, 11].

In the past 5 years, robotic surgery has emerged as a field with significant promise for increasing the accuracy and reducing the morbidity of many surgical procedures.

HNC surgeons at MD Anderson are exploiting the advantages of robotic surgery in the management of tumors of the oropharynx, larynx, and thyroid [12]. In a preclinical study, Dr. Hanna and colleagues [8, 13] described the first robot-assisted endoscopic approach to the anterior skull base and the pituitary gland. In their report of this novel approach, they describe the feasibility of repairing dural defects without the need for a craniotomy, which has the potential for reducing morbidity and improving outcome in minimally invasive cranial base surgery.

Advances in Nonsurgical Therapy and Organ Preservation

Generally, early primary tumors of the head and neck (stages I–II) can be effectively treated with either surgery or radiotherapy. For example, patients with early glottic (T1 or T2) cancer can be successfully treated with either transoral microsurgical or laser resection or definitive radiotherapy with good oncologic and functional outcomes. In contrast, locoregionally advanced HNC (stages III–IV) usually requires multimodality therapy. For several decades, radical resection followed by radiotherapy was the cornerstone of treatment of locoregionally advanced HNC. Patients with advanced cancer of the larynx or hypopharynx were usually treated with total laryngectomy or total laryngopharyngectomy, respectively. This resulted in loss of the normal laryngeal voice, and patients had to either rely on an electrolarynx or esophageal voice for speech. The permanent anterior neck stoma added a significant deformity and impaired quality of life.

In 1979, Dr. Ki Hong and colleagues [14] explored the role of neoadjuvant (induction) chemotherapy and reported a high (76%) response rate in advanced, previously untreated HNC. They found that a major response to chemotherapy may predict the response to subsequent radiotherapy; they also demonstrated the feasibility of avoiding surgical resection in selected patients who experience complete tumor regression after receiving induction chemotherapy followed by definitive radiotherapy [15]. Their findings formed the basis for the Department of Veterans Affairs Laryngeal Cancer Study Group, a landmark phase III clinical trial of induction chemotherapy to select patients with advanced laryngeal cancer for either radiotherapy or total laryngectomy [16]. The findings from this trial defined a new role for chemotherapy in patients with advanced laryngeal cancer and indicated that a treatment strategy involving induction chemotherapy and definitive radiotherapy can be effective in preserving the larynx in approximately two-thirds (65%) of patients without compromising overall survival. This started a new era of "organ preservation" in patients treated for advanced HNC, but the value of adding chemotherapy to radiotherapy and the optimal timing of chemotherapy were unknown. For this reason, the Radiation Therapy Oncology Group (RTOG), led by Dr. Helmuth Goepfert and others, launched a three-arm randomized clinical trial comparing induction cisplatin plus fluorouracil followed by radiotherapy, radiotherapy with concurrent administration of cisplatin, or radiotherapy alone [17]. This landmark study demonstrated that radiotherapy with concurrent administration

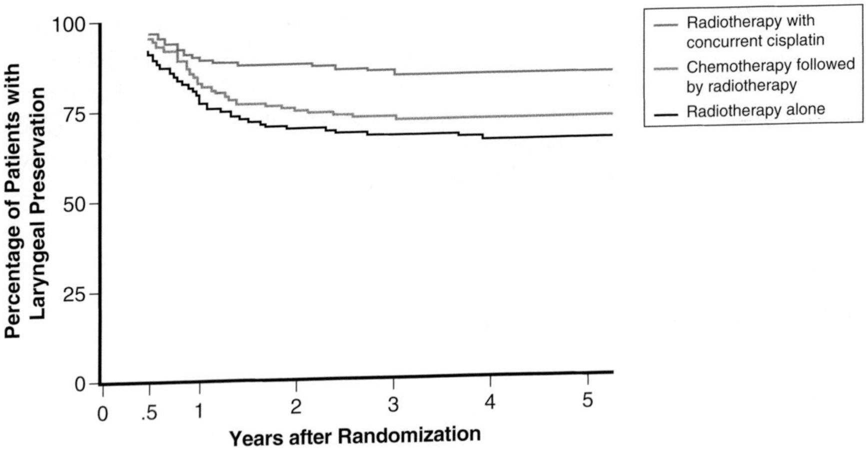

Fig. 25.5 Rates of laryngeal preservation according to treatment group in RTOG trial [16].

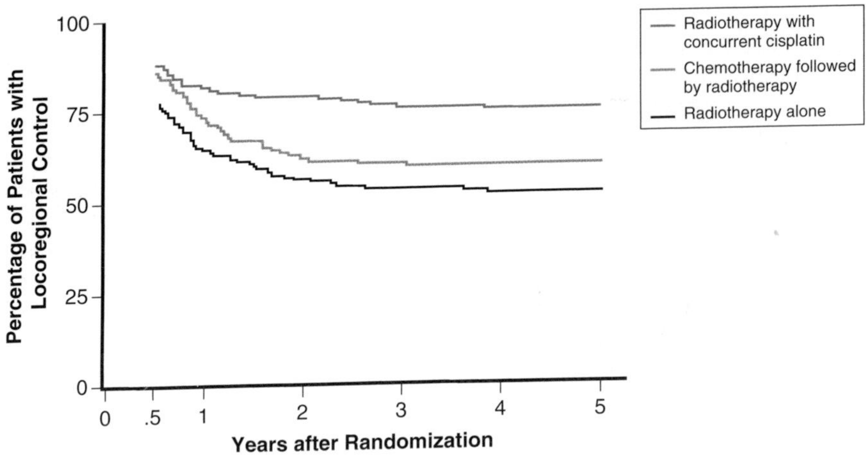

Fig. 25.6 Rates of locoregional control according to treatment group in RTOG trial [16].

of cisplatin is superior to induction chemotherapy followed by radiotherapy or radiotherapy alone for laryngeal preservation and locoregional control (Figs. 25.5 and 25.6). The findings from this and other studies established concurrent chemoradiotherapy as a new "standard of care" for organ preservation in patients treated for advanced HNC.

The improved rates of locoregional control and organ preservation associated with concurrent chemoradiotherapy came with a heavy price of increased toxicity, however, and alternative treatment strategies, particularly targeted therapy, were sought. To this end, Dr. Kian Ang and his colleagues focused their research efforts on studying the synergistic effects of cetuximab, a monoclonal antibody against the

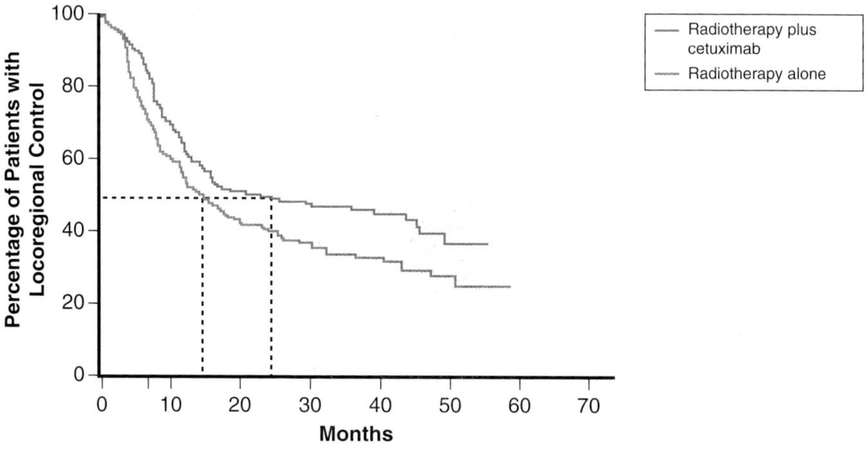

Fig. 25.7 Kaplan–Meier estimates of locoregional control among all patients randomly assigned to radiotherapy plus cetuximab or radiotherapy alone in phase III trial [19].

epidermal growth factor receptor (EGFR), and radiotherapy. Their findings from preclinical [18] and biomarker studies [19], for example, were the bases of a landmark phase III clinical trial that compared radiotherapy alone with radiotherapy plus cetuximab in the treatment of locoregionally advanced HNC [20]. This study demonstrated that treatment of locoregionally advanced HNC with concomitant high-dose radiotherapy plus cetuximab improves locoregional control and reduces mortality without increasing the common toxic effects associated with radiotherapy to the head and neck (Fig. 25.7).

Dr. Merrill Kies and colleagues [21] have also reported the results of a phase II clinical trial demonstrating the promising role of adding cetuximab to induction chemotherapy in the treatment of advanced HNC.

Ongoing clinical trials at MD Anderson are investigating the evolving role of targeted therapy in the multimodality treatment of advanced HNC. For example, Dr. Bonnie Glisson and colleagues are currently investigating the role of the insulin-like growth factor receptor (IGFR) targeting and co-targeting IGFR and EGFR in HNC. Other examples of promising targeting agents include the EGFR tyrosine kinase inhibitor erlotinib, which demonstrated modest single-agent activity in recurrent or metastatic head and neck squamous cell carcinoma and is currently being evaluated in combination with standard chemotherapy regimens and prior to surgery for advanced HNC. Bevacizumab, a monoclonal antibody against vascular endothelial growth factor (VEGF), is also currently being evaluated in combination with cetuximab in the treatment of recurrent disease. Dr. Vasiliki Papadimitrakopoulou has recently completed a phase I–II trial of vandetanib, a tyrosine kinase inhibitor of both EGFR and VEGF receptor 2 (VEGFR2), with radiotherapy and chemoradiotherapy. There is reason to believe that co-targeting of key drivers of the malignant phenotype, such as EGFR, VEGF/VEGFR, and IGFR, in biologic platforms with established radiotherapy and chemotherapy regimens may lead to more effective and less toxic therapy. Furthermore, through correlative assessment of biomarkers in tumor and blood, these studies should lead to increased personalization of treatment for patients with HNC.

Advances in Rehabilitation

With improvements in cure and survival rates, more emphasis is now being directed to rehabilitation and quality of life in patients with HNC. In addition to surgeons, medical and radiation oncologists, pathologists, and diagnostic radiologists, the MD Anderson head and neck multidisciplinary team includes outstanding rehabilitative and supportive services.

Dental oncologists provide comprehensive preventive and therapeutic oral and dental care for patients undergoing and recovering from intensive multimodality treatment of HNC. For example, Dr. Mark Chambers and his colleagues are investigating novel approaches to the management of treatment-associated xerostomia, mucositis, trismus, and osteoradionecrosis. Maxillofacial prosthodontists provide innovative techniques for dental, palatal, orbital, and facial restoration such as osteointegrated implants.

The Section of Speech and Language Pathology provides comprehensive and innovative services for assessment and rehabilitation of critical functions such as swallowing, voice, speech, hearing, and balance. With increasing trends of organ preservation, the function of the "preserved organ" has been the subject of much attention. For example, after intensive chemoradiotherapy for laryngeal and oropharyngeal preservation, a substantial number of patients experience significant dysphagia and may become dependent on tube feeding to meet their nutritional needs. Dr. Jan Lewin and her colleagues defined comprehensive measures of evaluation and rehabilitation of the swallowing function before, during, and after treatment. They also developed a world-class program in voice and speech rehabilitation after laryngectomy or other major head and neck resection. Novel treatments of postoperative and post-radiotherapy lymphedema of the head and neck are also currently being investigated. Chemotherapy and radiotherapy may have toxic effects on the auditory and vestibular systems affecting hearing and balance, respectively. Dr. Paul Gidley and his staff in the Section of Audiology developed a program that offers MD Anderson patients comprehensive assessment of and rehabilitation for hearing and balance disorders.

HNC and/or its treatment may have a profound effect on nutrition due to difficulty eating, chewing, and swallowing and altered taste perception. Nutritionists in the Head and Neck Center developed algorithms for nutritional support of patients with HNC throughout their treatment and recovery. Patients with HNC also have significant psychosocial burdens, and social services are provided throughout the cycle of care. Physical and occupational therapists are integrated into the multidisciplinary team to help patients recover as they return to their daily activity and employment. Dr. Michelle Fingeret and her colleagues are currently conducting intensive research in "body image" perceptions of patients with HNC and are evaluating methods of intervention to reduce the psychological burden that cancer or its treatment has left on these patients.

Advances in Outcome Measurement and Reporting

In 2006, Michael Porter, Professor of Economics in the Harvard Business School, published a book titled *Redefining Health Care: Creating Value-Based Competition on Results*. Porter defines *value in health care* as "the health outcome divided by the cost expended." To test this definition in cancer care, Porter and his team analyzed the care provided at MD Anderson's Head and Neck Center as a case study of a value-based system. The study focused on the multidisciplinary care center concept of our clinic system where patients are treated within a highly specialized integrated care model. Under the leadership of Drs. Randal Weber, Tom Burke, Ron Walters, and Tom Feeley, the case study offered our organization an opportunity to partner with Porter and the Harvard Business School to critically examine the value proposition as it relates to cancer care delivery.

The study evaluated the outcomes of care for 2,467 patients with previously untreated cancers of the oral cavity, larynx, and oropharynx. In addition to traditional oncologic outcomes such as survival, the study sought to evaluate some basic functional outcomes, which included the absence of a tracheostomy or feeding tube after treatment. We also evaluated selected care process metrics such as the timing from referral to completion of multidisciplinary evaluation, presentation at the treatment planning conference, and treatment completion time.

The results of this study demonstrated that more than 80% of patients were alive at 2 years after treatment for laryngeal and oropharyngeal cancer and that nearly 75% of patients with cancer of the oral cavity survived at least 2 years. In the entire cohort, 98% of patients were eating without a feeding tube at 1 year, and 91% were tracheostomy-free at 1 year. Of the process metrics, the average time from referral to evaluation by the multidisciplinary planning committee was 17 days, and 100% of patients were evaluated by the multidisciplinary planning committee and completed treatment within 100 days.

Cost measurement in health care is complex and is beyond the scope of this chapter. Under the leadership of Dr. Tom Feeley, the Institute for Cancer Care Excellence, whose mission and goal is to deliver improved value to cancer patients and individuals at risk of cancer, is using the Head and Neck Case Study to explore novel cost accounting systems that capture the entire cost of treating a medical condition throughout the whole cycle of care.

This study also demonstrated a critical need for an informatics infrastructure that can be queried for detailed clinical care events, interventions, and outcomes. Our current experience in this study of manual abstraction of key outcome information from medical records was both time- and labor-intensive and will not meet the needs of public reporting of outcomes, which is foundational to the "value" proposition and to improving the quality of care. The Head and Neck Center is currently piloting the use of a structured clinical documentation enhancement of the electronic medical record. It is our goal to continue to improve our outcome measurement and reporting to fulfill our unwavering commitment to improve the care we deliver to our patients.

Appendix

See Figs. 25.8 through 25.27.

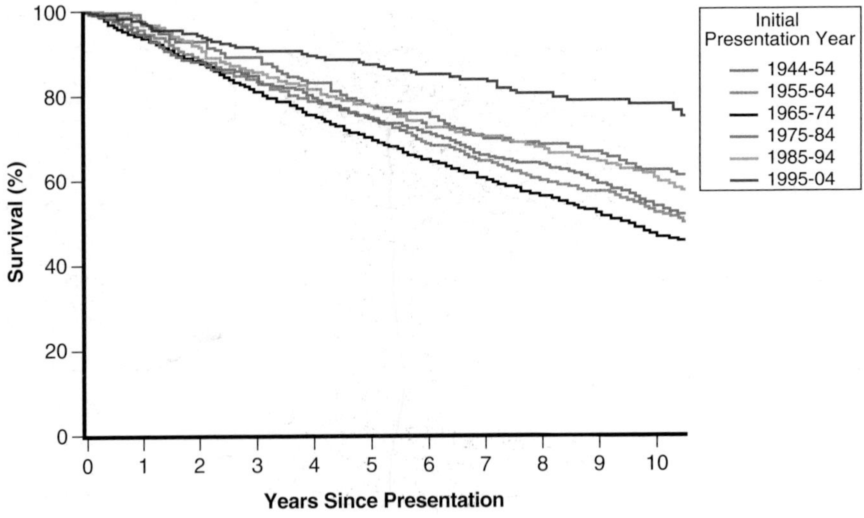

Fig. 25.8 Survival rates for patients with local (SEER stage) cancer of the head and neck with oral cavity primary sites (1944–2004) ($P<0.0001$, log-rank test for trend).

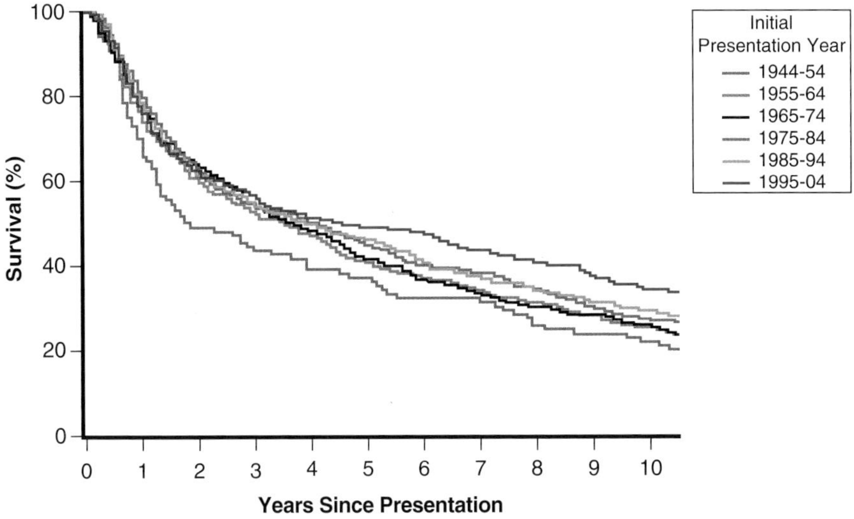

Fig. 25.9 Survival rates for patients with regional (SEER stage) cancer of the head and neck with oral cavity primary sites (1944–2004) ($P=0.001$, log-rank test for trend).

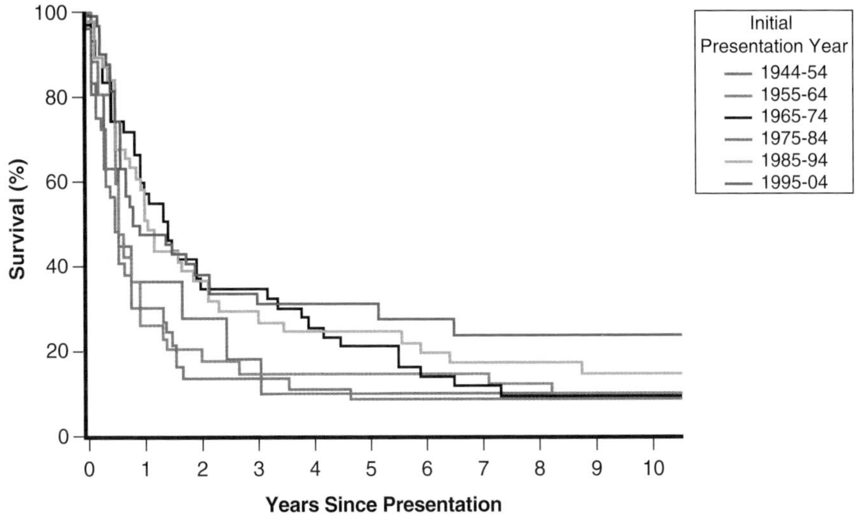

Fig. 25.10 Survival rates for patients with distant (SEER stage) cancer of the head and neck with oral cavity primary sites (1944–2004) ($P=0.062$, log-rank test for trend).

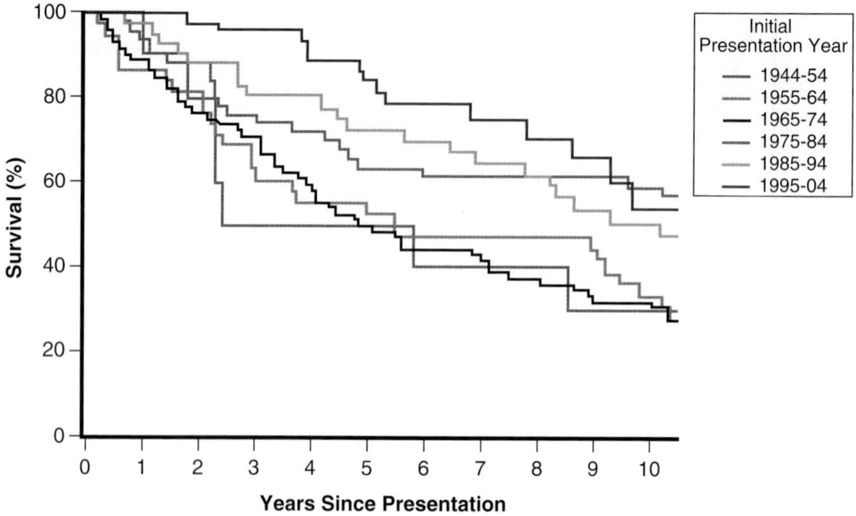

Fig. 25.11 Survival rates for patients with local (SEER stage) cancer of the head and neck with oropharyngeal primary sites (1944–2004) ($P<0.0001$, log-rank test for trend).

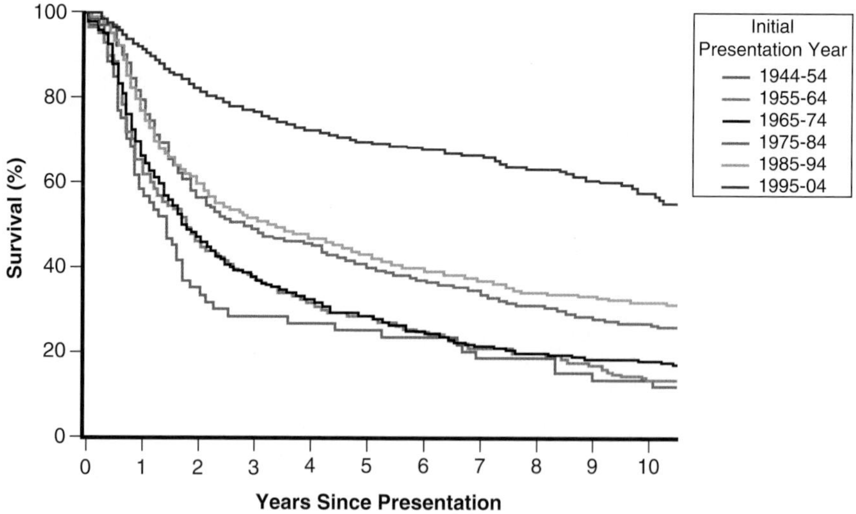

Fig. 25.12 Survival rates for patients with regional (SEER stage) cancer of the head and neck with oropharyngeal primary sites (1944–2004) ($P<0.0001$, log-rank test for trend).

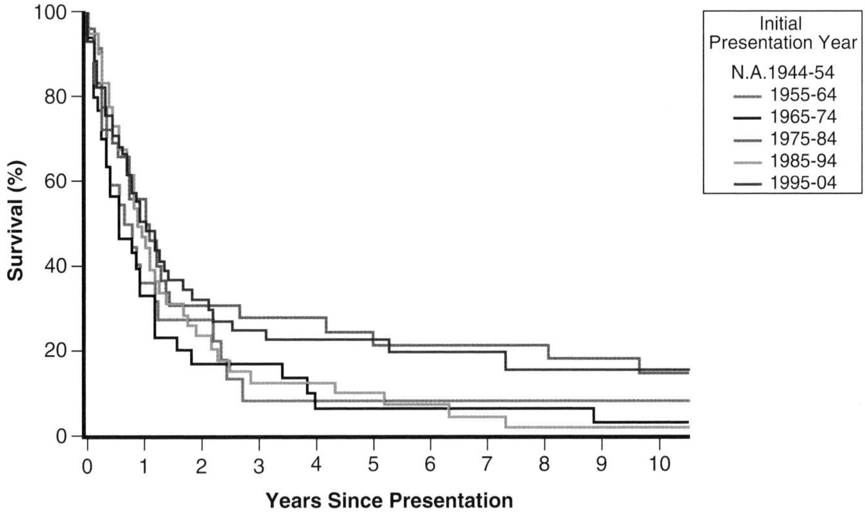

Fig. 25.13 Survival rates for patients with distant (SEER stage) cancer of the head and neck with oropharyngeal primary sites (1944–2004) ($P<0.159$, log-rank test for trend). Because of the very small number of individuals with distant cancer of the head and neck with oropharyngeal primary sites seen from 1944 to 1954, data from this period were excluded. *N.A.* not applicable.

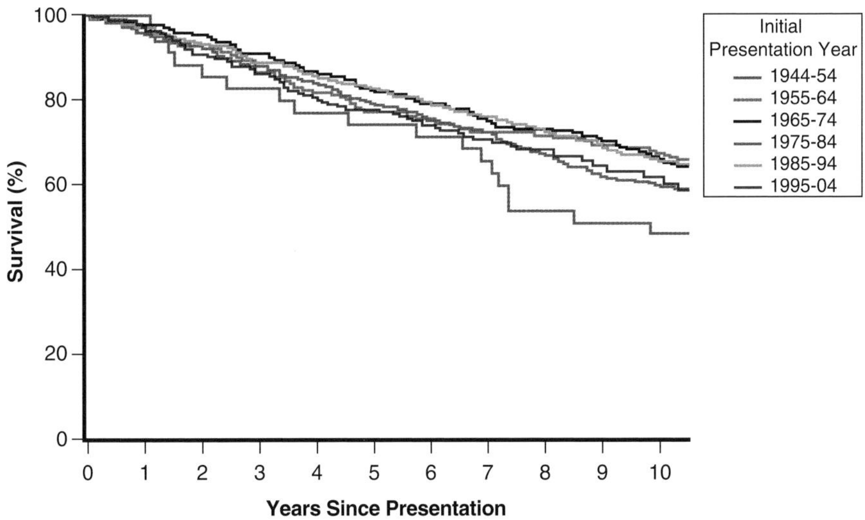

Fig. 25.14 Survival rates for patients with local (SEER stage) cancer of the head and neck with laryngeal primary sites (1944–2004) ($P=0.645$, log-rank test for trend).

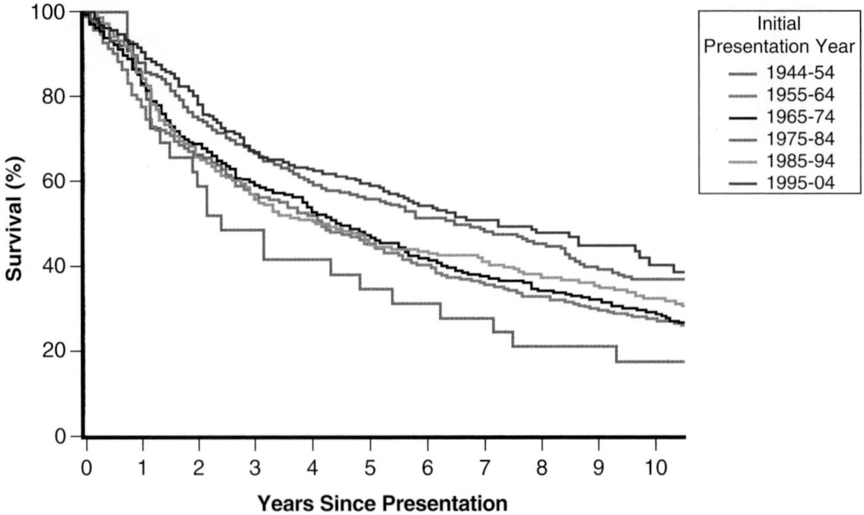

Fig. 25.15 Survival rates for patients with regional (SEER stage) cancer of the head and neck with laryngeal primary sites (1944–2004) ($P<0.0001$, log-rank test for trend).

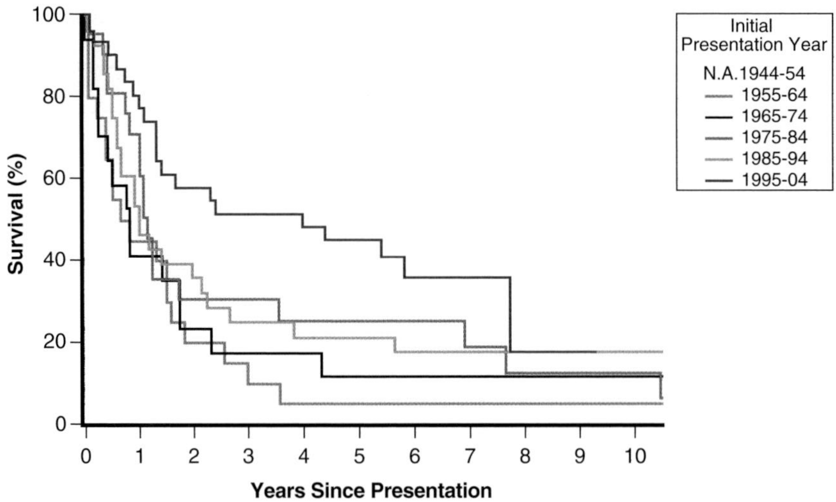

Fig. 25.16 Survival rates for patients with distant (SEER stage) cancer of the head and neck with laryngeal primary sites (1944–2004) ($P=0.027$, log-rank test for trend). Because of the very small number of individuals with distant cancer of the head and neck with laryngeal primary sites seen from 1944 to 1954, data from this period were excluded. *N.A.* not applicable.

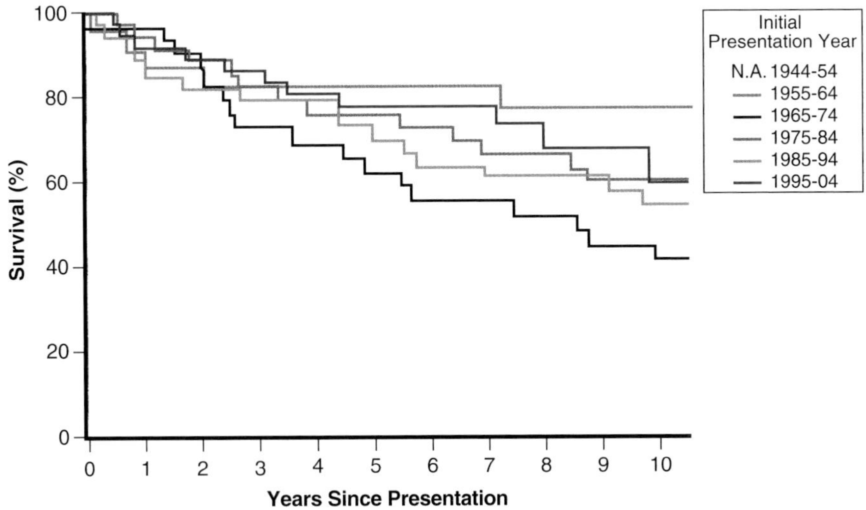

Fig. 25.17 Survival rates for patients with local (SEER stage) cancer of the head and neck with paranasal sinus and nasal cavity primary sites (1944–2004) ($P=0.166$, log-rank test for trend). Because of the very small number of individuals with local cancer of the head and neck with paranasal sinus and nasal cavity primary sites seen from 1944 to 1954, data from this period were excluded. *N.A.* not applicable.

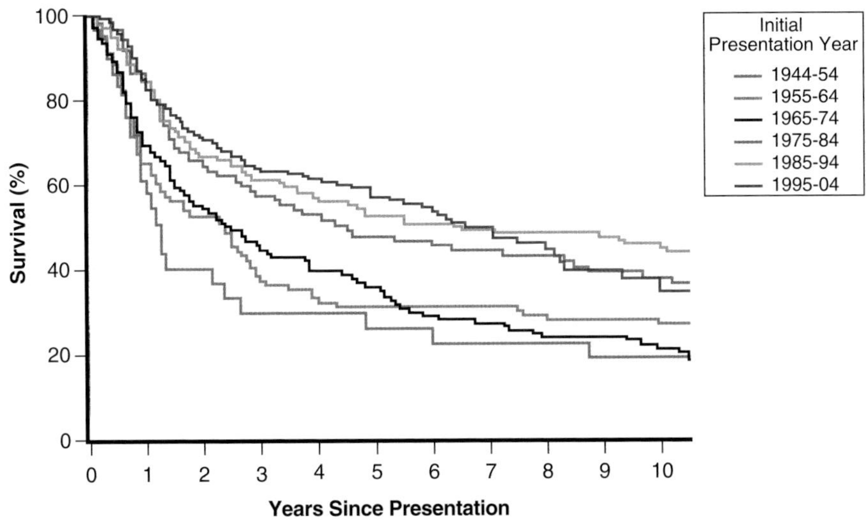

Fig. 25.18 Survival rates for patients with regional (SEER stage) cancer of the head and neck with paranasal sinus and nasal cavity primary sites (1944–2004) ($P<0.0001$, log-rank test for trend).

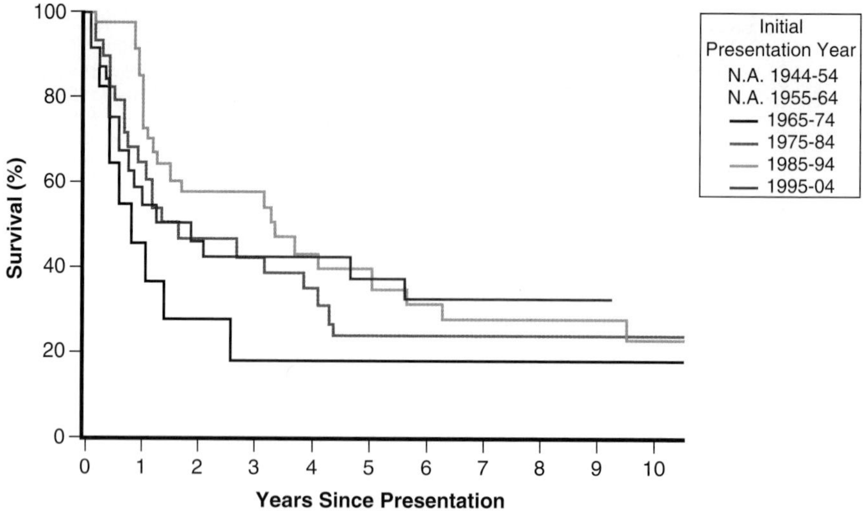

Fig. 25.19 Survival rates for patients with distant (SEER stage) cancer of the head and neck with paranasal sinus and nasal cavity primary sites (1944–2004) ($P = 0.001$, log-rank test for trend). Because of the very small number of individuals with distant cancer of the head and neck with paranasal sinus and nasal cavity primary sites seen from 1944 to 1954 and from 1955 to 1964, data from these periods were excluded. *N.A.* not applicable.

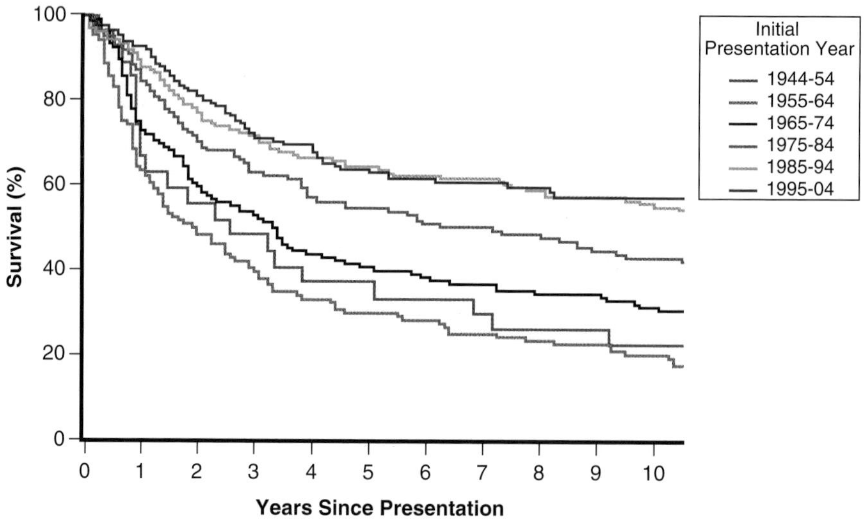

Fig. 25.20 Overall rates for patients with cancer of the head and neck with nasopharyngeal primary sites (1944–2004) ($P < 0.0001$, log-rank test for trend).

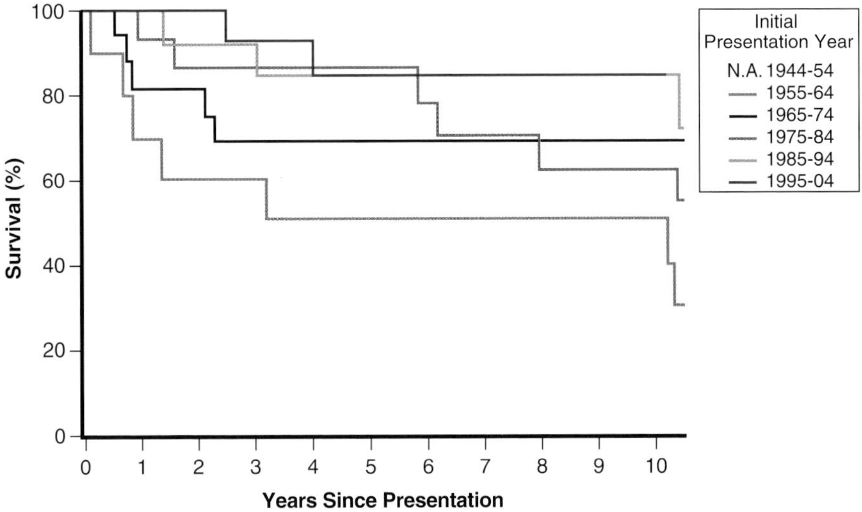

Fig. 25.21 Survival rates for patients with local (SEER stage) cancer of the head and neck with nasopharyngeal primary sites (1944–2004) ($P = 0.153$, log-rank test for trend). Because of the very small number of individuals with local cancer of the head and neck with nasopharyngeal primary sites seen from 1944 to 1954, data from this period were excluded. *N.A.* not applicable.

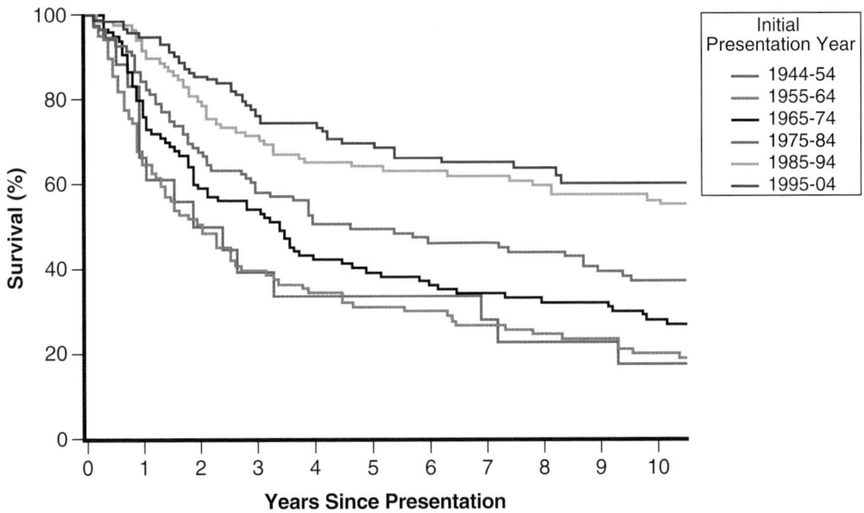

Fig. 25.22 Survival rates for patients with regional (SEER stage) cancer of the head and neck with nasopharyngeal primary sites (1944–2004) ($P < 0.0001$, log-rank test for trend).

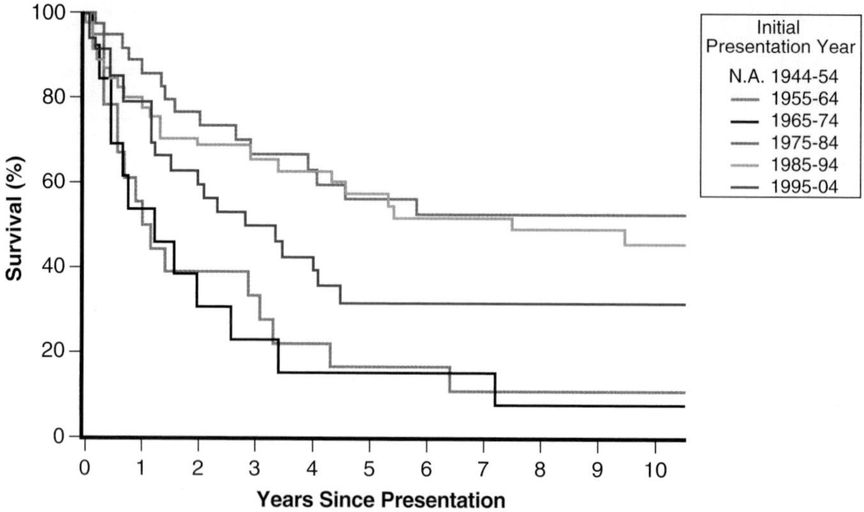

Fig. 25.23 Survival rates for patients with distant (SEER stage) cancer of the head and neck with nasopharyngeal primary sites (1944–2004) ($P<0.0001$, log-rank test for trend). Because of the very small number of individuals with distant cancer of the head and neck with nasopharyngeal primary sites seen from 1944 to 1954, data from this period were excluded. *N.A.* not applicable.

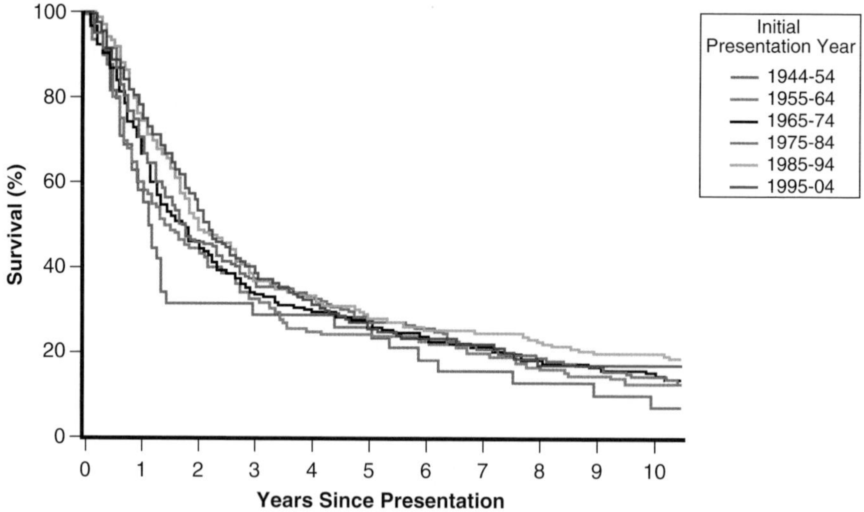

Fig. 25.24 Overall rates for patients with cancer of the head and neck with hypopharyngeal primary sites (1944–2004) ($P=0.020$, log-rank test for trend).

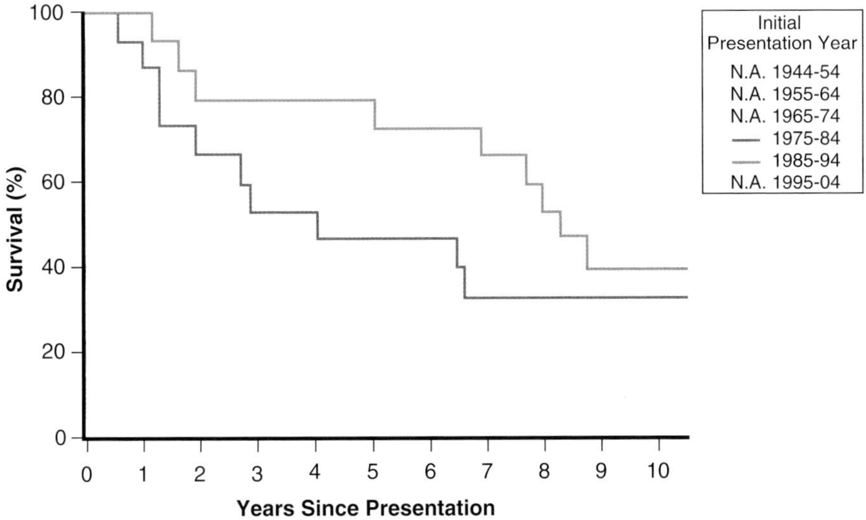

Fig. 25.25 Survival rates for patients with local (SEER stage) cancer of the head and neck with hypopharyngeal primary sites (1944–2004) ($P=0.375$, log-rank test for trend). Because of the very small number of individuals with local cancer of the head and neck with hypopharyngeal primary sites seen from 1944 to 1954, from 1955 to 1964, from 1965 to 1974, and from 1995 to 2004, data from these periods were excluded. *N.A.* not applicable.

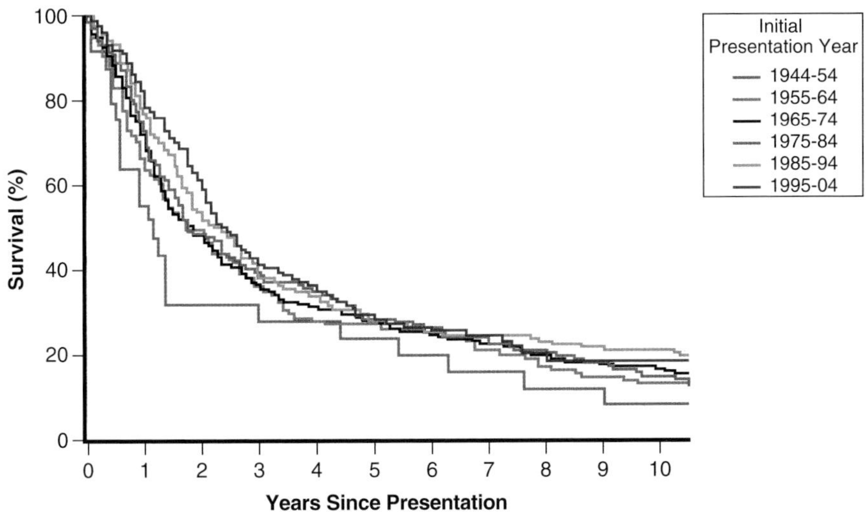

Fig. 25.26 Survival rates for patients with regional (SEER stage) cancer of the head and neck with hypopharyngeal primary sites (1944–2004) ($P=0.246$, log-rank test for trend).

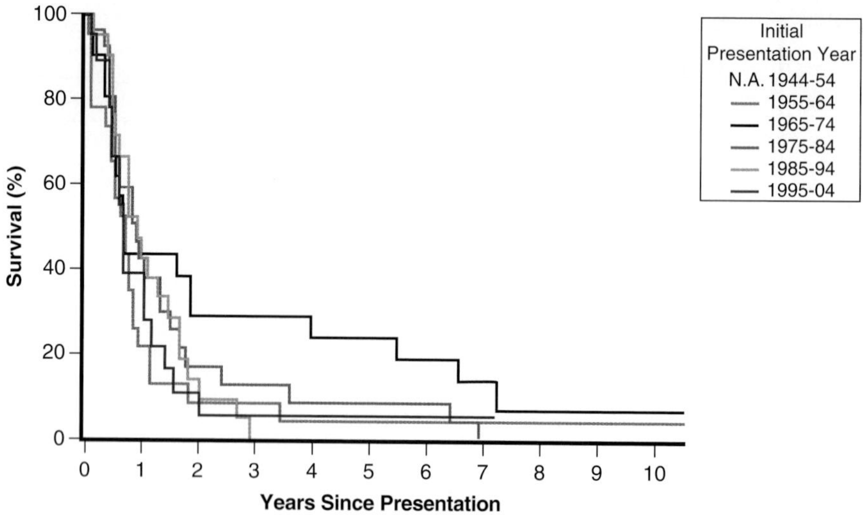

Fig. 25.27 Survival rates for patients with distant (SEER stage) cancer of the head and neck with hypopharyngeal primary sites (1944–2004) ($P = 0.358$, log-rank test for trend). Because of the very small number of individuals with distant cancer of the head and neck with hypopharyngeal primary sites seen from 1944 to 1954, data from this period were excluded. *N.A.* not applicable.

References

1. Siegel R, Ward E, Brawley O, Jemal A. The impact of eliminating socioeconomic and racial disparities on premature cancer deaths. CA Cancer J Clin. 2011;61(4):212–36.
2. Cognetti DM, Weber RS, Lai SY. Head and neck cancer. Cancer. 2008;113(S7):1911–32.
3. Ang KK, Harris J, Wheeler R, et al. Human papillomavirus and survival of patients with oropharyngeal cancer. N Engl J Med. 2010;363(1):24–35.
4. Sturgis EM, Dahlstrom KR. HPV vaccination. Inaccurate assumptions about oropharyngeal cancer. BMJ. 2009;339:b4525.
5. Lindberg R. Distribution of cervical lymph node metastases from squamous cell carcinoma of the upper respiratory and digestive tracts. Cancer. 1972;29(6):1446–9.
6. Moreno MA, Skoracki RJ, Hanna EY, Hanasono MM. Microvascular free flap reconstruction versus palatal obturation for maxillectomy defects. Head Neck. 2010;32(7):860–8.
7. Yu P, Clayman GL, Walsh GL. Long-term outcomes of microsurgical reconstruction for large tracheal defects. Cancer. 2011;117(4):802–8.
8. Hanna E, DeMonte F, Ibrahim S, Roberts D, Levine N, Kupferman M. Endoscopic resection of sinonasal cancers with and without craniotomy: oncologic results. Arch Otolaryngol Head Neck Surg. 2009;135(12):1219–24.
9. Holsinger FC, Nussenbaum B, Nakayama M, et al. Current concepts and new horizons in conservation laryngeal surgery: an important part of multidisciplinary care. Head Neck. 2010;32(5):656–65.
10. Laccourreye L, Garcia D, Ménard M, Brasnu D, Laccourreye O, Holsinger FC. Horizontal supraglottic partial laryngectomy for selected squamous carcinoma of the vallecula. Head Neck. 2008;30(6):756–64.

11. Laccourreye O, Seccia V, Ménard M, Garcia D, Vacher C, Holsinger FC. Extended lateral pharyngotomy for selected squamous cell carcinomas of the lateral tongue base. Ann Otol Rhinol Laryngol. 2009;118(6):428–34.
12. Lewis CM, Chung WY, Holsinger FC. Feasibility and surgical approach of transaxillary robotic thyroidectomy without CO2 insufflation. Head Neck. 2010;32(1):121–6.
13. Kupferman M, DeMonte F, Holsinger FC, Hanna E. Transantral robotic access to the pituitary gland. J Otolaryngol Head Neck Surg. 2009;141(3):413–5.
14. Hong WK, Shapshay SM, Bhutani R, et al. Induction chemotherapy in advanced squamous head and neck carcinoma with high-dose cis-platinum and bleomycin infusion. Cancer. 1979;44(1):19–25.
15. Hong WK, O'Donoghue GM, Sheetz S, et al. Sequential response patterns to chemotherapy and radiotherapy in head and neck cancer: potential impact of treatment in advanced laryngeal cancer. Prog Clin Biol Res. 1985;201:191–7.
16. Induction chemotherapy plus radiation compared with surgery plus radiation in patients with advanced laryngeal cancer. N Engl J Med. 1991;324(24):1685–90.
17. Forastiere AA, Goepfert H, Maor M, et al. Concurrent chemotherapy and radiotherapy for organ preservation in advanced laryngeal cancer. N Engl J Med. 2003;349(22):2091–8.
18. Milas L, Mason K, Hunter N, et al. In vivo enhancement of tumor radioresponse by C225 antiepidermal growth factor receptor antibody. Clin Cancer Res. 2000;6(2):701–8.
19. Ang KK, Berkey BA, Tu X, et al. Impact of epidermal growth factor receptor expression on survival and pattern of relapse in patients with advanced head and neck carcinoma. Cancer Res. 2002;62(24):7350–6.
20. Bonner JA, Harari PM, Giralt J, et al. Radiotherapy plus cetuximab for squamous-cell carcinoma of the head and neck. N Engl J Med. 2006;354(6):567–78.
21. Kies MS, Holsinger FC, Lee JJ, et al. Induction chemotherapy and cetuximab for locally advanced squamous cell carcinoma of the head and neck: results from a phase II prospective trial. J Clin Oncol. 2010;28(1):8–14.

Chapter 26
Thyroid Cancer

Steven I. Sherman, Nancy Perrier, and Gary L. Clayman

Introduction

An estimated 56,460 persons in the USA will be diagnosed with various forms of thyroid cancer in 2012, the ninth most commonly diagnosed cancer overall [1]. With 76% of cases now identified in women, thyroid cancer has become the fifth most commonly diagnosed malignancy in that gender, up from the tenth most common only 10 years ago. Between 1998 and 2007, the most recent period for which Surveillance, Epidemiology, and End Results program (SEER) data are available, the average annual percent change in age-adjusted incidence of thyroid cancer in the USA—6.1%—was the highest among all cancers [2]. Worldwide, the incidence of thyroid cancer has been increasing as well [3]. The reasons underlying this marked increase are likely multiple, with one being the increasing number of diagnoses of incidental small cancers resulting from improved sensitivity of diagnostic imaging procedures such as ultrasound [4]. Mortality rates in patients with thyroid cancer have also been rising in the USA, albeit far more slowly. Although only 1,780 deaths from thyroid cancer are expected in 2012, the average age-adjusted mortality increased 0.6% per year between 1998 and 2007, most notably among men, who experienced a striking 1.6% increase per year [2]. In Texas, the mortality rates have been increasing faster than those in the rest of the USA.

S.I. Sherman (✉)
Department of Endocrine Neoplasia and Hormonal Disorders, The University of Texas MD Anderson Cancer Center, Houston, TX, USA
e-mail: sisherma@mdanderson.org

N. Perrier
Department of Surgical Oncology, The University of Texas MD Anderson Cancer Center, Houston, TX, USA

G.L. Clayman
Department of Head and Neck Surgery, The University of Texas MD Anderson Cancer Center, Houston, TX, USA

M.A. Rodriguez et al. (eds.), *60 Years of Survival Outcomes at The University of Texas MD Anderson Cancer Center*, DOI 10.1007/978-1-4614-5197-6_26,

Thyroid cancer is subdivided into four major histologic subtypes: papillary thyroid carcinoma (PTC), follicular thyroid carcinoma (FTC), medullary thyroid carcinoma (MTC), and anaplastic thyroid carcinoma (ATC) (see Table 26.1 [5] for the American Joint Committee on Cancer (AJCC)-TNM staging system criteria and Table 26.2 [6] for SEER staging criteria). Of these, both PTC and FTC derive from the thyroid follicular epithelium, cells normally responsible for the uptake of iodine

Table 26.1 AJCC-TNM staging of thyroid carcinoma, 7th edition [5]

Primary tumor (T)	
TX	Primary tumor cannot be assessed
T0	No evidence of primary tumor
T1	Tumor 2 cm or less in greatest dimension limited to the thyroid
T1a	Tumor 1 cm or less, limited to the thyroid
T1b	Tumor more than 1 cm but not more than 2 cm in greatest dimension, limited to the thyroid
T2	Tumor more than 2 cm but not more than 4 cm in greatest dimension limited to the thyroid
T3	Tumor more than 4 cm in greatest dimension limited to the thyroid or any tumor with minimal extrathyroid extension (e.g., extension to sternothyroid muscle or perithyroid soft tissues)
T4a	Moderately advanced disease: Tumor of any size extending beyond the thyroid capsule to invade subcutaneous soft tissues, larynx, trachea, esophagus, or recurrent laryngeal nerve
T4b	Very advanced disease: Tumor invades prevertebral fascia or encases carotid artery or mediastinal vessels
All anaplastic carcinomas are considered T4 tumors	
T4a	Intrathyroidal anaplastic carcinoma
T4b	Anaplastic carcinoma with gross extrathyroid extension
Regional lymph nodes (N)	
Regional lymph nodes are the central compartment, lateral cervical, and upper mediastinal lymph nodes	
NX	Regional lymph nodes cannot be assessed
N0	No regional lymph node metastasis
N1	Regional lymph node metastasis
N1a	Metastasis to Level VI (pretracheal, paratracheal, and prelaryngeal/Delphian lymph nodes)
N1b	Metastasis to unilateral, bilateral, or contralateral cervical (Levels I, II, III, IV, or V) or retropharyngeal or superior mediastinal lymph nodes (Level VII)
Distant metastasis (M)	
M0	No distant metastasis
M1	Distant metastasis

(continued)

Table 26.1 (continued)

Anatomic stage/prognostic groups			
Differentiated			
		Under 45 years	
Stage I	Any T	Any N	M0
Stage II	Any T	Any N	M1
		45 years and older	
Stage I	T1	N0	M0
Stage II	T2	N0	M0
Stage III	T3	N0	M0
	T1	N1a	M0
	T2	N1a	M0
	T3	N1a	M0
Stage IVA	T4a	N0	M0
	T4a	N1a	M0
	T1	N1b	M0
	T2	N1b	M0
	T3	N1b	M0
	T4a	N1b	M0
Stage IVB	T4b	Any N	M0
Stage IVC	Any T	Any N	M1
Medullary carcinoma (all age groups)			
Stage I	T1	N0	M0
Stage II	T2	N0	M0
	T3	N0	M0
Stage III	T1	N1a	M0
	T2	N1a	M0
	T3	N1a	M0
Stage IVA	T4a	N0	M0
	T4a	N1a	M0
	T1	N1b	M0
	T2	N1b	M0
	T3	N1b	M0
	T4a	N1b	M0
Stage IVB	T4b	Any N	M0
Stage IVC	Any T	Any N	M1
Anaplastic carcinoma			
All anaplastic carcinomas are considered Stage IV			
Stage IVA	T4a	Any N	M0
Stage IVB	T4b	Any N	M0
Stage IVC	Any T	Any N	M1

Note: All categories may be subdivided: (s) solitary tumor and (m) multifocal tumor (the largest determines the classification)

for use in the production of thyroid hormone, under the influence of thyroid-stimulating hormone (TSH). PTC and FTC, collectively referred to as differentiated thyroid carcinomas (DTC), currently account for 96.5% of all incident thyroid cancers [2]. In addition to more extensive disease, the major risk factors for mortality

Table 26.2 SEER summary staging of thyroid carcinoma [6]

Stage	Description
Local	Confined to one lobe and/or isthmus; both lobes involved; thyroid gland capsule involved; multiple foci but confined to thyroid gland; through capsule of gland, but not beyond
Regional	Direct extension to pericapsular tissues, strap muscle(s), nerve(s), major blood vessels, soft tissue of neck, esophagus, larynx including thyroid and cricoid cartilages, sternocleidomastoid muscle, OR lymph nodes (anterior deep cervical, internal jugular, retropharyngeal, cervical NOS)
Distant	Direct extension to trachea, mediastinal tissues, skeletal muscle other than strap muscles and sternocleidomastoid, bone, OR other distant involvement, OR submandibular, submental, or other distant nodes

SEER Surveillance, Epidemiology, and End Results program

from DTC include age greater than 45 years at diagnosis. MTC, on the other hand, arises from the calcitonin-secreting neuroendocrine-derived C cells within the upper portions of the thyroid lobes and represents 1.6% of incident thyroid malignancies. About 20% of patients with MTC have an inherited form of the disease, either multiple endocrine neoplasia type II or familial MTC; almost all inherited cases are due to autosomal dominant germline mutations of the *RET* proto-oncogene [7]. ATC likely develops as a consequence of multiple dedifferentiating mutations occurring in DTC and accounts for only about 1% of thyroid cancers. Although the 10-year relative survival rate for patients with DTC is greater than 90%, 10-year survival rates are worse for patients with MTC (80%) and ATC (13%) [8].

Historical Perspective

Unlike most other forms of cancer, no data exist from randomized controlled trials of any of the primary treatments commonly used for thyroid carcinoma (surgery, radioiodine, and thyroid hormone suppression for DTC; surgery for MTC; and chemotherapy and external beam radiation with or without surgery for ATC). Thus, current consensus guidelines for primary therapy are still based on a combination of large retrospective studies and expert opinion [7, 9, 10]. Investigators at The University of Texas MD Anderson Cancer Center have contributed extensively both to the body of retrospective studies and to the development of guidelines for therapy.

Since the early twentieth century, surgical resection of the thyroid gland has been the mainstay of treatment for thyroid malignancies, but debate has long focused on the optimal extent of primary surgery, i.e., partial versus total thyroidectomy. Early publications from MD Anderson Cancer Center emphasized the need for total thyroidectomy (removal of both lobes of the thyroid as well as the middle portion) in patients with DTC because of the high frequency of bilateral multifocal disease and provided some of the first evidence suggesting improved outcomes [11–13].

Radioactive iodine (131-I) was introduced for scanning and treatment of metastatic DTC in the mid-1940s. Use of radioactive iodine for adjuvant therapy after total thyroidectomy gained momentum after study findings were published in the early 1980s, including a seminal report from the MD Anderson multidisciplinary thyroid cancer treatment group describing a multivariate analysis that demonstrated improved disease-free survival in 706 patients with DTC [14]. Recently, analyses from a multicenter thyroid cancer registry led by MD Anderson investigators have provided the strongest evidence to date for improved survival among DTC patients presenting with National Thyroid Cancer Treatment Cooperative Study stages II, III, and IV treated with total thyroidectomy and adjuvant radioactive iodine [15]. TSH-suppressive thyroid hormone therapy was also found to improve survival, with greater degrees of suppression associated with optimal survival in patients with stages III and IV disease.

For patients with MTC, total thyroidectomy was established by the 1980s as the standard initial surgical procedure, with subsequent refinements focusing on the extent of nodal dissection [16, 17]. Early adoption of *RET* genotype-driven treatment strategies based on prospective testing in children and adults with inherited forms of MTC has resulted in personalized surgical management [18]. The role of external beam radiotherapy in both DTC and MTC has remained contentious, although recent retrospective studies have suggested durable disease control in patients at high risk of locoregional recurrence who receive adjuvant radiotherapy [19, 20]. One of the earliest publications describing a possible role for chemotherapy in patients with advanced or metastatic thyroid carcinoma contributed to the FDA approval of doxorubicin [21]. Traditionally, however, cytotoxic chemotherapies have been rarely used for DTC or MTC because of their limited efficacy and intolerable adverse effects. With the introduction of novel therapies targeting oncogenic mutant kinases and tumor angiogenesis, MD Anderson physicians have led a resurgence of clinical interest in systemic therapies for patients with disease refractory to standard approaches [22, 23].

The MD Anderson Cancer Center Experience

The MD Anderson Tumor Registry data set was derived from 6,460 men and women with a diagnosis of thyroid cancer who were seen between 1944 and 2004. Of this group, 1,677 patients who had received no previous treatment for their malignancy received definitive primary treatment at MD Anderson. After excluding patients with other primary malignancies except for superficial skin cancers, 1,232 patients remained and formed the basis of this report. Within this cohort, 1,028 (83.4%) had DTC, 111 (9.0%) had MTC, and 62 (5.0%) had ATC (Table 26.3). Thus, a disproportionate number of newly diagnosed patients with either MTC or ATC have been seen at our institution compared with the historical U.S. distribution of these histologies (9.0% vs. 1.6% for MTC, 5.0% vs. about 1% for ATC, respectively), suggesting that patients with more aggressive histologic variants may have been more likely to be referred.

Table 26.3 Histologic subtypes of thyroid cancer in 1,232 patients seen at MD Anderson between 1944 and 2004

	Histologic subtype				
	DTC[a]	MTC	ATC	Other	Total
Decade	[No. of patients]				
1944–1954	28	1	3	0	32
1955–1964	85	7	5	5	102
1965–1974	110	12	10	3	135
1975–1984	104	19	3	4	125
1985–1994	218	18	13	4	253
1995–2004	483	54	28	15	580
Total	*1,028*	*111*	*62*	*31*	*1,232*

ATC anaplastic thyroid carcinoma, *DTC* differentiated thyroid carcinoma, *MTC* medullary thyroid carcinoma

[a]Papillary thyroid carcinoma and follicular thyroid carcinoma are collectively known as differentiated thyroid carcinomas

Table 26.4 SEER stages for 1,028 patients with differentiated thyroid carcinoma who were treated at MD Anderson, 1944–2004

	SEER stage				
	Local	Regional	Distant	Unstaged	Total
Decade	[No. of patients]				
1944–1954	4	17	7	0	28
1955–1964	23	47	15	0	85
1965–1974	30	56	24	0	110
1975–1984	35	45	23	1	104
1985–1994	69	106	42	1	218
1995–2004	189	219	70	5	483
Total	*350*	*490*	*181*	*7*	*1,028*

SEER Surveillance, Epidemiology, and End Results program

Among patients with DTC, 34% presented with local disease, 48% with regional extension, and 18% with distant metastases (Table 26.4). Between the first three and the last three decades, the proportion of patients who presented with regional and distant metastatic disease decreased from 74% to 63%, reaching a nadir in the last 10 years at 60%. Nonetheless, the frequency of patients with regional or distant metastatic disease at presentation was markedly higher than the 40% reported nationally between 1988 and 2005 [24].

Among MTC patients, 30% presented with localized disease, whereas 43% presented with regional disease and 25% with distant metastatic disease (Table 26.5). No major trend over time was identified, except for increased detection of localized disease in the last decade; the introduction of genetic testing for *RET* mutations to facilitate early diagnosis may have contributed to this recent stage migration [25]. Similar to our experience with DTC, the proportion of patients who presented with regional or distant metastatic MTC was considerably higher than the 52% reported from a national SEER dataset [26].

Table 26.5 SEER stages for 111 patients with medullary thyroid carcinoma who were treated at MD Anderson, 1944–2004

	SEER stage				
	Local	Regional	Distant	Unstaged	Total
Decade	[No. of patients]				
1944–1954	1	0	0	0	1
1955–1964	1	2	4	0	7
1965–1974	3	5	3	1	12
1975–1984	3	11	5	0	19
1985–1994	4	10	4	0	18
1995–2004	21	20	12	1	54
Total	*33*	*48*	*28*	*2*	*111*

SEER Surveillance, Epidemiology, and End Results program

Table 26.6 SEER stages for 62 patients with anaplastic thyroid carcinoma who were treated at MD Anderson, 1944–2004

	SEER stage				
	Local	Regional	Distant	Unstaged	Total
Decade	[No. of patients]				
1944–1954	0	0	3	0	3
1955–1964	0	0	3	2	5
1965–1974	0	4	6	0	10
1975–1984	0	1	2	0	3
1985–1994	1	1	8	3	13
1995–2004	0	12	15	1	28
Total	*1*	*18*	*37*	*6*	*62*

SEER Surveillance, Epidemiology, and End Results program

Among patients with ATC, 60% presented with distant metastatic disease, also higher than the 43% reported nationally (Table 26.6) [27].

Overall, the higher proportions of patients who presented with more advanced disease likely reflect referral patterns to the institution, although more extensive use of cross-sectional and functional imaging might also bias toward increased identification of regional and distant metastatic disease.

Kaplan–Meier survival analyses for the entire cohort of 1,232 patients demonstrate a significant trend toward improved outcomes over the 60-year period (Figs. 26.1, 26.2, 26.3, and 26.4), but visual inspection indicates that major survival advances began in the 1975–1984 decade (Fig. 26.1). Five-year survival estimates improved from 72–74% for the first three decades to 86–88% in the latter three decades, with corresponding 10-year survival estimates increasing from 59–62% to 76–80%. Significant trends in improved survival were observed in two subgroups: patients with localized disease (Fig. 26.2) and patients with distant metastases (Fig. 26.4), whereas the trend was similar but not significant for patients with regional disease (Fig. 26.3). These survival improvements may correspond to the broader adoption of adjuvant radioactive iodine for DTC and of total thyroidectomy as the standard primary treatment for all forms of thyroid cancer.

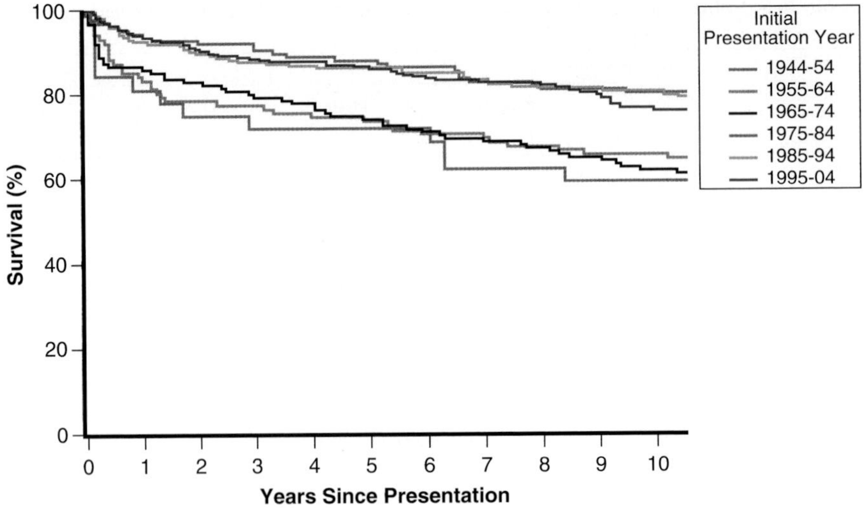

Fig. 26.1 Overall survival rates for 1,232 patients with thyroid cancer (all histologies and disease extent) (1944–2004) ($P<0.0001$, log-rank test for trend).

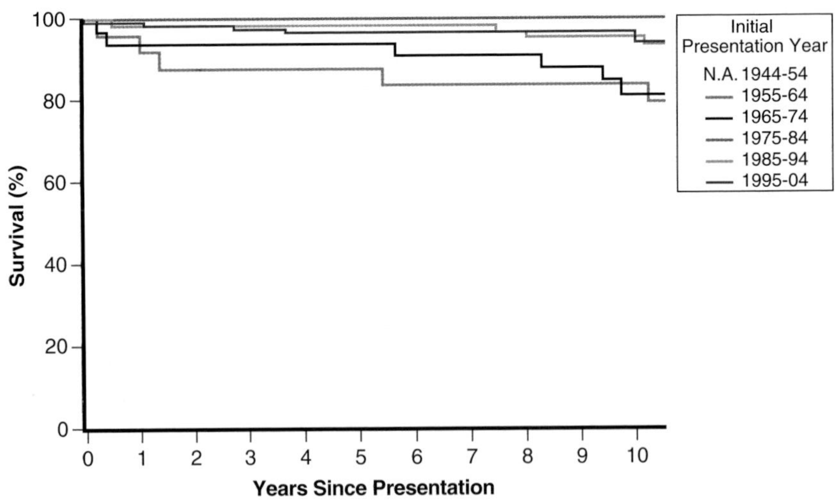

Fig. 26.2 Overall survival rates for 390 patients with local (SEER stage) thyroid cancer (all histologies) (1944–2004) ($P=0.017$, log-rank test for trend). Because of the very small number of individuals with local thyroid cancer seen from 1944 to 1954, data from this period were excluded. *N.A.* not applicable.

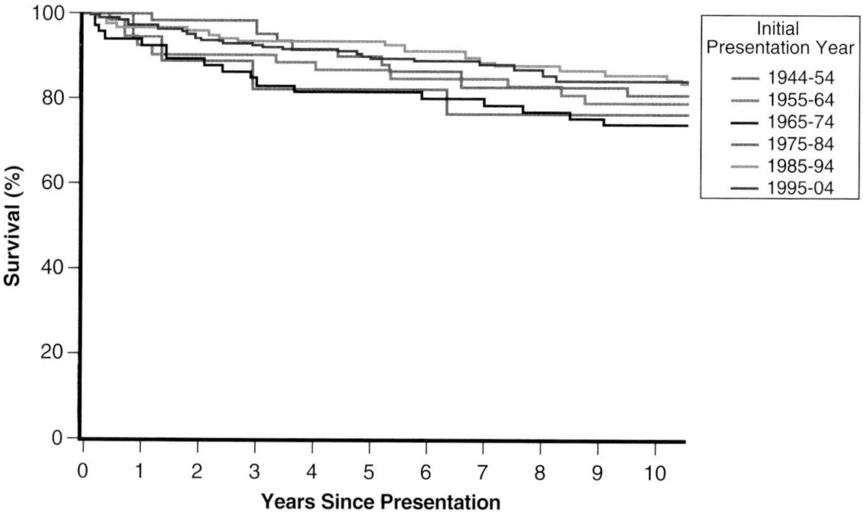

Fig. 26.3 Overall survival rates for 569 patients with regional (SEER stage) thyroid cancer (all histologies) (1944–2004) ($P=0.225$, log-rank test for trend).

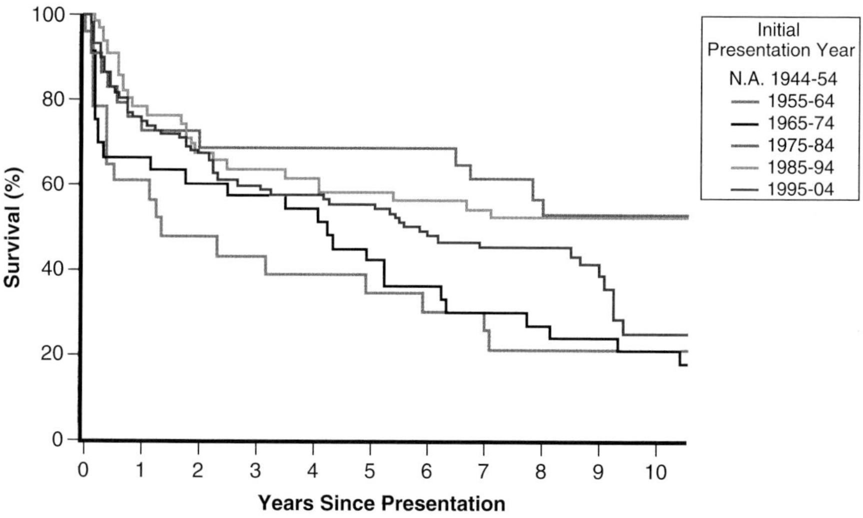

Fig. 26.4 Overall survival rates for 252 patients with distant (SEER stage) metastatic thyroid cancer (all histologies) (1944–2004) ($P=0.003$, log-rank test for trend). Because of the very small number of individuals with distant thyroid cancer seen from 1944 to 1954, data from this period were excluded. *N.A.* not applicable.

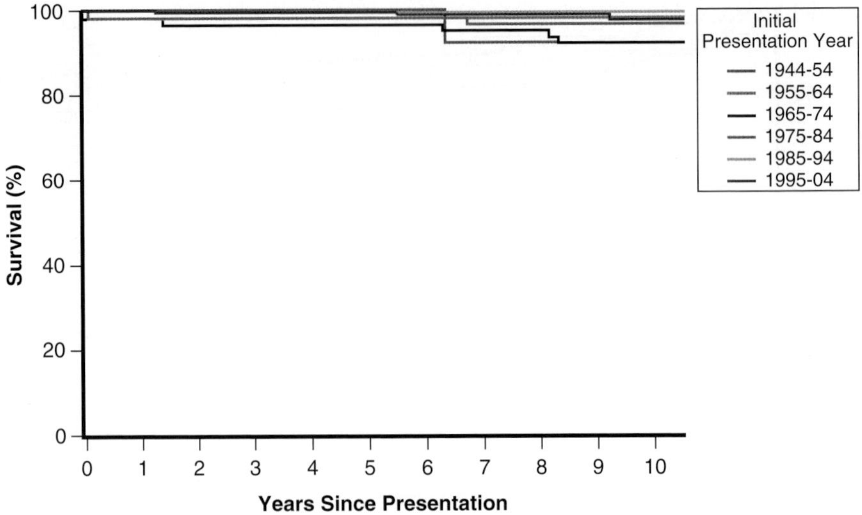

Fig. 26.5 Overall survival rates for 573 patients with differentiated thyroid carcinoma who were <45 years of age at diagnosis (1944–2004).

Analysis of the outcomes of DTC patient subgroups confirms and extends these overall survival findings. Because of the excellent relative survival rates associated with patient age of <45 years at diagnosis, only about 20% of patient deaths have occurred in this subgroup; however, no major trend can be observed due to the small number of events (Fig. 26.5). In contrast, improvement in survival rates in patients 45 years or older at diagnosis was seen beginning in the 1975–1984 decade (Fig. 26.6). When this older subgroup is evaluated on the basis of initial disease extent, a general trend toward improved outcomes in the later decades can be identified as well (Figs. 26.7, 26.8, and 26.9). The small number of cases and patient deaths limits the ability to evaluate time trends in outcomes in the MTC and ATC subgroups.

One important caveat must be considered in evaluating changes in patient outcomes over this 60-year period. If a secular trend existed in the use of imaging procedures for disease staging, leading to increased imaging in the latter decades, caution would have to be applied to interpreting any improvements in patient outcomes without considering a possible "Will Rogers phenomenon" associated with stage migration [28]. As with any other retrospective analysis spanning several decades, improvements in supportive care and management of comorbid diseases may also have contributed to increased survival.

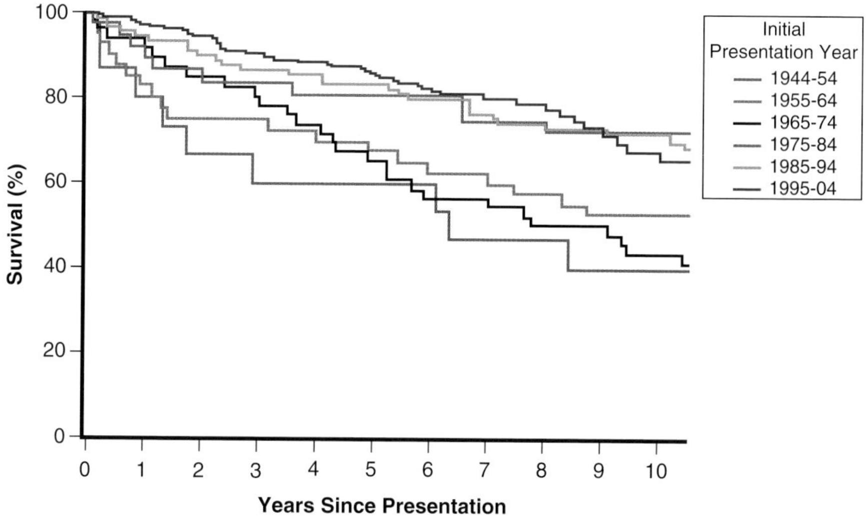

Fig. 26.6 Overall survival rates for 455 patients with differentiated thyroid carcinoma who were ≥45 years of age at diagnosis (1944–2004).

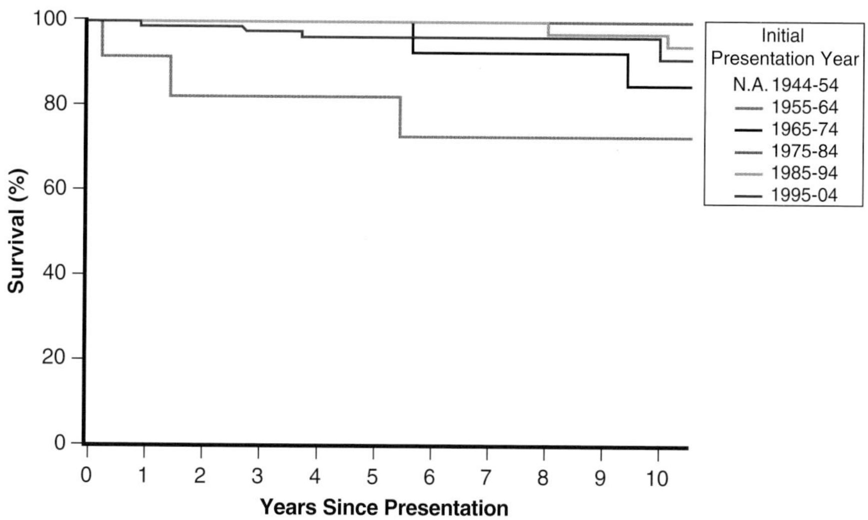

Fig. 26.7 Overall survival rates for 158 patients with local (SEER stage) differentiated thyroid carcinoma who were ≥45 years of age at diagnosis (1944–2004). Because of the very small number of individuals with local thyroid cancer seen from 1944 to 1954, data from this period were excluded. *N.A.* not applicable.

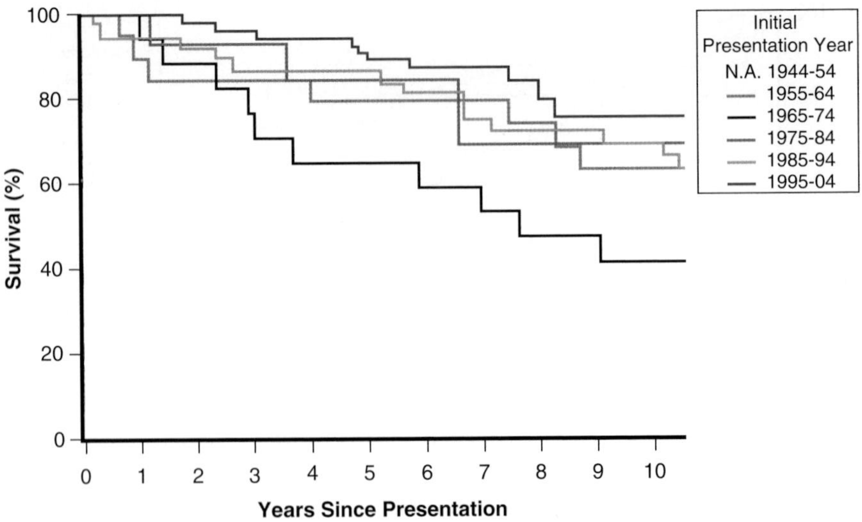

Fig. 26.8 Overall survival rates for 179 patients with regional (SEER stage) differentiated thyroid carcinoma who were ≥45 years of age at diagnosis (1944–2004). Because of the very small number of individuals with regional thyroid cancer seen from 1944 to 1954, data from this period were excluded. *N.A.* not applicable.

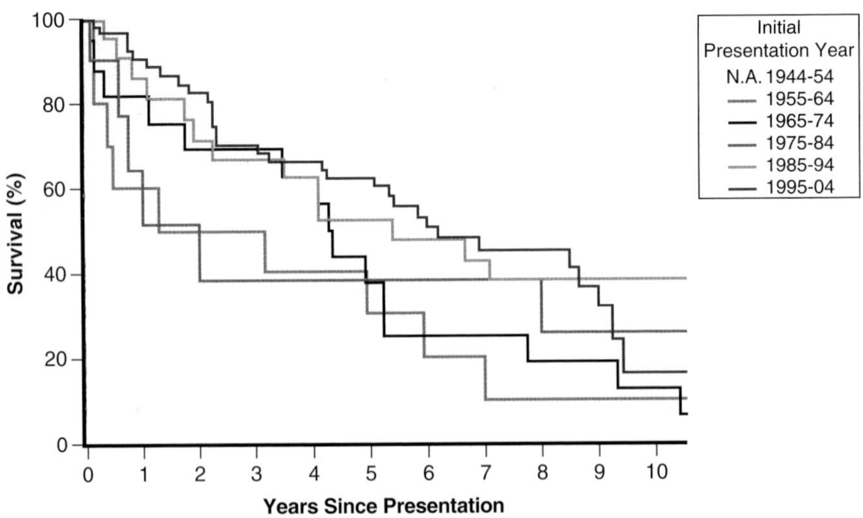

Fig. 26.9 Overall survival rates for 113 patients with distant (SEER stage) metastatic differentiated thyroid carcinoma who were ≥45 years of age at diagnosis (1944–2004). Because of the very small number of individuals with distant thyroid cancer seen from 1944 to 1954, data from this period were excluded. *N.A.* not applicable.

Current Management Approach

Our current multidisciplinary approach to treating patients with thyroid carcinoma is based on disease histology combined with disease extent and prognosis. Because death and morbidity can result from uncontrolled neck disease, even in patients with distant metastases, priority is also placed on interventions to prevent locoregional complications. Given the role of MD Anderson physicians in developing national consensus guidelines, there is extensive overlap between our disease-management approach and the approach recommended in the recently published national guidelines [7, 9, 10].

Patients with either DTC or MTC undergo comprehensive neck ultrasound as the primary staging procedure for locoregional disease [29]. Cross-sectional imaging with computed tomography or magnetic resonance imaging is indicated if grossly invasive disease is suspected or extensive regional metastases are appreciated on ultrasound. Although thyroid lobectomy with isthmusectomy is appropriate for patients with T1a N0 M0 DTC, we generally perform total thyroidectomy for most other patients with DTC and for all patients with MTC. A regional neck dissection should be performed if there is clinical, ultrasonographic, or intraoperative evidence of nodal involvement in the lateral neck compartments in patients with DTC, whereas a prophylactic central neck (level VI) dissection is generally performed along with the thyroidectomy in MTC patients and in those patients with DTC when central compartment nodal disease is noted intraoperatively. For patients with invasion of neck structures such as the esophagus, trachea, or strap muscles, more comprehensive resection of all gross disease should be performed whenever feasible while preserving and/or reconstructing structures to maintain functional voice and swallowing if possible.

The basis for selection of patients with DTC for adjuvant radioiodine continues to evolve. According to analyses from the National Thyroid Cancer Treatment Cooperative Study Group [15], improvements in overall survival are associated with adjuvant radioiodine treatment (also known as "remnant ablation") in the following patient groups:

- PTC in patients younger than 45 years, with tumor greater than 4 cm, or in the presence of macroscopic extrathyroidal extension
- PTC at age 45 years or older, with tumor of at least 1 cm, or in the presence of multifocal tumors, extrathyroidal extension, or metastases to locoregional nodes
- FTC in patients younger than 45 years, with tumor greater than 4 cm, or in the presence of macroscopic multifocality, macroscopic invasion of either the tumor capsule or extrathyroidal tissues, poor differentiation
- FTC at age 45 years or older

Despite the absence of specific analyses demonstrating improved outcomes, radioiodine treatment is also recommended for those patients with more aggressive variants, such as tall cell, columnar cell, insular, or poorly differentiated histologies. In addition, we consider radioiodine therapy for younger PTC patients with tumors less than 4 cm who demonstrate either microscopic extrathyroidal extension or cervical metastases, although no survival advantage was reported for this subgroup in this analysis. Patients with DTC and known residual or extracervical disease are also treated with higher therapeutic doses of radioiodine. Selection of the administered activity of 131-I is generally based on evaluation of tracer uptake on a diagnostic radioiodine scan performed several weeks after thyroidectomy, combined with the intraoperative and surgical pathology findings. Adjuvant external beam radiotherapy is considered only for those patients at very high risk of recurrent disease that would not be amenable to further organ-sparing surgical intervention.

Postoperative thyroid hormone therapy is necessary for both DTC and MTC patients to treat postsurgical hypothyroidism. In DTC patients, however, higher doses sufficient to suppress TSH levels are generally used initially to reduce the risk of disease recurrence or disease-related mortality. Concern for thyrotoxic complications provides a counterbalancing influence on the aggressiveness of therapy. For stage I and II disease, the serum TSH concentration should be at or slightly below the lower half of the reference range. However, for stage III and IV disease, the target concentration for serum TSH should be less than 0.1 mU/L. The presence of heart disease or low bone density may necessitate a lower level of TSH suppression with smaller doses of thyroid hormone. The dose also may be decreased in patients who remain disease-free for 5–10 years after primary therapy.

The treatment of metastatic DTC usually begins with high-dose radioiodine and is based on documentation of uptake on a pretherapy diagnostic scan. However, disease not visualized on a diagnostic scan is highly unlikely to receive a sufficiently effective radiation dose from therapy. In the setting of radioiodine-refractory disease, TSH-suppressive thyroid hormone therapy is sufficient to maintain asymptomatic stability or a minimal rate of progression in many patients. The development of symptomatic or bulky distant metastases, growing significantly over a 6- to 12-month interval, is an indication for consideration of systemic therapy, preferably within a clinical trial. Similar considerations for initiating systemic therapy are applied to patients with MTC, in whom radioiodine therapy has no beneficial role. Surgery, radiotherapy, cryotherapy, or other palliative localized interventions can be used to reduce symptoms secondary to bone or selected other distant metastases.

Management of ATC is rarely curative. Although surgery can occasionally completely resect small, localized ATC lesions, the high rate of recurrence justifies postoperative external beam radiotherapy. On the other hand, most patients do not benefit from cytoreductive surgery, and therefore the primary treatment is usually chemoradiation. Full course chemotherapy is generally initiated as soon as distant metastases are identified, but the prognosis remains quite bleak.

Further improvements in patient outcomes will require better approaches to the selection of appropriate patients and therapies. Improved prognostication should permit identification of patients who do not require initial treatments as aggressive as those currently used, thus reducing unnecessary risks and morbidity. At the other end of the disease spectrum, the development of more effective systemic therapies that target critical signaling pathways within these malignancies will lead to improved survival and reduced symptoms related to metastatic disease.

References

1. Siegel R, Naishadham D, Jemal A. Cancer statistics, 2012. CA Cancer J Clin. 2012;62: 10–29.
2. Altekruse SF, Kosary CL, Krapcho M, et al., editors. Seer cancer statistics review, 1975-2007. Bethesda: National Cancer Institute; 2010.
3. Kilfoy BA, Zheng T, Holford TR, et al. International patterns and trends in thyroid cancer incidence, 1973-2002. Cancer Causes Control. 2009;20:525–31.
4. Enewold L, Zhu K, Ron E, et al. Rising thyroid cancer incidence in the United States by demographic and tumor characteristics, 1980-2005. Cancer Epidemiol Biomarkers Prev. 2009;18:784–91.
5. Edge SB, Byrd DR, Compton CC, Fritz AG, Greene FL, Trotti III A, editors. AJCC cancer staging handbook. 7th ed. Chicago: American Joint Committee on Cancer; 2010.
6. Shambaugh EM, Weiss MA, Axtell LM, editors. The 1977 Summary staging guide for the Cancer Surveillance, Epidemiology and End Results Reporting Program. Bethesda, MD: National Cancer Institute, SEER Program; 1977.
7. Kloos RT, Eng C, Evans DB, et al. Medullary thyroid cancer: management guidelines of the American Thyroid Association. Thyroid. 2009;19:565–612.
8. Gilliland FD, Hunt WC, Morris DM, Key CR. Prognostic factors for thyroid carcinoma: a population-based study of 15,698 cases from the Surveillance, Epidemiology and End Results (SEER) program 1973-1991. Cancer. 1997;79:564–73.
9. National Comprehensive Cancer Network. NCCN clinical practice guidelines in oncology: thyroid carcinoma. Updated 2010. http://www.nccn.org/professionals/physician_gls/PDF/thyroid.pdf. Accessed 15 Sep 2010.
10. Cooper DS, Doherty GM, Haugen BR, et al. Revised American Thyroid Association management guidelines for patients with thyroid nodules and differentiated thyroid cancer. Thyroid. 2009;19:1167–214.
11. Clark Jr RL, White EC, Russell WO. Total thyroidectomy for cancer of the thyroid: significance of intraglandular dissemination. Ann Surg. 1959;149:858–66.
12. Rose RG, Kelsey MP, Russell WO, Ibanez ML, White EC, Clark RL. Follow-up study of thyroid cancer treated by unilateral lobectomy. Am J Surg. 1963;106:494–500.
13. Clark RL, Ibanez ML, White EC. What constitutes an adequate operation for carcinoma of the thyroid? Arch Surg. 1966;92:23–6.
14. Samaan NA, Maheshwari YK, Nader S, et al. Impact of therapy for differentiated carcinoma of the thyroid: an analysis of 706 cases. J Clin Endocrinol Metab. 1983;56:1131–8.
15. Jonklaas J, Sarlis NJ, Litofsky D, et al. Outcomes of patients with differentiated thyroid carcinoma following initial therapy. Thyroid. 2006;16:1229–42.
16. Saad MF, Ordonez NG, Rashid RK, et al. Medullary carcinoma of the thyroid: a study of the clinical features and prognostic factors in 161 patients. Medicine. 1984;63:319–42.
17. Evans DB, Fleming JB, Lee JE, Cote G, Gagel RF. The surgical treatment of medullary thyroid carcinoma. Semin Surg Oncol. 1999;16:50–63.
18. Kouvaraki MA, Shapiro SE, Perrier ND, et al. *RET* proto-oncogene: a review and update of genotype-phenotype correlations in hereditary medullary thyroid cancer and associated endocrine tumors. Thyroid. 2005;15:531–44.
19. Schwartz DL, Lobo MJ, Ang KK, et al. Postoperative external beam radiotherapy for differentiated thyroid cancer: outcomes and morbidity with conformal treatment. Int J Radiat Oncol Biol Phys. 2009;74:1083–91.
20. Schwartz DL, Rana V, Shaw S, et al. Postoperative radiotherapy for advanced medullary thyroid cancer-Local disease control in the modern era. Head Neck. 2008;30:883–8.
21. Gottlieb JA, Hill Jr CS. Chemotherapy of thyroid cancer with adriamycin: experience with 30 patients. N Engl J Med. 1974;290:193–7.
22. Sherman SI. Advances in chemotherapy of differentiated epithelial and medullary thyroid cancers. J Clin Endocrinol Metab. 2009;94:1493–9.

23. Cabanillas ME, Waguespack SG, Bronstein Y, et al. Treatment with tyrosine kinase inhibitors for patients with differentiated thyroid cancer: the MD Anderson experience. J Clin Endocrinol Metab. 2010;95:2588–95.
24. Chen AY, Jemal A, Ward EM. Increasing incidence of differentiated thyroid cancer in the United States, 1988-2005. Cancer. 2009;115:3801–7.
25. Wohllk N, Cote GJ, Evans DB, Goepfert H, Ordonez NG, Gagel RF. Application of genetic screening information to the management of medullary thyroid carcinoma and multiple endocrine neoplasia type 2. Endocrinol Metab Clin North Am. 1996;25:1–25.
26. Roman S, Lin R, Sosa JA. Prognosis of medullary thyroid carcinoma: demographic, clinical, and pathologic predictors of survival in 1252 cases. Cancer. 2006;107:2134–42.
27. Kebebew E, Greenspan FS, Clark OH, Woeber KA, McMillan A. Anaplastic thyroid carcinoma. Treatment outcome and prognostic factors. Cancer. 2005;103:1330–5.
28. Feinstein AR, Sosin DM, Wells CK. The Will Rogers phenomenon. Stage migration and new diagnostic techniques as a source of misleading statistics for survival in cancer. N Engl J Med. 1985;312:1604–8.
29. Kouvaraki MA, Shapiro SE, Fornage BD, et al. Role of preoperative ultrasonography in the surgical management of patients with thyroid cancer. Surgery. 2003;134:946–54.

Chapter 27
Soft Tissue Sarcomas

Vinod Ravi, Raphael Pollock, and Shreyaskumar R. Patel

Introduction

Soft tissue sarcomas are a group of tumors that arise from any extraskeletal nonepithelial tissue, including adipose and fibrous tissues, as well as muscle, tendon, nerve, lymphatic, and vascular tissues. Hence, these neoplasms are heterogeneous in nature, and although they are generally classified histopathogically according to the tissue they most resemble, such classification is difficult (and in some cases impossible) because of the tendency of tumors to lose histologic differentiation [1]. The World Health Organization classification of tumors currently lists more than 50 different histopathologic subtypes of soft tissue sarcomas [2]. Soft tissue sarcomas are also rare. Of the more than 1.5 million cancers expected to be diagnosed in the USA in 2010, The American Cancer Society expects only 10,520 of them to be soft tissue sarcomas. Of the more than 500,000 expected cancer deaths, about 3,920 will be from this cancer [3]. The heterogeneity of these tumors poses both a diagnostic and therapeutic challenge, especially in the setting of a rare disease.

Because the tissues from which these tumors arise are distributed throughout the body, the tumors can arise in any anatomic location. Most (60%) are seen in the extremities, and 10% occur in the head and neck. Another 30% of these neoplasms are found in the torso, including retroperitoneal and intra-abdominal tumors, where they can grow extensively before causing symptoms and are therefore often associated with delayed diagnosis [4].

V. Ravi (✉) • S.R. Patel
Department of Sarcoma Medical Oncology, The University of Texas MD Anderson Cancer Center, 1515 Holcombe Blvd, Unit 450, Houston, TX 77025, USA
e-mail: vravi@mdanderson.org

R. Pollock
Department of Surgical Oncology, The University of Texas MD Anderson Cancer Center, Houston, TX, USA

M.A. Rodriguez et al. (eds.), *60 Years of Survival Outcomes at The University of Texas MD Anderson Cancer Center*, DOI 10.1007/978-1-4614-5197-6_27,

Historical Perspective

Management of Nonmetastatic Disease

In the absence of metastasis, surgical resection has been and remains the standard of care in the management of soft tissue sarcomas. From a historical standpoint, large soft tissue sarcomas arising in the extremities managed by local surgical excision resulted in high recurrence rates (30–60%). For this reason, radical compartmental excisions or amputations were performed in an attempt to achieve better local control, which successfully brought down recurrence rates to 5–20%, albeit at the expense of functional outcomes [1].

Subsequently, these radical procedures for tumor management were replaced by limb-sparing procedures that incorporated radiotherapy and chemotherapy. The first randomized clinical trial that incorporated multidisciplinary care in the treatment of patients with extremity sarcoma was a phase 3 trial that enrolled patients with high-grade soft tissue sarcoma to receive amputation or limb-sparing resection plus adjuvant radiotherapy, with both groups receiving adjuvant chemotherapy. Disease-free survival rates at 5 years were equivalent in both groups; therefore, clinical practice changed from amputation to multidisciplinary care that incorporated limb-sparing surgery, with comparable outcomes [2]. Over time, with the use of multimodality treatment strategies, amputation rates have decreased to less than 10%, with limb-sparing treatment predominating in the majority of patients [3]. Surgery is also integral to the management of localized soft tissue sarcomas occurring in other parts of the body. Historically, dissection along the tumor pseudocapsule (enucleation or "shelling out") has been associated with local recurrence in one-third to two-thirds of patients. On the other hand, wide local excision with a margin of normal tissue around the lesion has resulted in local recurrence rates of 10–31%.

The role of radiotherapy in the treatment of patients with resectable disease was well illustrated by Yang et al. [4] when they randomized 91 patients with high-grade extremity lesions following limb-sparing surgery to receive adjuvant chemotherapy alone or concurrent chemotherapy and radiotherapy. In the same trial, 50 patients with low-grade sarcomas were also randomized to receive adjuvant radiotherapy or no further treatment after limb-sparing surgery. The local control rate for those who received radiotherapy was 99% compared with 70% in the non-radiotherapy group, with similar results in the low-grade and high-grade tumors. Pisters et al. evaluated the role of adjuvant brachytherapy in a randomized trial of 126 cases who were randomized to receive surgery alone or surgery followed by brachytherapy. Local control rates were 70% in the surgery-alone group but were 91% in the brachytherapy group. Both of these clinical trials showed the significant role of radiotherapy along with surgery in the treatment of nonmetastatic soft tissue sarcoma.

The role of adjuvant chemotherapy in the treatment of resectable soft tissue sarcomas has been investigated by several individual clinical trials, and in 1997, a meta-analysis of 14 individual trials was conducted to further investigate outcomes in a larger sample of patients. Results of the meta-analysis showed improved local and distant recurrence-free survival but failed to show a difference in overall survival except in the subset of extremity sarcomas. Modern-day adjuvant chemotherapy for soft tissue sarcomas of the extremity incorporates a combination of an anthracycline with ifosfamide. The utility of this approach was best demonstrated in a randomized clinical trial by an Italian Sarcoma Study Group who showed that the combination of ifosfamide and epirubicin with growth factor support resulted in a median disease-free survival duration of 48 months in patients who received chemotherapy as opposed to 16 months in the control group. Median overall survival was 75 months for patients who received chemotherapy but was 46 months for those who received no chemotherapy [5]. With longer follow-up (median, 7.5 years), the distant metastases-free survival curves have shown convergence, suggesting some loss of chemotherapy benefit over time and the need for better agents with a curative potential [6].

Unresectable Soft Tissue Sarcoma

MD Anderson Cancer Center has played a pivotal role in the development of chemotherapeutic options for soft tissue sarcoma. Doxorubicin, the single most effective and widely used drug in the treatment of soft tissue sarcomas, was first used to treat soft tissue sarcomas [7] at this institution in 1971. Subsequently, results from clinical trials at MD Anderson in 1972 showed that the combination of doxorubicin and dacarbazine was effective in the treatment of sarcomas [8]. This combination continues to be used in the treatment of leiomyosarcomas and other unresectable/metastatic soft tissue sarcomas. The addition of cyclophosphamide to the doxorubicin/dacarbazine combination was investigated in a phase III Southwestern Oncology Group (SWOG) trial that failed to demonstrate any significant differences in response rates [9]. Superiority of ifosfamide over cyclophosphamide was suggested by a phase 2 randomized study of the two agents that showed a higher response rate for patients treated with ifosfamide [10]. This subsequently led to the deletion of dacarbazine, a weak agent with overlapping myelosuppression, and the adoption of combined dose-intense doxorubicin and ifosfamide as the standard for treatment of adult soft tissue sarcomas [11].

The MD Anderson Cancer Center Experience

The data set used for this discussion was derived from a total of 6,907 patients who presented at MD Anderson with soft tissue sarcomas between 1944 and 2004. Excluding those with other primary cancers and those who were treated elsewhere prior to presentation here, our data set included 1,382 patients who received their initial definitive treatment at this institution. Survival data were calculated from initial presentation.

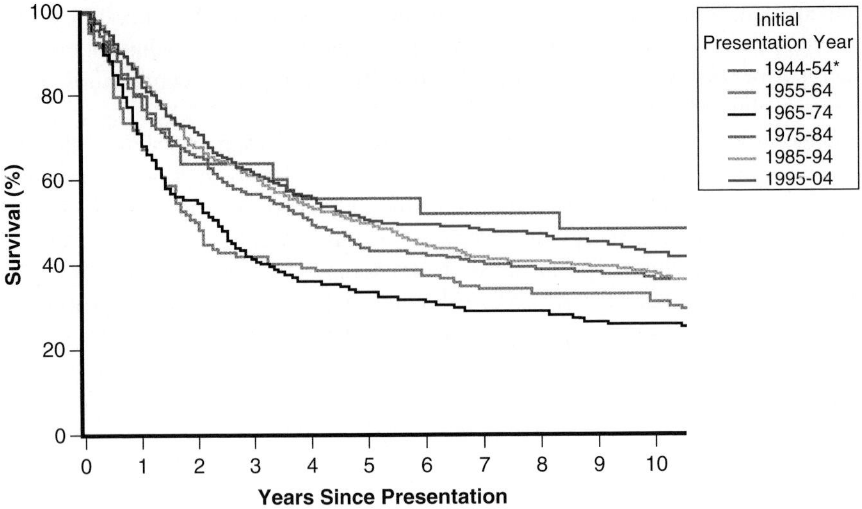

Fig. 27.1 Overall survival rates for patients with soft tissue sarcoma (1944–2004) ($P<0.0001$, log-rank test for trend). *Note: 88% of 1944–1954 patients had local-stage disease.

Table 27.1 Kaplan–Meier overall survival

Decade	Percent survival	
Year	5 years	10 years
1944–1954[a]	56.5	48.0
1955–1964	38.5	31.3
1965–1974	33.6	25.7
1975–1984	43.7	36.5
1985–1994	49.8	38.1
1995–2004	50.4	42.7

[a]88% of 1944–1954 patients had local-stage disease.

The overall survival trends reflected in Fig. 27.1 and Table 27.1 indicate improvements in both 5- and 10-year survival rates over the 60-year time span. During the 1944–1954 timeframe, overall survival was higher than in any of the following decades, most likely a function of the small sample size and a larger proportion of localized disease (88%) during that period. From 1965 to 1974, we see a lower (rather than higher) overall survival rate than that of the preceding decade. This difference in trend may be explained by a higher proportion of patients with metastatic disease during that time period. Interestingly, among patients with metastatic disease, there is a marked increase in the percentage of patients surviving 5 years: from 6.7% in

Table 27.2 Kaplan–Meier survival by SEER stage

	Percent survival by SEER stage					
	Local (years)		Regional (years)		Distant (years)	
Year	5	10	5	10	5	10
1944–1954	59.1	50.0	NA	NA	NA	NA
1955–1964	56.5	47.7	38.6	28.3	4.8	0.0
1965–1974	50.5	38.9	29.6	18.5	6.7	6.7
1975–1984	61.8	52.6	39.2	33.5	11.5	8.2
1985–1994	69.7	54.2	45.0	35.1	13.7	6.8
1995–2004	68.3	57.6	51.0	44.5	14.4	10.9

SEER Surveillance, Epidemiology, and End Results program

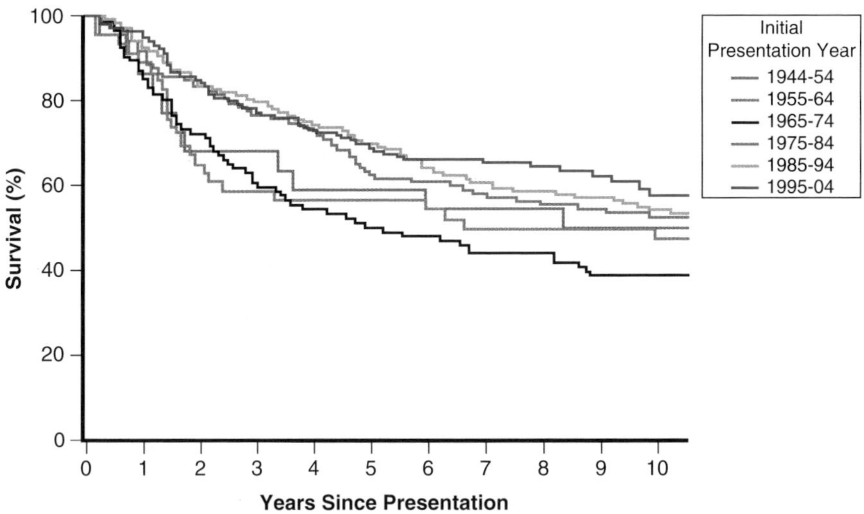

Fig. 27.2 Survival rates for patients with local (SEER stage) soft tissue sarcoma (1944–2004) ($P=0.049$, log-rank test for trend).

1965–1974 to 11.5% in 1975–1984. The latter period saw a sharp increase in the use of systemic treatment options for the management of metastatic disease such as doxorubicin, whereas effective chemotherapy options were virtually absent before 1975 (Table 27.2) (Figs. 27.2, 27.3, and 27.4).

Finally, there are other treatment advances that should not go unmentioned: even though they did not increase survival, they significantly affected its quality. These include limb-sparing surgical techniques, palliative radiation, and surgery to relieve symptoms, and better management of adverse effects from chemotherapy and radiotherapy.

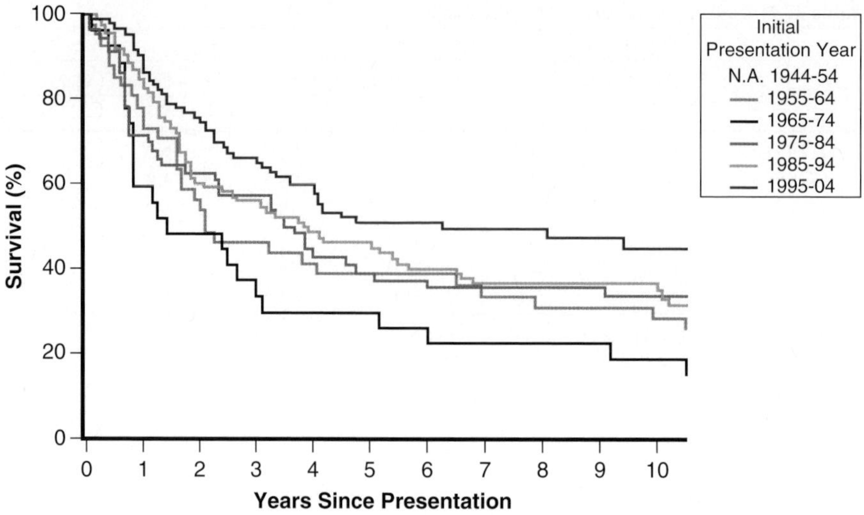

Fig. 27.3 Survival rates for patients with regional (SEER stage) soft tissue sarcoma (1944–2004) ($P=0.025$, log-rank test for trend). Because no individuals with regional soft tissue sarcoma were seen from 1944 to 1954, data from this period were excluded. *N.A.* not applicable.

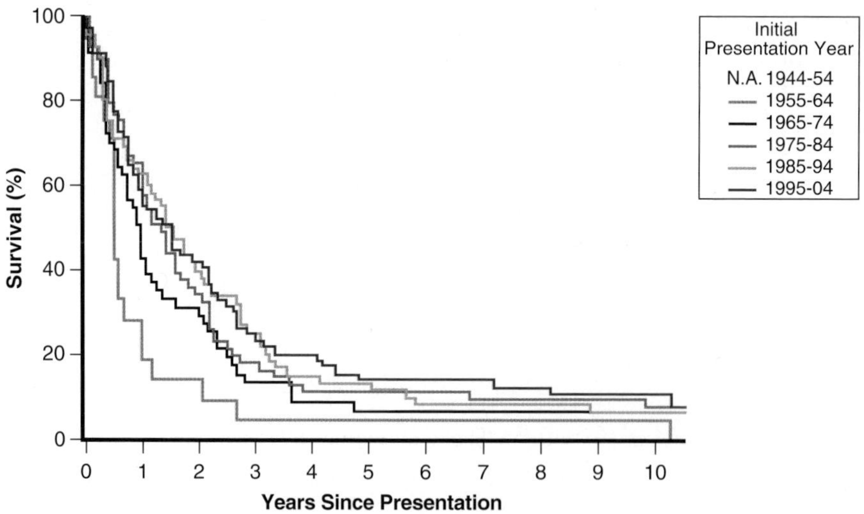

Fig. 27.4 Survival rates for patients with distant (SEER stage) soft tissue sarcoma (1944–2004) ($P=0.014$, log-rank test for trend). Because of the very small number of individuals with distant soft tissue sarcoma seen from 1944 to 1954, data from this period were excluded. *N.A.* not applicable.

Current Management Approach

The National Comprehensive Cancer Network (NCCN) currently publishes standard treatment guidelines for four broad categories of soft tissue sarcoma: tumors of the extremity or trunk, retroperitoneal or intra-abdominal tumors, gastrointestinal stromal tumors, and desmoid tumors. This is a disease for which there are many histologic variants, a myriad of anatomic manifestations, and pathologic tumor grades that pose greater risks than others in terms of advancement or metastasis.

Given this complexity, it is possible to state generally that for most patients, the definitive treatment is surgery (when the tumors are resectable), and chemotherapy and radiotherapy may be used singly or in combination as adjuncts either preoperatively or postoperatively. In general, our approach to all of these tumors relies on multidisciplinary assessment of the risk posed by both the tumor and treatment.

For low-grade sarcomas, the risk of metastatic disease is considered to be low and they are primarily managed by surgery with or without radiotherapy. High-grade sarcomas larger than 5 cm have a higher likelihood of micrometastases; therefore, a multidisciplinary approach incorporating chemotherapy and preoperative radiotherapy followed by surgery is often necessary. Since there is considerable variability in the response to chemotherapy within various histologic subtypes, preoperative chemotherapy is preferred because it enables assessment of the patient's disease response to treatment. On the other hand, the effectiveness of postoperative adjuvant chemotherapy is almost impossible to determine in real time because of the absence of any visible disease to follow. Sarcomas that fall into the intermediate-grade category tend to metastasize later in their course and often merit systemic therapy if larger than 8–10 cm. In this category, risk of recurrence and risk of chemotherapy have to be weighed carefully before finalizing the plan of care.

For patients with advanced or metastatic disease, systemic therapy becomes the primary modality for treatment. These patients may qualify for surgical procedures with curative intent, depending on the response to chemotherapy, extent of disease, and durability of the response to systemic therapy. For the most part, surgery and radiotherapy in a patient with uncontrolled metastatic disease have only a palliation role in treating tumor-related symptoms.

We expect these approaches to bring continued improvement in survival and quality of life for patients with soft tissue sarcomas. More significant improvements in survival will depend on continued research in the following areas:

- Identification of genomic and proteomic aberrations in soft tissue sarcomas that would help us understand the key pathogenic pathways that drive these rare tumors.
- Identification of targeted drugs and drug combinations that specifically inhibit the key pathogenic pathways.

The use of imatinib in patients with gastrointestinal stromal tumors (GISTs) is an excellent example of how application of the above-mentioned principles results in improved survival. Gastrointestinal stromal tumors are generally resistant to conventional chemotherapy, and before the advent of imatinib had an extremely poor clinical course. Identification of the key molecular aberration in GISTs, i.e., activating a mutation in the *KIT* or *PDGFRA* gene, was a critical step in developing effective therapies for this tumor. We hope that application of similar principles in other sarcoma subtypes will result in treatments that are specific and highly effective while limiting adverse effects to a minimum.

References

1. Shiu M, Castro E, Hajdu S, et al. Surgical treatment of 297 soft tissue sarcomas of the lower extremity. Ann Surg. 1975;182:597–602.
2. Rosenberg S, Tepper J, Glatstein E, et al. The treatment of soft-tissue sarcomas of the extremities: prospective randomized evaluations of (1) limb-sparing surgery plus radiation therapy compared with amputation and (2) the role of adjuvant chemotherapy. Ann Surg. 1982;196: 305–15.
3. Milliard W, Hajdu S, Casper E, et al. Comparison of amputation with limb-sparing operations for adult soft tissue sarcoma of the extremity. Ann Surg. 1992;215:269–75.
4. Yang JC, Chang AE, Baker AR, et al. Randomized prospective study of the benefit of adjuvant radiation therapy in the treatment of soft tissue sarcomas of the extremity. J Clin Oncol. 1998;16:197–203.
5. Frustaci S, Gherlinzoni F, De Paoli A, et al. Adjuvant chemotherapy for adult soft tissue sarcomas of the extremities and girdles: results of the Italian randomized cooperative trial. J Clin Oncol. 2001;19:1238–47.
6. Frustaci S, De Paoli A, Bidoli E, et al. Ifosfamide in the adjuvant therapy of soft tissue sarcomas. Oncol. 2003;65 Suppl 2:80–4.
7. Middleman E, Luce J, Frei III E. Clinical trials with adriamycin. Cancer. 1971;28:844–50.
8. Gottlieb JA, Baker LH, Quagliana JM, et al. Chemotherapy of sarcomas with a combination of adriamycin and dimethyl triazeno imidazole carboxamide. Cancer. 1972;30:1632–8.
9. Baker LH, Frank J, Fine G, et al. Combination chemotherapy using adriamycin, DTIC, cyclophosphamide, and actinomycin D for advanced soft tissue sarcomas: a randomized comparative trial. A phase III, Southwest Oncology Group Study (7613). J Clin Oncol. 1987;5: 851–61.
10. Bramwell VH, Mouridsen HT, Santoro A, et al. Cyclophosphamide versus ifosfamide: final report of a randomized phase II trial in adult soft tissue sarcomas. Eur J Cancer Clin Oncol. 1987;23:311–21.
11. Patel SR, Vadhan-Raj S, Burgess MA, et al. Results of two consecutive trials of dose-intensive chemotherapy with doxorubicin and ifosfamide in patients with sarcomas. Am J Clin Oncol. 1998;21:317–21.

Chapter 28
Sarcomas of Bone

Valerae Lewis

Introduction

Sarcomas of bone are a rare and diverse set of tumors that, although related in their primary location (bone), vary in their etiology, behavior, and treatment. In 2011, approximately 2,890 new cases of bone and joint cancers were diagnosed in the USA. Osteosarcoma, chondrosarcoma, and Ewing sarcoma are the most common primary tumors of bone, representing 30%, 15%, and 6%, respectively, of all bone sarcomas. The remainder of bone sarcomas are made up of malignant fibrous histiocytoma, chordoma, adamantinoma, hemangioendothelioma, hemangiopericytoma, and low-grade fibrosarcoma of the bone.

This review will concentrate on advances in treatment for osteosarcoma and Ewing sarcoma at The University of Texas MD Anderson Cancer Center because the treatment algorithms and oncologic outcomes of these two tumors have undergone significant evolution and improvement over the years (Figs. 28.1, 28.2, 28.3, 28.4, 28.5, 28.6, 28.7, and 28.8). However, for chondrosarcoma of the bone, neither the treatment algorithm (surgery-based) nor the oncologic outcome has significantly changed over the years [1].

V. Lewis (✉)
Department of Orthopaedic Oncology, The University of Texas MD
Anderson Cancer Center, 1400 Pressler St., Unit 1448, Houston, TX 77030, USA
e-mail: volewis@mdanderson.org

M.A. Rodriguez et al. (eds.), *60 Years of Survival Outcomes at The University of Texas MD Anderson Cancer Center*, DOI 10.1007/978-1-4614-5197-6_28,

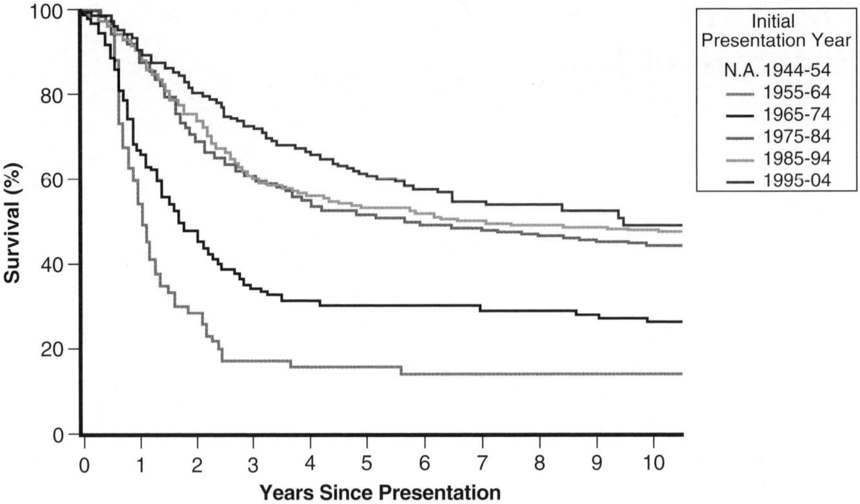

Fig. 28.1 Overall survival rates for patients with osteosarcoma (1944–2004) ($P<0.0001$, log-rank test for trend). Because of the very small number of individuals with osteosarcoma seen from 1944 to 1954, data from this period were excluded. *N.A.* not applicable.

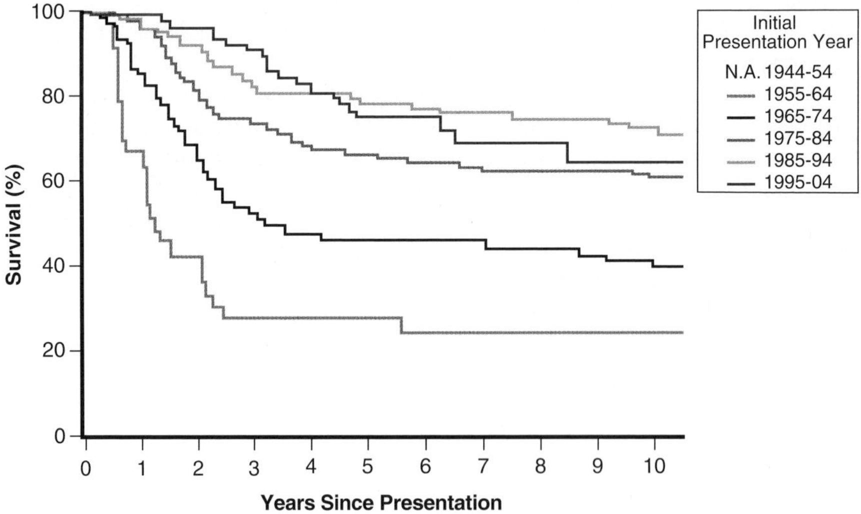

Fig. 28.2 Survival rates for patients with local (SEER stage) osteosarcoma (1944–2004) ($P<0.0001$, log-rank test for trend). Because of the very small number of individuals with local osteosarcoma seen from 1944 to 1954, data from this period were excluded. *N.A.* not applicable.

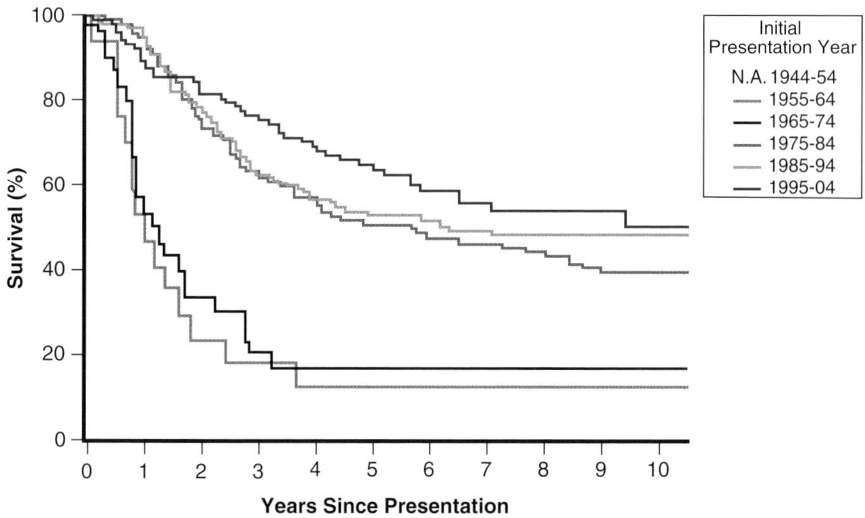

Fig. 28.3 Survival rates for patients with regional (SEER stage) osteosarcoma (1944–2004) (P<0.0001, log-rank test for trend). Because of the very small number of individuals with regional osteosarcoma seen from 1944 to 1954, data from this period were excluded. *N.A.* not applicable.

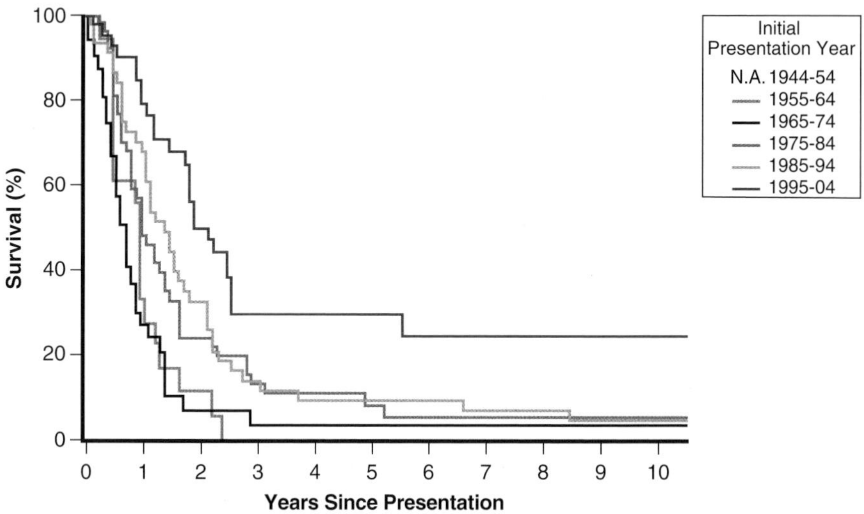

Fig. 28.4 Survival rates for patients with distant (SEER stage) osteosarcoma (1944–2004) (P<0.0001, log-rank test for trend). Because of the very small number of individuals with distant osteosarcoma seen from 1944 to 1954, data from this period were excluded. *N.A.* not applicable.

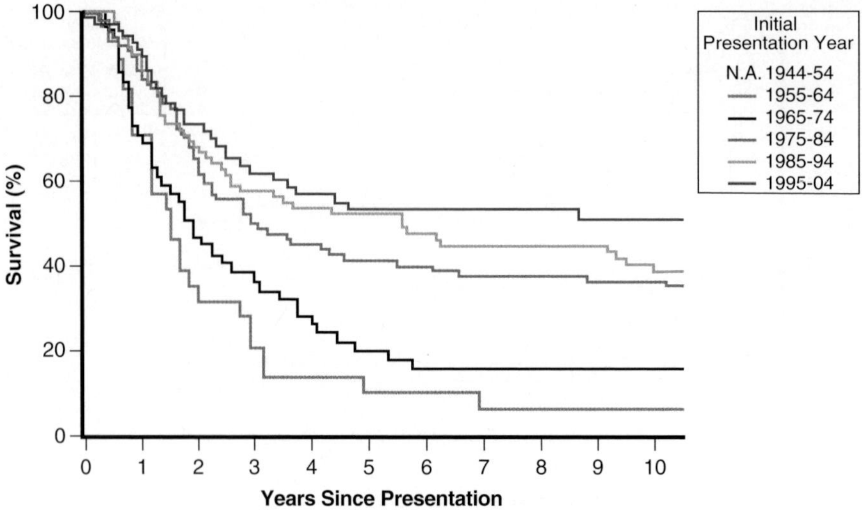

Fig. 28.5 Overall survival rates for patients with Ewing sarcoma (1944–2004) ($P<0.0001$, log-rank test for trend). Because of the very small number of individuals with Ewing sarcoma seen from 1944 to 1954, data from this period were excluded. *N.A.* not applicable.

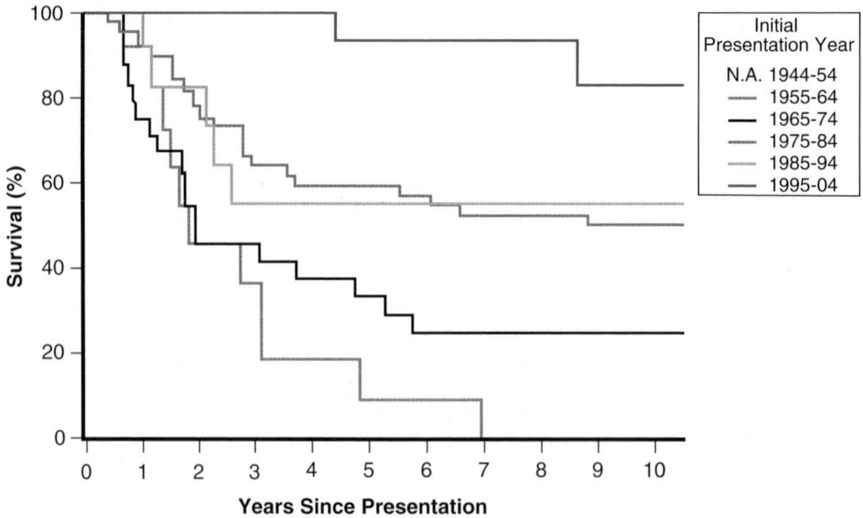

Fig. 28.6 Survival rates for patients with local (SEER stage) Ewing sarcoma (1944–2004) ($P<0.0001$, log-rank test for trend). Because of the very small number of individuals with local Ewing sarcoma seen from 1944 to 1954, data from this period were excluded. *N.A.* not applicable.

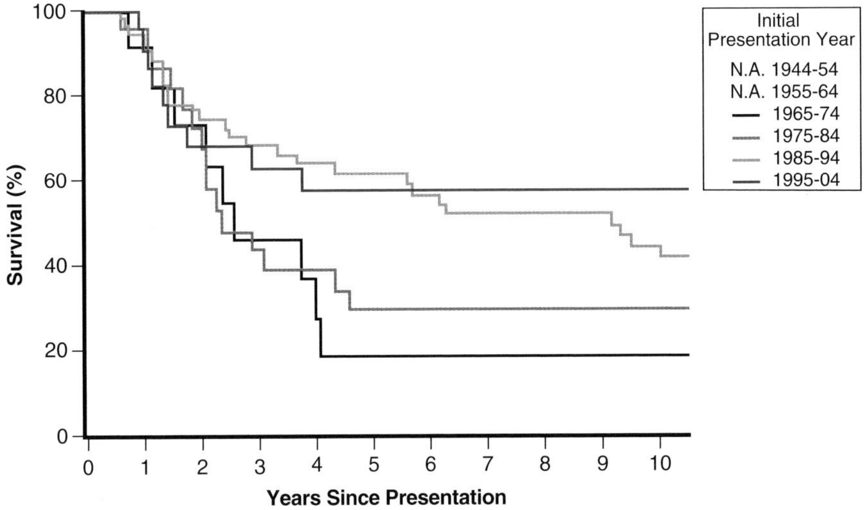

Fig. 28.7 Survival rates for patients with regional (SEER stage) Ewing sarcoma (1944–2004) ($P=0.065$, log-rank test for trend). Because of the very small number of individuals with regional Ewing sarcoma seen from 1944 to 1954 and from 1955 to 1964, data from these periods were excluded. *N.A.* not applicable.

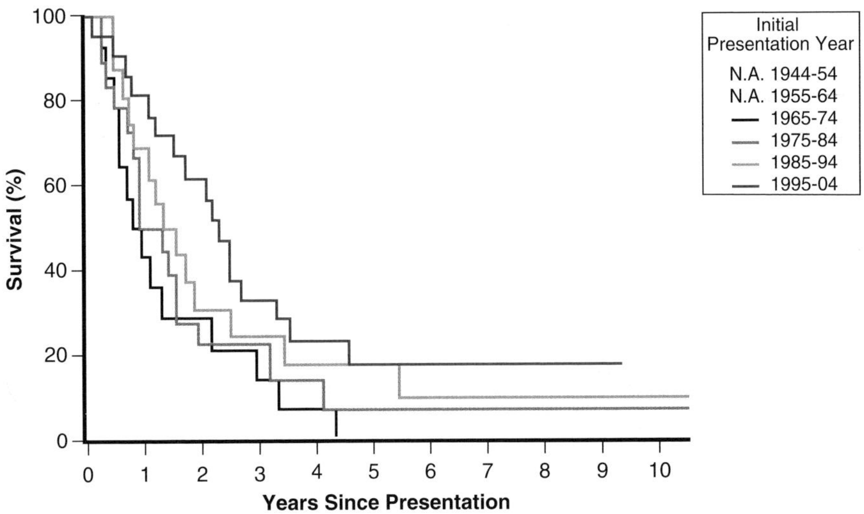

Fig. 28.8 Survival rates for patients with distant (SEER stage) Ewing sarcoma (1944–2004) ($P=0.017$, log-rank test for trend). Because of the very small number of individuals with distant Ewing sarcoma seen from 1944 to 1954 and from 1955 to 1964, data from these periods were excluded. *N.A.* not applicable.

Osteosarcoma

Historical Perspective

Osteosarcoma is the most common primary malignant tumor of bone [2, 3]. The incidence of osteosarcoma has not changed in recent years. Approximately 900 new cases are diagnosed each year in the USA, of which 400 arise in children and adolescents younger than 20 years of age [4, 5]. Osteosarcoma, rare in children younger than 5 years, has a bimodal age distribution, with one peak in adolescence and a second peak in the seventh to eighth decade. Osteosarcomas generally occur in children during the years of rapid growth (most commonly at ages 13–16 years) and in the areas of rapid growth (most commonly in the metaphysis of long bones, especially distal femur, proximal tibia, and proximal humerus). For unknown reasons, osteosarcoma in children is more common in males than in females, and the incidence is slightly higher in African Americans than in Caucasians [6]. However, osteosarcoma in adults is as common in males as in females and is more common in Caucasians than in African Americans.

Most cases of osteosarcoma are sporadic. However, several predisposing factors have been identified including prior irradiation and several genetic conditions, including retinoblastoma, Li–Fraumeni syndrome, Rothmund–Thomson syndrome, Bloom syndrome, and Werner syndromes. In these circumstances, obtaining a thorough medical history is a very important component to staging and workup.

Staging

Obtaining two orthogonal radiographs of the entire bone is the first step in the workup. Magnetic resonance imaging (MRI) of the entire bone defines the intraosseous extent of the tumor as well as the soft tissue extension and the relationship of the tumor to the neurovascular bundle and the joint. A bone scan is taken to evaluate the entire skeleton for the presence of metastatic disease or skip lesions. Computed tomography (CT) of the chest is used to evaluate the thorax, the most common location of metastatic disease. Positron emission tomography (PET)/CT is becoming more popular and has been helpful in assessing the response of the tumor to treatment. However, several studies have noted that the ability of PET/CT for detecting pulmonary metastases and other osseous lesions in the skeleton may be inferior to the imaging capabilities of spiral CT of the chest and bone scan.

To classify osteosarcomas, the staging system first developed by Enneking, the Musculoskeletal Tumor Society staging system (Table 28.1) [7], is used most commonly. This system classifies tumors by grade (low-grade versus high-grade) and location (intracompartmental versus extracompartmental). The most common presentation of osteosarcomas is at stage IIB.

Table 28.1 Musculoskeletal Tumor Society staging system

Stage	Description
I	Low grade
A	Intracompartmental
B	Extracompartmental
II	High grade
A	Intracompartmental
B	Extracompartmental
III	Distal metastases
A	Intracompartmental
B	Extracompartmental

Osteosarcomas are bone-forming tumors. Histologically, osteosarcomas can be classified as conventional and then subclassified according to the predominant cellular component (osteoblastic, fibroblastic, or chondroblastic), according to location (parosteal or periosteoteal), by varying histology (small cell or telangiectactic), or by predisposing factors (post-radiation sarcoma or Paget sarcoma). The oncologic outcome varies, depending on grade and histologic subtype.

Historically, the prognosis for patients with osteosarcoma was bleak. Surgery alone, which in most cases was amputation, resulted in a 5-year survival rate of 20%. Micrometastases are presumed to be present at diagnosis in most patients. This was based on the fact that despite achieving local control, 80% of patients with osteosarcoma treated with surgery alone developed metastatic disease. Chemotherapy has the potential to eradicate microscopic disease. With the advent and implementation of modern chemotherapy, 5-year survival rates improved significantly [8, 9]. The treatment of osteosarcoma became multidisciplinary, consisting chemotherapy and surgery. Two randomized trials by Link et al. [10] and Eilber et al. [11] demonstrated the benefits of adjuvant chemotherapy in patients presenting with localized high-grade osteosarcoma compared with surgery alone.

The concept of neoadjuvant chemotherapy was first proposed by Rosen and Nirenberg [12]. Neoadjuvant chemotherapy allows one to define prognostic groups on the basis of tumor response. It can also decrease the size of the tumor and facilitate resection. In addition, from a technical and functional standpoint, preoperative chemotherapy allows time for operative planning and the construction of custom megaprostheses (if needed). Although most endoprostheses are now modular, and readily available, this time delay to surgery from diagnosis was particularly helpful in the early stages of limb salvage surgery. Thus, chemotherapy not only improved survival but also facilitated the advent of and advances in limb salvage surgery.

Although adjuvant chemotherapy is now standard in the treatment of osteosarcoma, the choice of regimen (drug algorithm) and route of administration remain controversial. Chemotherapy can be given intra-arterially or intravenously. Intra-arterial (IA) administration was first reported by Mavligit et al. [13] in 1981. The theory is that IA administration increases the concentration of chemotherapy at the site of the primary tumor but that healthy tissues receive lower chemotherapeutic doses. Studies have shown that when comparing drug levels after IA chemotherapy versus intravenous (IV) administration, the levels were equivalent in the peripheral blood but were two to five times higher in the draining vein of an arterially infused area [14]. Surgically, tumors that have received IA chemotherapy tend to have a thick fibrotic rind. However, no significant difference in overall survival has been noted between IA and IV chemotherapy. Jaffe et al. [15] used IA cisplatin (CDDP) (150 mg/m^2) as a single agent every 2–3 weeks and reported that 16 of 42 patients had at least 90% tumor necrosis; in another study, Jaffe and colleagues [16] compared IA cisplatin with IV high-dose methotrexate as primary treatment for osteosarcoma and found that the response rate of patients treated with IA cisplatin was higher ($P=0.065$) than that of patients treated with high-dose methotrexate (60% versus 27%). Intra-arterial chemotherapy became the standard for treatment of adult and pediatric osteosarcoma at MD Anderson in 1980 and has continued to be the standard in the adult setting.

The MD Anderson Cancer Center Experience: Osteosarcoma

The MD Anderson data set was derived from 3,869 patients who presented between 1944 and 2004 with sarcoma of bone. Of these patients, 2,339 had no previous treatment, and 2,078 received definitive treatment at MD Anderson Cancer Center. Of this total group, 1,043 patients had a diagnosis of osteosarcoma. As expected, the majority of those who presented with osteosarcoma had high-grade intramedullary osteosarcoma.

The survival curves in Figs. 28.1, 28.2, 28.3, 28.4, 28.5, 28.6, 28.7, and 28.8 represent the clinical outcomes for patients who received definitive treatment for osteosarcoma or Ewing sarcoma at MD Anderson.

There has been significant improvement in outcome of osteosarcoma over the past 60 years, which is reflected in our data by significant improvement in 5-year survival rates: from 0% to 61.3%. As seen in other published data, at least two-thirds of children, adolescents, and adults younger than age 40 years with nonmetastatic extremity osteosarcomas who received current chemotherapy regimens will be long-term survivors [17]. This is also reflected in our data by the significant improvement in 5-year survival rates in patients with local disease: from 0% to 74.5% (Fig. 28.2).

However, as our data reflect, the outcome of patients with metastatic disease, although improving over time, is less optimal. Only 35–40% of patients with pulmonary metastases are cured with multimodality therapy, and long-term survival is less than 20% for patients who present with overt disease or develop metastatic disease after initiation of treatment.

The survival curves for patients with localized disease demonstrate little improvement in 5-year outcome (78.3% versus 74.5% from 1985 to 1994) or in 10-year outcome (71% versus 64.5% from 1995 to 2004). After the initial improvement in oncologic outcome, additional changes in chemotherapy regimens and agents have not resulted in further improvements.

Despite the favorable response of osteosarcomas to chemotherapy, surgery is a necessary component of curative therapy [18]. With the advent of new technologies and advances in reconstruction, significant emphasis is now placed on limb-sparing procedures and functional outcome [19]. Patient selection remains important because every patient is not a candidate for limb salvage: oncologic outcome must not be sacrificed for function. Tumor location, extent of disease, and patient age are the most important determinants of the feasibility of limb-sparing surgery. Among the relative contraindications for limb-sparing surgery are nerve and/or vessel encasement by tumor, the presence of a large biopsy-related hematoma, and the presence of a pathologic fracture. However, the only absolute indication for amputation at this time is progression of the tumor on chemotherapy.

Current Management Approach: Osteosarcoma

Once a bone lesion is identified, a thorough medical history is obtained, and a physical examination is performed. Blood laboratory analyses and blood chemistries that include a complete blood cell count with differential, platelets, total protein, albumin, calcium, total bilirubin, alkaline phosphatase, lactate dehydrogenase (LDH), aspartate transaminase, phosphate, sodium, potassium, chloride, CO_2, and coagulation battery should be obtained. Plain films and MRI of the primary lesion, along with a bone scan, are used to identify the osseous extent of the disease. Chest radiography, CT of the chest, +/− PET are used to identify metastatic lesion disease. Biopsy (open versus needle) of the lesion confirms the diagnosis. Before initiation of systemic therapy, a baseline echocardiogram, audiology examination, and pregnancy test (if clinically indicated) are obtained, and sperm banking/fertility is discussed. Doxorubicin, cisplatin, and methotrexate are considered standard first-line therapy [20].

At MD Anderson, the chemotherapy regimens differ in the adult and pediatric population. In adults, preoperative therapy involves 4 cycles of doxorubicin and cisplatin given at 21-day intervals. In patients with localized disease, cisplatin may be delivered intra-arterially at a dose of 120 mg/m^2 in combination with doxorubicin given as a continuous IV infusion at 90 mg/m^2. Treatment response is assessed after the first 2 cycles, a clinical examination is performed, and the primary lesion is often reimaged. If no progression of disease is observed, chemotherapy is continued for two more cycles and then surgical resection is performed. The response to therapy is then assessed by using the percentage of tumor necrosis. If the tumor has ≥90% necrosis, 4 additional cycles of doxorubicin at 75 mg/m^2 and ifosfamide at 10 g/m^2 are given. If the tumor has <90% necrosis, 6 cycles of high-dose ifosfamide and 6 cycles of high-dose methotrexate are given sequentially (if tolerated).

In the pediatric population, doxorubicin plus dexrazoxane (for cardioprotection), cisplatin, and high-dose methotrexate are the first-line treatment. In some older protocols, doxorubicin (37.5 mg/m^2/day) as continuous infusion (to try to reduce cardiotoxicity, although not as effective as dexrazoxane and associated with more mucositis) and cisplatin (60 mg/m^2/day) were given over 2 days in the first week of chemotherapy. It has been noted that there is less ototoxicity if cisplatin is given over 2 days instead of 1 day. Thus, a 750 mg/m^2 bolus of dexrazoxane (administered over 15–30 min) followed by a 75 mg/m^2 bolus of doxorubicin, which has excellent cardioprotection and less mucositis, and then cisplatin (60 mg/m^2/day × 2 days) may be considered the state-of-the-art option. Methotrexate (12 g/m^2; max = 20 g) is then given with hydration and leucovorin rescue from 24 h until methotrexate concentration is less than 0.1 μM in weeks 4 and 5. The treatment response is then assessed. If there has been no progression of disease, chemotherapy is continued and the regimen repeated. The patient is ready for definitive surgical resection at about week 10–12. Once the primary bone lesion (e.g., tumor in distal femur) is resected, the response to therapy is then assessed by using percent necrosis. Good responders (≥90% necrosis) continue with the regimen of dexrazoxane (750 mg/m^2)/doxorubicin (75 mg/m^2) + cisplatin (120 mg/m^2), and methotrexate (12 g/m^2), whereas poor responders (<90% necrosis) receive dexrazoxane (750 mg/m^2)/doxorubicin (75 mg/m^2) and cisplatin (120 mg/m^2), methotrexate (12 g/m^2), followed by a cycle of ifosfamide (2.8 g/m^2/dose × 5 days) +/− etoposide (100 mg/m^2/day × 5 days). Some patients with very low percent necrosis (e.g., <30%) to the initial regimen may receive high-dose ifosfamide (14 g/cycle) × 6–8 cycles.

Several new treatment options are being investigated in clinical trials at MD Anderson. One promising agent is muramyl tripeptide phosphatidyl-ethanolamine (MTP-PE). MTP-PE is a synthetic lipophilic analog of muramyl dipeptide. MTP-PE, encapsulated in liposomes, is delivered selectively to monocytes and macrophages, causing these cells to become activated and tumoricidal. The addition of MTP to chemotherapy has resulted in improved 6-year overall survival rates: from 70% to 78% (P < 0.03; relative risk <0.71) [21]. In addition, in the pediatric population, an outpatient regimen is being used that has had good oncologic and emotional results.

Promising new investigational drugs are now being tested in metastatic and/or relapsed osteosarcomas. These agents will likely be tested soon with active chemotherapy ± radiotherapy. However, to demonstrate significantly meaningful clinical activity, we will need to look at potential synergy with chemotherapy effects on necrosis of primary tumors and/or effects on lung metastases.

Ewing Sarcoma

Historical Perspective

Ewing sarcoma was first described by James Ewing as a distinct clinical entity in 1921. In the past several decades, the diagnosis has grown to include a group of neoplastic tumor diseases known as the Ewing family of tumors (EFT). This group includes primitive neuroectodermal tumors (PNETs), Askin tumors, and atypical Ewing sarcoma. Ewing sarcoma, which can occur in the bone or soft tissues, is the second most common primary bone tumor in children and adolescents [2]. However, it represents less than 5% of all cancers affecting children. Approximately 200 new cases are diagnosed each year in the USA. It is most commonly seen in patients younger than age 30 years, with the peak incidence between ages 10 and 15 years. Fewer than 5% of cases of Ewing sarcoma arise in adults older than age 40 years [22]. There is a slight male predominance, and for unknown reasons, Ewing sarcoma is extremely rare in African Americans [23–25]. There are no predisposing factors, and Ewing sarcoma has not been consistently associated with any familial or congenital syndromes.

Ewing sarcoma can develop in almost any bone or soft tissue. However, it has a predilection for the flat (pelvic and scapula) and long bones of the skeleton. Patients typically present with pain and swelling and often a soft tissue mass. Pathological fracture is seen in 15% of cases on presentation. Constitutional symptoms, such as fever, fatigue, weight loss, or anemia, are present in about 10–20% of patients. Although less than 25% of patients present with overt metastases, subclinical metastases are presumed to be present at diagnosis in most patients, as is the case with osteosarcoma. This is based on the fact that 80–90% of patients experience relapse after local therapy alone.

Staging

The diagnostic workup begins with obtaining radiographs of the affected site. MRI of the entire bone defines the intraosseous extent of the tumor, the soft tissue extension, and the relationship of the tumor to the joint and neurovascular bundles. Often the radiographs are subtle, but MRI reveals a large soft tissue mass. A bone scan is performed to evaluate the entire skeleton for the presence of metastatic or skip lesions. CT of the chest is used to evaluate the thorax for metastatic disease. PET/CT can be performed, but its use is still investigational in this subgroup of sarcomas. Ewing sarcoma has a predilection to spread to bone marrow; thus, some advocate bone marrow biopsy or scanning MRI of the spine to exclude widespread metastatic disease. A bone marrow biopsy is more sensitive and specific than a screening MRI for determining the possibility of bone marrow metastases.

Unlike osteosarcoma and other solid tumors, no commonly used staging system exists for the Ewing family of tumors. Although the staging system from the Musculoskeletal Tumor Society is available, it is not routinely used because it does not specify the site, which is an important prognostic factor. Thus, these staging systems cannot effectively stratify patients in terms of outcome and therefore lack clinical relevance.

Several prognostic factors for Ewing have been identified, including the presence or absence of metastatic disease, primary tumor location and size, patient age, response to therapy, and the presence of certain chromosomal translocations [26, 27]. One of the most important prognostic factors is the presence or absence of metastases.

The presence or absence of metastasis at diagnosis is a critical factor in guiding initial treatment. Disseminated disease carries a very poor prognosis, although it has been shown that patients with metastases limited to the lung may have better survival rates than do those with multisite metastases [27]. Approximately 30% of patients with metastases limited to the lungs survive 5 years, compared with only 10% of those with bone or bone marrow involvement [27]. This can be partially attributed to the fact that bone or bone marrow involvement tends to be larger and more extensive when discovered and thus more difficult to resect. Patients with large (>100 ml) or axial primary tumors (i.e., pelvis, rib, spine, scapula, skull, clavicle, sternum) have a worse prognosis than do those with extremity lesions [27]. Constitutional symptoms, elevated serum LDH, and viable tumor in the resected specimen are also associated with poor prognosis.

Morphologically, classic Ewing sarcoma is a primitive, undifferentiated neoplasm. Histologically, it displays sheets of small, round, blue cells with hyperchromatic nuclei and scant cytoplasm. Atypical Ewing and PNET can differ histologically from classic Ewing sarcoma since they can appear poorly differentiated, tend to have a higher mitotic rate, and may have spindle cells; also, the neoplastic cells themselves can be arranged in an organoid or lobular pattern. Since the histologic differential can be broad, immunohistochemistry and molecular studies such as RT-PCR and fluorescent in situ hybridization (FISH) play a critical role in confirming the diagnosis. Ewing sarcoma tumor cells strongly express a cell surface glycoprotein, p30/32 MIC2 antigen, which is encoded by the *MIC2* gene [7]. Immunohistochemical staining can identify this antigen, and although there is false-positive reactivity with lymphoblastic lymphoma, MIC2 analysis has a sensitivity of up to 95% and thus has become very useful in the diagnosis of Ewing sarcoma. Ewing sarcoma is also associated with distinct translocations. Cytogenetic studies are able to identify these translocations and thus have become another very useful method for confirming the diagnosis.

The MD Anderson Cancer Center Experience: Ewing Sarcoma

Historically, the prognosis for patients with Ewing sarcoma was bleak. As with osteosarcoma, however, advances in multidisciplinary management over the past 20–30 years have resulted in marked improvement in long-term survival. Advances in chemotherapy have increased the 5-year survival rate from 5–10% to 70–80% [7–9]. Several advances in systemic therapy have occurred since 1981, largely due to the efforts of several cooperative studies: (1) The First Intergroup Ewing's Sarcoma Study (IESS-I) demonstrated that the combination of vincristine, doxorubicin, cyclophosphamide, and actinomycin D (VDCA or VACA) was associated with a significantly better 5-year relapse-free survival rate (60%) than was vincristine, actinomycin D, and cyclophosphamide (VAC) alone (24%) or VAC plus adjuvant bilateral pulmonary irradiation (44%) [28]. (2) The Second Intergroup Study

(IESS-II) demonstrated that intensity of dosage of the drug administered during the early months of therapy was critical for relapse-free survival [29]. (3) The Third Intergroup Study (IESS-III) demonstrated that the addition of ifosfamide and etoposide to VDCA was associated with a significantly better 5-year relapse-free survival rate (69%) than was VDCA alone (54%) in patients with nonmetastatic EFT or PNET [30]. Several other studies confirmed the benefit of adding alternating cycles of ifosfamide and etoposide to a VDC backbone [30–32]. The current standard chemotherapy for EFT in the USA includes vincristine, doxorubicin, and cyclophosphamide, alternating with ifosfamide and etoposide. The current trend is to intensify the dosing of alkylating agents and to attempt to administer them over a shorter period of time.

Classically, the treatment for Ewing sarcoma consisted of chemotherapy and irradiation, with surgery reserved for expendable bones [33]. However, the current trend, and the treatment currently used at MD Anderson, is chemotherapy and surgical resection when the primary tumor can be completely removed. Several studies have shown that surgery improves survival [34, 35]. It must be noted that the favorable results seen in these studies may also be due in part to a selection bias because surgery is performed on more favorable lesions (small, local, and accessible) and thus results in better outcome. However, one explanation is that surgery removes all cells that may have become chemoresistant before they have a chance to recur and/or metastasize. It is not unusual to see disease recur after irradiation [36]. Radiotherapy is now reserved for tumors in anatomic sites where total resection cannot be performed, when significant metastatic disease is present, when the functional deficit is unacceptable to the patient, or when there has been resection with positive or close (<1 cm) margins [33]. However, because advances in chemotherapy have increased long-term survival, the problems of late recurrence after irradiation, functional impairment secondary to radiation complications (soft tissue fibrosis, avascular necrosis, and growth disturbances) and radiation-induced sarcomas have become more apparent.

The MD Anderson data set was derived from 3,869 patients who presented between 1944 and 2004 with sarcoma of bone. Of these patients, 2,339 had no previous treatment, and 2,078 received definitive treatment at MD Anderson Cancer Center. Of this total group, 319 patients had a diagnosis Ewing sarcoma and received their complete and definitive treatment at MD Anderson.

Outcome in Ewing sarcoma has improved significantly, and this is reflected in our data by the incremental improvement in 5-year survival: from 0% to 53.7%. The overall survival curve is depicted in Fig. 28.5. This improvement was especially noted in patients with localized disease, whose survival rates increased from 9.1% to 93.8% (Fig. 28.6). Although survival rates for patients with metastatic disease have improved over the decades (0.0–19.0%), outcome for these patients unfortunately remains gloomy (Fig. 28.8). However, all patients with metastases do not share the same prognosis. Patients with a limited number of lung metastases do not share the same dismal prognosis as do those with metastatic disease at other sites (e.g., bone or bone marrow).

Current Management Approach: Ewing Sarcoma

The current MD Anderson approach to the treatment of patients with Ewing sarcoma is multidisciplinary. At presentation, after review of the radiographic images, proper staging is performed. A thorough medical history is obtained, and a physical examination is performed. Blood laboratory analyses and blood chemistries that include a complete blood cell count with differential, platelets, total protein, albumin, calcium, total bilirubin, alkaline phosphatase, LDH, aspartate transaminase, phosphate, sodium, potassium, chloride, CO_2, and coagulation battery are obtained. Plain films and MRI of the primary lesion, bone scan, +/– scanning MRI of the spine, chest radiograph, CT of the chest, and +/– PET scan complete the radiographic staging. Biopsy (open versus needle) of the lesion then confirms the diagnosis. Once the diagnosis is confirmed, systemic therapy is initiated. Before the initiation of systemic therapy, a baseline echocardiogram, audiology examination, and pregnancy test are obtained (if clinically indicated), and sperm banking/fertility is discussed. If the patient has localized (solitary) disease, neoadjuvant chemotherapy is begun. At MD Anderson Cancer Centre, treatment of localized Ewings varies depending on patient age.

In the pediatric population, the chemotherapy regimen includes vincristine (2 mg/m^2, maximum 2 mg), doxorubicin (37.5 mg/m^2/day × 2 days; 75 mg/m^2/cycle), and cyclophosphamide (1,200 mg/m^2, given with mesna on day 1 only) alternating with ifosfamide (9 g/m^2/cycle divided over 5 days, given with mesna) and etoposide (500 mg/m^2/cycle divided over 5 days) for 6 weeks. Once again, dexrazoxane is given with doxorubicin for cardioprotection. Recent data have shown that, at least for pediatric patients, delivery of chemotherapy every 2 weeks rather than every 3 weeks (compressed timing) resulted in superior outcome, so this timing is preferred in patients who can tolerate it. Tumor response is assessed after 6 weeks, with reimaging of the primary tumor and clinical examination. If there has been a response to chemotherapy, neoadjuvant chemotherapy is continued for an additional 4–6 weeks, and then the primary tumor is resected. If the margins are clear, chemotherapy is resumed to complete 17 cycles. If the margins are close, the patient receives radiotherapy to the tumor bed for 5–6 weeks, followed by chemotherapy for a total of 17 cycles. If the tumor progresses on chemotherapy, the patient is a candidate for immediate resection, and salvage chemotherapy (i.e., temozolomide plus trinotecan) is begun.

In the adult population, doxorubicin (75 mg/m^2/cycle), ifosfamide (10 g/m^2/cycle), and vincristine (2 mg/cycle) is given for up to 6 cycles. As stated above, the tumor response to chemotherapy is assessed during the course of the treatment and will help determine the number of cycles given. After the sixth cycle, the patient is evaluated for definitive surgical resection. Once resected, the tumor is assessed for viability. If there is viable tumor, the patient is a candidate for additional chemotherapy, possibly with higher-dose ifosfamide and etoposide (total duration of therapy, approximately 12 months). If there is total or near total tumor necrosis, the patient will receive 2–4 cycles of high-dose ifosfamide. If the tumor is not resectable, the patient will receive definitive irradiation to the site and then chemotherapy up to maximal tolerance.

Surgical Management of Bone Sarcomas

The advent and implementation of chemotherapy, as well as advances in imaging, have facilitated the advancement of surgical management of bone sarcomas. Although amputation was the treatment of choice 20 years ago, to maintain cosmesis and function, the emphasis is now on limb salvage. For extremity lesions, chemotherapy and limb salvage (complete tumor resection and reconstruction) can improve cosmesis and functional outcome without significantly sacrificing local disease control [37, 38]. Limb salvage procedures, however, are usually associated with narrower surgical margins, which can potentially increase the likelihood of local failure. Several multicenter series have suggested an increased risk of local recurrence with limb salvage versus amputation, even in patients with good response to chemotherapy; however, other (single institution) studies have indicated similar local recurrence rates [39–41]. Although the overall data are somewhat controversial, the trend has been to perform limb salvage surgery when oncologically feasible.

Attempts have been made to compare functional outcome of limb salvage patients and amputation patients. The data do not support findings that limb salvage versus amputation significantly improves quality of life or long-term psychosocial outcome [41–43]. The functional restrictions and additional surgeries needed after limb salvage can take a toll on many limb salvage patients. Although limb salvage has become the popular treatment of choice, appropriate patient selection is of utmost importance. If there is any doubt that a wide local excision cannot be accomplished, amputation is the oncologic treatment of choice.

Surgical techniques have evolved in parallel with the evolution of chemotherapy. Many methods of reconstruction are available, including metal endoprostheses (modular and expanding), allografts, arthrodeses, vascularized fibular transfers, and rotationplasty. Metal megaprostheses are now modular, off-the-shelf, and readily available when needed. Noninvasive expandable endoprostheses are particularly useful in children, and although designed on a custom basis, are readily available and quite popular. To choose the appropriate surgical option requires an understanding of the capabilities and limitations of each of these reconstructive options as well as careful evaluation of the patient and their support system. A discussion of these limitations is out of the scope of this chapter; however, suffice it to say that each reconstructive technique has its own advantages and disadvantages, and the appropriate method for surgical reconstruction must be individualized. Several factors need to be considered when choosing a reconstructive option, including anatomic location, stage of disease, extent of the needed resection, likelihood and nature of complications associated with a particular type of reconstruction, and the patient's age, size, expectations, and anticipated functional demands.

MD Anderson has considerable experience in novel techniques for reconstruction of the pelvis and in treatment of extremity tumors in children and adults. This expertise offers valuable options for our patients when the success of their treatment depends on both systemic and local control.

References

1. Giuffrida AY, Burgueno JE, Koniaris LG, Gutierrez JC, Duncan R, Scully SP. Chondrosarcoma in the United States (1973 to 2003): an analysis of 2890 cases from the SEER database. J Bone Joint Surg Am. 2009;91:1063–72.
2. Smith MA, GJ, Ries LA. Cancer in adolescents 15 to 19 years old. In: Cancer incidence and survival among children and adolescents: United States SEER Program 1975–1997 (NIH Pub. No. 99-4649). Bethesda, MD: National Cancer Institute; 1999.
3. Stiller CA, Bielack SS, Jundt G, Steliarova-Foucher E. Bone tumours in European children and adolescents, 1978-1997. Report from the Automated Childhood Cancer Information System project. Eur J Cancer. 2006;42:2124–35.
4. Ries LAG, SM, Gurney JG, et al. Cancer incidence and survival among children and adolescents: United States SEER Program 1975–1995 (NIH Pub. No. 99-4649). Bethesda, MD: National Cancer Institute; 1999. p. 99–110.
5. Data from the American Cancer Society. American Cancer Society. http://www.cancer.org/docroot/home/index.asp. Accessed 23 May 2012.
6. Mirabello L, Troisi RJ, Savage SA. Osteosarcoma incidence and survival rates from 1973 to 2004: data from the Surveillance, Epidemiology, and End Results Program. Cancer. 2009;115:1531–43.
7. Enneking WF. A system of staging musculoskeletal neoplasms. Clin Orthop Relat Res. 1986;204:9–24.
8. Benjamin R, Chawla S, Murray J, et al. Preoperative chemotherapy for osteosarcoma: a treatment approach facilitating limb salvage with major prognostic indications. In: Jones S, Salmon S, editors. Adjuvant therapy of cancer IV. Philadelphia: Grune and Stratton; 1984. p. 601–10.
9. Hudson M, Jaffe MR, Jaffe N, et al. Pediatric osteosarcoma: therapeutic strategies, results, and prognostic factors derived from a 10-year experience. J Clin Oncol. 1990;8:1988–97.
10. Link MP, Goorin AM, Miser AW, et al. The effect of adjuvant chemotherapy on relapse-free survival in patients with osteosarcoma of the extremity. N Engl J Med. 1986;314:1600–6.
11. Eilber F, Giuliano A, Eckardt J, Patterson K, Moseley S, Goodnight J. Adjuvant chemotherapy for osteosarcoma: a randomized prospective trial. J Clin Oncol. 1987;5:21–6.
12. Rosen G, Nirenberg A. Neoadjuvant chemotherapy for osteogenic sarcoma: a five year follow-up (T-10) and preliminary report of new studies (T-12). Prog Clin Biol Res. 1985;201:39–51.
13. Mavligit GM, Calvo 3rd DB, Patt YZ, Hersh EM. Immune restoration and/or augmentation of local xenogeneic graft versus host reaction by Cimetidine in vitro. J Immunol. 1981; 126:2272–4.
14. Stewart DJ, Benjamin RS, Zimmerman S, et al. Clinical pharmacology of intraarterial cis-diamminedichloroplatinum(II). Cancer Res. 1983;43:917–20.
15. Jaffe N, Raymond AK, Ayala A, et al. Effect of cumulative courses of intraarterial cis-diamminedichloroplatin-II on the primary tumor in osteosarcoma. Cancer. 1989;63:63–7.
16. Jaffe N, Robertson R, Ayala A, et al. Comparison of intra-arterial cis-diamminedichloroplatinum II with high-dose methotrexate and citrovorum factor rescue in the treatment of primary osteosarcoma. J Clin Oncol. 1985;3:1101–4.
17. Bacci G, Ferrari S, Donati D, et al. Neoadjuvant chemotherapy for osteosarcoma of the extremity in patients in the fourth and fifth decade of life. Oncol Rep. 1998;5:1259–63.
18. Jaffe N, Carrasco H, Raymond K, Ayala A, Eftekhari F. Can cure in patients with osteosarcoma be achieved exclusively with chemotherapy and abrogation of surgery? Cancer. 2002;95:2202–10.
19. Peabody TD, Gibbs Jr CP, Simon MA. Evaluation and staging of musculoskeletal neoplasms. J Bone Joint Surg Am. 1998;80:1204–18.
20. Link M, Meyers P, Gebhardt M. Osteosarcoma. In: Pizzo P, Poplack DG, editors. Principles and practice of pediatric oncology. Philadelphia: Lippincott, Williams, & Wilkins; 2006. p. 1074–115.

21. Meyers PA, Schwartz CL, Krailo MD, et al. Osteosarcoma: the addition of muramyl tripeptide to chemotherapy improves overall survival – a report from the Children's Oncology Group. J Clin Oncol. 2008;26:633–8.
22. Glass AG, Fraumeni Jr JF. Epidemiology of bone cancer in children. J Natl Cancer Inst. 1970;44:187–99.
23. Fraumeni Jr JF, Glass AG. Rarity of Ewing's sarcoma among U.S. Negro children. Lancet. 1970;1:366–7.
24. Parkin DM, Stiller CA, Nectoux J. International variations in the incidence of childhood bone tumours. Int J Cancer. 1993;53:371–6.
25. Jawad MU, Cheung MC, Min ES, Schneiderbauer MM, Koniaris LG, Scully SP. Ewing sarcoma demonstrates racial disparities in incidence-related and sex-related differences in outcome: an analysis of 1631 cases from the SEER database, 1973-2005. Cancer. 2009;115:3526–36.
26. Bacci G, Ferrari S, Bertoni F, et al. Prognostic factors in nonmetastatic Ewing's sarcoma of bone treated with adjuvant chemotherapy: analysis of 359 patients at the Istituto Ortopedico Rizzoli. J Clin Oncol. 2000;18:4–11.
27. Cotterill SJ, Ahrens S, Paulussen M, et al. Prognostic factors in Ewing's tumor of bone: analysis of 975 patients from the European Intergroup Cooperative Ewing's Sarcoma Study Group. J Clin Oncol. 2000;18:3108–14.
28. Nesbit Jr ME, Gehan EA, Burgert Jr EO, et al. Multimodal therapy for the management of primary, nonmetastatic Ewing's sarcoma of bone: a long-term follow-up of the First Intergroup study. J Clin Oncol. 1990;8:1664–74.
29. Burgert Jr EO, Nesbit ME, Garnsey LA, et al. Multimodal therapy for the management of nonpelvic, localized Ewing's sarcoma of bone: intergroup study IESS-II. J Clin Oncol. 1990;8:1514–24.
30. Grier HE, Krailo MD, Tarbell NJ, et al. Addition of ifosfamide and etoposide to standard chemotherapy for Ewing's sarcoma and primitive neuroectodermal tumor of bone. N Engl J Med. 2003;348:694–701.
31. Ferrari S, Mercuri M, Rosito P, et al. Ifosfamide and actinomycin-D, added in the induction phase to vincristine, cyclophosphamide and doxorubicin, improve histologic response and prognosis in patients with non metastatic Ewing's sarcoma of the extremity. J Chemother. 1998;10:484–91.
32. Kolb EA, Kushner BH, Gorlick R, et al. Long-term event-free survival after intensive chemotherapy for Ewing's family of tumors in children and young adults. J Clin Oncol. 2003;21:3423–30.
33. Gibbs CP, Weber KL, Scarborough MT. Malignant bone tumors. In: Beaty JH, editor. AAOS instructional course lectures, vol. 51. Rosemont: American Academy of Orthopaedic Surgeons; 2002. p. 413–28.
34. Bacci G, Toni A, Avella M, et al. Long-term results in 144 localized Ewing's sarcoma patients treated with combined therapy. Cancer. 1989;63:1477–86.
35. Wilkins RM, Pritchard DJ, Burgert Jr EO, Unni KK. Ewing's sarcoma of bone. Experience with 140 patients. Cancer. 1986;58:2551–5.
36. Horowitz ME, Neff JR, Kun LE. Ewing's sarcoma. Radiotherapy versus surgery for local control. Pediatr Clin North Am. 1991;38:365–80.
37. Bacci G, Forni C, Longhi A, et al. Local recurrence and local control of non-metastatic osteosarcoma of the extremities: a 27-year experience in a single institution. J Surg Oncol. 2007;96:118–23.
38. Wittig JC, Bickels J, Kellar-Graney KL, Kim FH, Malawer MM. Osteosarcoma of the proximal humerus: long-term results with limb-sparing surgery. Clin Orthop Relat Res. 2002;156–76
39. Lindner NJ, Ramm O, Hillmann A, et al. Limb salvage and outcome of osteosarcoma. The University of Muenster experience. Clin Orthop Relat Res. 1999;83–9
40. Picci P, Sangiorgi L, Rougraff BT, Neff JR, Casadei R, Campanacci M. Relationship of chemotherapy-induced necrosis and surgical margins to local recurrence in osteosarcoma. J Clin Oncol. 1994;12:2699–705.

41. Rougraff BT, Simon MA, Kneisl JS, Greenberg DB, Mankin HJ. Limb salvage compared with amputation for osteosarcoma of the distal end of the femur. A long-term oncological, functional, and quality-of-life study. J Bone Joint Surg Am. 1994;76:649–56.
42. Nagarajan R, Clohisy DR, Neglia JP, et al. Function and quality-of-life of survivors of pelvic and lower extremity osteosarcoma and Ewing's sarcoma: the Childhood Cancer Survivor Study. Br J Cancer. 2004;91:1858–65.
43. Barr RD, Wunder JS. Bone and soft tissue sarcomas are often curable–but at what cost?: a call to arms (and legs). Cancer. 2009;115:4046–54.

Index

A
ABVD *vs.* MOPP therapy, 227
Acute myeloid leukemia (AML)
  ARA-C activity, 206
  cured, 206
  metastatic, 205
  prognoses and outcomes, 207
  prototype illness, 205
  randomized clinical trials, 206
  remission, 208
  survival rates, 207–208
  systemic therapy, 206
  therapeutic agents, 206
Adjuvant chemotherapy, 49, 51, 122
AJCC Version 7.0 stage, 136
Alexanian, R., 264
Allen, O., 121
American College of Surgeons (ACoS), 6
American College of Surgeons Oncology Group (ACOSOG), 31
American Joint Committee on Cancer (AJCC), 135, 136, 154, 156, 158, 163, 179, 180, 190, 196, 296
Anaplastic thyroid carcinoma (ATC), 296
Androgen ablative therapy, 38
Androgen deprivation therapy, 40, 43
Ang, K.K., 278
Anti-CD52 monoclonal antibody, 220
Arimidex, tamoxifen, alone or in combination (ATAC), 22
Axillary lymph node dissection (ALND), 26, 27

B
Barlogie, B., 264
Barrett's esophagus, 178
Bergsagel, D.E., 264
Bevacizumab, 52
Biliary carcinoma, 167
Bladder cancer
  advanced-stage disease, 150
  clinical stage, 145
  cT1 disease, 148
  cystoscopy and biopsy, 143
  distant disease, 149
  gemcitabine plus cisplatin, 151
  grade, stage, and variant histology, 149, 150
  high-grade disease, 143–144
  historical perspective, 144
  intermediate-stage disease, 150
  local disease, 145, 147
  low-grade disease, 150
  muscularis, urothelium/lamina propria, 143
  M-VAC, 151
  pathologic stage, 145
  regional disease, 146, 148
  re-resection, 150
  SEER stage, 145, 146
  survival rate, 145–147
Blokhin, N., 264
Bloom syndrome, 324
Bone sarcomas
  Bloom syndrome, 324
  Ewing sarcoma
    bone marrow biopsy, 329
    FISH, role of, 330
    historical perspective, 328–329
    IESS-I/II/III, 330, 331
    MIC2 gene, 330
    PET/CT, 329

M.A. Rodriguez et al. (eds.), *60 Years of Survival Outcomes at The University of Texas MD Anderson Cancer Center*, DOI 10.1007/978-1-4614-5197-6,

Bone sarcomas (*cont.*)
prognostic factors, 329
survival rates, 322, 323, 331
systemic therapy, 330, 332
treatment of, 331
osteosarcoma
biopsy, 327
clinical outcomes of, 326
definition, 324
diagnosis of, 326
distal femur, 328
drug algorithm, 325
historical perspective, 324
limb-sparing procedure, 327
osseous lesions, 324
PET/CT, 324
physical examination, 327
potential synergy, 328
staging, 324–326
survival rates, 320–323
Rothmund–Thomson syndrome, 324
surgical management, 333
Werner syndrome, 324
Brachytherapy, 100, 106
BRCA1/BRCA2, 85–86
Breast cancer
breast-preserving surgery, 19
combined modality therapy, 31
disease stage, 22
distant disease
bisphosphonates, 30
chemotherapy, 27–29
endocrine therapy, 29–30
HER-2-positive disease, 31
historical perspective, 20–21
localized disease
adjuvant therapy, 22–23
biologic therapy, 24
locoregional disease
inflammatory carcinoma, 24–25
local therapy, 24
preservation, 25–26
regional nodal treatment, 26–27
paclitaxel and FAC chemotherapy, 31
patients and methods, 21–22
radiation treatment, 30–31
SEER staging system, 19–23
treatment, 19
Bureaus of Vital Statistics (BVS), 9
Burke, T., 281
Byers, 275

C
Cabanillas, F., 259
Cancer and Leukemia Group B/Radiation Therapy Oncology Group (CALGB/RTOG), 69
Cancer treatment
frontline chemotherapy (*see* Frontline chemotherapy) salvage treatment, 259–260
Care-delivery design, 2
CDH1 gene, 190
CD20-positive lymphocytic and histiocytic (LH) cells, 225
CD30-positive Reed–Sternberg (RS) cells, 225
Celiac axis neurolysis, 123
Cervical cancer
brachytherapy, 106
definitive treatment, 99
external beam therapy, 106
historical perspective, 97–98
local disease
brachytherapy, 100
concurrent cisplatin-based chemotherapy, 101
laparoscopic surgical technique, 102
locally advanced disease, 99
megavoltage radiation, 99
outcome of, 101
ovarian function, 100
SEER, 100
surgical techniques, 102
metastatic disease, 104–105
multidisciplinary, 107
preinvasive disease, 97
radical hysterectomy, 106
regional disease, 102–104
stages, 99
Chambers, M., 280
Chemotherapy and radiation therapy (CRT), 122
Chronic lymphocytic leukemia (CLL)
American Cancer Society, 211
B-cell lymphoproliferative disorder, 211
benign monoclonal B-lymphocytosis, 212
biology and pathogenesis of, 221
clinical trial, fludarabine, 213–214
database, 213
diagnosis of, 213
epidemiology, 212–213
guidelines, 221
lymph nodes, 211
patient evaluation, 222
peripheral blood or bone marrow, 211

Richter syndrome, 212
risk stratification, 222
smoldering CLL, 212
survival rates of
cytogenetic treatment, 217, 218
diagnosis and classification of, 216–217
first and second-line chemotherapy, 217, 219, 220
fludarabine, 217
IGHV treatment, 217, 218
novel agent, 220
refractory disease treatment, 219–220
supportive care, 221
ZAP-70 treatment, 217, 219
treatment pattern, 214–216
Clark, R.L., 1, 6, 206
Colon cancer
cause of, 77
diagnosis, 82, 83
distant disease, 78, 80
historical perspective, 78
local disease, 78, 79
regional disease, 78, 79
risk factors
HNPCC syndrome, 78–79
immunohistochemical analysis, 80
microsatellite DNA, 79
MSI testing, 80
polymerase chain reaction, 81
sporadic MSI, 80
surgical approach, 83
treatment, 81–83
Computed tomography (CT), 324, 329
Concurrent chemotherapy, 52
Concurrent cisplatin chemotherapy, 103, 104
Cutaneous melanoma
analytic case, 157, 161
distant disease, 158, 160, 163
historical perspective
AJCC anatomic stage, 154, 156
elective lymph node dissection, 155
FDA, 157
refine treatment, 156
"revolutionary" technique, 155–156
staging and prognosis, 154
systemic approaches, 156–157
TNM stage, 154, 155
incidence of, 153
ipilimumab and vemurafenib, 164
local disease, 158, 159, 163
localized tumors, 159, 161, 162
morphogenetic classification, 154
pathology-based stage, 158–159
radiotherapy, 164
regional disease, 158, 160, 162, 163
SEER stage, 158
SLNB, 161, 162
stage I/II disease, 162, 163
tumor registry methodology, 158

D

Definitive primary therapy, 90
Definitive radiation therapy, 54
Dicke, K., 259
Disease-based model, 1–2
Doxorubicin (Adriamycin), bleomycin, vinblastine, and dacarbazine (ABVD), 227

E

Eaton–Lambert myasthenic syndrome, 65
E-cadherin protein, 190
Eilber, F., 325
Elective lymph node dissection, 155
Endocrine therapy, 29–30
Endometrial cancer
carcinoma, 109
computed tomography, 112
definitive treatment, 112
distant tumors, 115–116
historical perspective, 110–111
localized tumors, 113–114
low-risk disease, 116
outcome of, 116
postmenopausal, 109–110
prior assessment, 111–112
regional tumors, 114–115
systemic therapy, 116
tumor registry methodology, 112
types, 109
Endoscopic retrograde cholangiopancreatography (ERCP), 121
Epidermal growth factor receptor (EGFR), 52, 122, 279
Epithelial ovarian cancer, 93
Esophageal cancer
epidemiology, 178–179
esophagectomy, 182
historical perspective
gold standard, 183, 184
non-regional lymph node, 179
perioperative mortality, 182–183
surgical techniques, 183

Esophageal cancer (*cont.*)
survival rates, 180–182
TNM staging system, 179
local disease, 177, 178
lymphatics spanning network, 177
molecular and genetic profile, 185
novel drugs, 186
pancreaticoduodenectomy, 182
patients presentation, 178, 184
randomized phase 2 trial, 186
staging technique, 186
surgical technique, 186
survival data, 180, 184–185
Whipple resection, 182
European Organisation for Research and Treatment of Cancer (EORTC), 71
Ewing, J., 328
Ewing sarcoma
bone marrow biopsy, 329
FISH, role of, 330
historical perspective, 328–329
IESS-I/II/III, 330, 331
MIC2 gene, 330
PET/CT, 329
prognostic factors, 329
survival rates, 322, 323, 331
systemic therapy, 330, 332
treatment of, 331
Exocrine cancer. *See* Pancreatic cancer
Extensive-stage disease, 63–64
External beam radiotherapy, 42
External beam therapy, 106

F
Familial adenomatous polyposis (FAP), 78
Feeley, T., 281
Fingeret, M., 281
First intergroup Ewing's sarcoma study (IESS-I), 330
First-line chemotherapy and radiotherapy (XRT), 63
Fletcher, G., 98, 100, 107
Fluorescent in situ hybridization (FISH), 330
5-Fluorouracil (5-FU), 80, 82
5-Fluorouracil, epirubicin, and cyclophosphamide (FEC), 24, 27
Follicular Lymphoma International Prognostic Index (FLIPI), 243, 245
Follicular thyroid carcinoma (FTC), 296, 297
Food and Drug Administration (FDA), 52
Frei, E., 206
Freireich, E.J., 206
Frontline chemotherapy
Ann Arbor stage III–IV disease, 251, 257
intensified-dose chemotherapy, 258–259
lymphosarcoma, 255
medical oncology, 256
radiation therapy, 258
rituximab, 256
synergy of immunotherapy, 257

G
Gastric cancer
adenocarcinoma, 189
AJCC staging, 196
CDH1 gene, 190
distant disease, 192
distant survival treatment, 197, 200
E-cadherin protein, 190
Helicobacter pylori infection, 190
local survival treatment, 197, 198
locoregional disease, 196
multidisciplinary approach, 198
obesity, 189
outcomes of, 196
patient distribution, 195
perioperative therapy, 193–194
personalized therapy, 201
randomized phase 3 trials, 194
regional disease, 192
regional survival treatment, 197, 199
retrospective data, 194
SEER database, 192, 196–197
surgical staging system, 190–192
survival rates, 192–193, 197
symptoms, 190
systemic therapy, 194
TNM staging, 200
treatment pattern, 195–196
tumor registry data, 194
Gastroesophageal reflux disease (GERD), 178
Gastro-Intestinal Study Group (GITSG), 122
Gemcitabine plus cisplatin (GC), 151
Gidley, P., 280
Glisson, B., 279
Goepfert, H., 277
Gottlieb, J.A., 257
Granulosa cell tumor, 95
Gynecologic Oncology Group (GOG), 89

H
Hanna, E., 276, 277
Head and neck cancer (HNC)
devastating disease, 271
epidemiology, 272

human papilloma virus, role of, 272
organ preservation
bevacizumab, 279
clinical trials, 279
glottic cancer, 277
induction chemotherapy, 277
larynx or hypopharynx, 277
phase III clinical trial, 279
RTOG trial, 278
synergistic effects, 278
targeted therapy, 279
outcome measurement, 281–282
paranasal sinus and nasal cavity site, 272, 274, 287
rehabilitation, 280–281
surgery
clinical presentation, 275
endoscopic approach, 277
goal of, 275
intracranial/extracranial approach, 276
mandible and maxilla, 276
nasal cavity tumors, 274, 276
outcomes of, 275
soft tissue defects, 276
surgical management of, 276
vascularized bone flaps, 276
survival rate of
hypopharyngeal site, 290–292
laryngeal site, 272, 274, 285–286
nasopharyngeal site, 288–289
oral cavity site, 272, 273, 282–283
oropharyngeal site, 272, 273, 284–285
paranasal sinus and nasal cavity site, 272, 274, 287
Helicobacter pylori infection, 179, 190
Hepatocellular carcinoma, 167
Hereditary non-polyposis colorectal cancer (HNPCC), 78–80
HER-2-positive breast cancer, 24
High-dose interleukin 2 (HD IL-2), 137
Historical perspective
frontline management
ABVD *vs.* MOPP therapy, 227
BEACOPP-based treatment approach, 228
chemotherapy regimen, 229
HD10 trial, 228
IFRT *vs.* STNI, 227
lymphatic system, 227
rituximab, 228
stable of, 229
relapsed/refractory
anti-CD30 antibody, 231
bortezomib, 230
clinical trial, 231
mini transplant, 232
NF-kβ pathway, 230
novel therapy, 231
phase 1/2 trial, 231, 232
prevention and treatment of, 233
salvage or second-line chemotherapy, 229–230
secondary myelodysplastic syndrome, 231
systemic or organ toxicity, 232
in vitro study, 230
History of tumor registry
ACoS, 6
coding section
abstracting, 7–8
identification and processing, 7
pathology report codes, 8
quality assurance, 8–9
reabstracting, 8
registry operations, 7
data utilization activity, 10–11
epidemiologist, 5
follow-up section
ACoS criteria, 10
BVS, 9
computer-generated letter, 9
criteria, 9–10
death processing, 10
hold file, 10
IBM data processing unit, 6
Hodgkin lymphoma
advances in treatment (*see* Historical perspective)
classic HL (cHL) type, 225
Costwold's modification, 226
diagnosed of, 236
future aspects, 237
histologic features of, 234
NLPHL patients, 225–226
survival rates of, 235–236
time interval, 234
Hofstetter, W., 184
Hong, W.K., 277
Hormone receptor-positive disease, 23

I

Ifosfamide, 259
Image-guided radiation therapy, 50
Immunohistochemical (IHC), 80
Induction chemotherapy, 49

Inflammatory carcinoma, 24–25
Insulin-like growth factor receptor (IGFR), 279
Intensity-modulated radiation therapy (IMRT), 50, 56–57, 228
Intensive therapy, 267
Internal target volume (ITV), 57
International prognostic index (IPI), 243, 253, 254, 257
International Union Against Cancer (UICC), 6
Intraperitoneal techniques, 86
Iressa Pan-Asian Study (IPASS), 52
Irinotecan, 72

J
Jaffe, N., 326

K
Kantarjian, H., 258
Kaplan, H., 227
Kaplan–Meier product-limit method, 15
Kaplan–Meier survival, 145–146
Kaplan–Meier survival curve, 137, 138
Khouri, I.F., 258
Kidney cancer
  cross-sectional imaging, 137
  distant disease, 137, 139
  FDA-approved treatments, 137
  HD IL-2 therapy, 140
  historical perspective, 134
  Kaplan–Meier survival curve, 137, 138
  localized/regional disease, 137, 139
  metastatic disease, 141
  oncologic, 140
  partial *vs.* radical nephrectomy, 140
  RCC, 133
  risk factors, 134–135
  stages, 135–136
  systemic disease, 141
  types, 133
Kies, M.S., 279
KIT or *PDGFRA* gene, 318

L
Laparoscopic technique, 81–82, 102
Lewin, J., 280
Limited-stage disease, 63–64
Lindberg, R., 275
Link, M.P., 325
Liver cancer
  biliary carcinoma, 167
  chronic hepatitis C virus infection, 168
  diagnosis of, 168, 172–173
  distant disease, 171, 172
  hepatocellular carcinoma, 167
  historical perspective, 168–169
  radiotherapy, 173
  screening, 171–172
  surgical resection, 173
  survival rates, 169–171
  unresectable disease, 174
  Wilson's disease, 167
Localized pancreatic cancer, 124–128
Locally advanced disease, 51–52, 99
Locoregional disease
  inflammatory carcinoma, 24–25
  local therapy, 24
  preservation, 25–26
  regional nodal treatment, 26–27
Log-rank test, 15
Lymphadenectomy, 81, 103
Lymphangiograms, 37

M
Magnetic resonance imaging (MRI), 324, 329
Mavligit, G.M., 325
McElwain, T.J., 264
McLaughlin, P., 257
Mean lung dose (MLD), 55
Mechlorethamine, vincristine (oncovin), procarbazine, and prednisone (MOPP), 227
Medullary thyroid carcinoma (MTC), 296, 298
Metastatic disease, 52–53, 104–105, 324, 325
Methotrexate, vinblastine, adriamycin, and cisplatin (M-VAC), 151
MIC2 gene, 330
Micropapillary urothelial cell carcinoma, 148
Monoclonal protein, 263
Mucosa-associated lymphoid tissue [MALT] lymphoma, 241
Multidisciplinary care, 271, 281, 312
Multidisciplinary treatment, 98, 169
Multiple myeloma
  historical perspective, 264
  intensive therapy, 267
  malignant proliferation, 263
  monoclonal protein, 263
  novel therapy, 268
  stem cell collection, 268
  survival rates, 265–267

treatment of, 268
tumor registry, 265
Murphy, S., 258
Musculoskeletal tumor society staging system, 324–325

N

National Cancer Institute-sponsored Working Group (NCI-WG), 217
National Comprehensive Cancer Network (NCCN), 51
National Thyroid Cancer Treatment Cooperative Study Group, 307
Neelapu, S., 253
Neoadjuvant chemotherapy, 51–52, 325
Neoplastic tumor diseases, 328
Neurologic paraneoplastic syndrome, 65
Nirenberg, A., 325
Nodular lymphocyte predominant Hodgkin lymphoma (NLPHL), 225
Non-Hodgkin lymphomas (NHLs)
aggressive B cell
adverse effects of, 260
B-cell origin, 254
Burkitt-like lymphomas, 254
cancer treatment (*see* Frontline chemotherapy)
definition, 253
diagnosis and classification of, 252–253
doxorubicin, 256
epidemiology, 252
histology, 254–255
lymphosarcoma, 251
mantle cell, 254
molecular and genetic profiles, 260–261
Reed–Sternberg cells, 251
salvage treatment, 259–260
second-line therapies, 260
survival, 255, 256
T-cell or NK-cell, 254
indolent B-cell
Ann Arbor staging system, 243, 245
B-cell origin, 241
bulky and/symptomatic disease, 249
classification system, 242–244
diagnosis of, 245
FLIPI, 243, 245
follicular lymphoma, 241–242
high sensitive, 244
histologic feature, 246
MALT, 241
salvage therapy, 249
survival rates, 246–247
therapeutic agents, 248
vital signaling pathway, 249
Non–small cell lung cancer (NSCLC)
cause of, 45
disease stage, 50
IMRT, 56–57
localized disease, 49
locally advanced disease, 49–50
locoregional/distant disease, 46
multidisciplinary planning, 50–51
proton beam therapy, 57–58
radiation (*see* Radiation/proton beam therapy)
risk factors, 46
SEER stage, 46–48
smoking, 45
systemic chemotherapy
locally advanced disease, 51–52
metastatic disease, 52–53
treatment, 46

O

Obesity, 178, 179, 189
Oral fluoropyrimidine capecitabine (XELOX), 82
Osler, W., 255
Osteosarcoma
biopsy, 327
clinical outcomes of, 326
definition, 324
diagnosis of, 326
distal femur, 328
drug algorithm, 325
historical perspective, 324
limb-sparing procedure, 327
osseous lesions, 324
PET/CT, 324
physical examination, 327
potential synergy, 328
staging, 324–326
survival rates, 320–323
Ovarian cancer
adjuvant therapy, 93
advanced-stage disease, 94
BRCA1/BRCA2, 85–86
chemotherapy, 94
COX2 inhibitors, 86
definitive primary therapy, 90
distant disease, 92–93
epithelial ovarian cancer, 93
genomic profiling, 86
granulosa cell tumor, 95

historical perspective
AcFuCy/VAC, 88
alkylating agent chemotherapy, 87
BEP chemotherapy, 89
cytoreductive surgery, 89
intraperitoneal techniques, 86
melphalan *vs.* 5-fluorouracil *vs.* hexamethylmelamine, 88
paclitaxel, 89
postoperative therapy, 86
second-line chemotherapy, 87
surgical cytoreduction, 89
treatment, 87
VBP, 88
local and regional disease, 91
localized disease, 91–92
low malignant potential, 85
malignant transformation, 86
postoperative therapy, 94
regional disease, 92
risk factors, 85
targeted therapy, 94
taxane/platinum chemotherapy, 93
tumor registry methodology, 91
Oxaliplatin, 82

P

Pancreatic cancer
borderline resectable, 129
CA19-9 levels, 120
computed tomography, 120–121
curative treatment, 120
ERCP, 129
grim statistics, 120
historical perspective
adjuvant chemotherapy, 122
ascites, 123
celiac axis neurolysis, 123
CRT, 122
FDA approval, 122
FOLFIRINOX, 122–123
morbidity and mortality, 121
preoperative stage, 122
radiotherapy, 122
surgery, 121
neoplasms, 119
novel methods, 130
post-ERCP acute pancreatitis, 121
preoperative therapy, 129
presentation, 123–124
risk factor, 119–120
stromal cells, 130
survival rates
local disease, 124, 126
localized, 124–128
metastatic, 124, 128
morbidity and mortality rates, 125
regional disease, 124, 127
transgenic mouse models, 130
types of, 119
Papadimitrakopoulou, V., 279
Papillary thyroid carcinoma (PTC), 296, 297
Partial nephrectomy techniques, 134
Pelvic lymph nodes, 37
Peutz–Jeghers syndrome, 120
Pisters, 312
Porter, M., 281
Positron emission tomography (PET), 324, 329
Positron emission tomography with computed tomography (PET/CT), 50
Postoperative radiation therapy, 55–56
Postoperative thyroid hormone therapy, 308
Post-radiation/Paget sarcoma, 325
Preinvasive disease, 97
Primitive neuroectodermal tumors (PNETs), 329
Prophylactic cranial irradiation (PCI), 69–71
Prostate cancer
androgen deprivation therapy, 40
cases of, 35
definition, 35, 36
diagnosis of, 39
distant disease, 40, 42
historical perspective, 37–38
localized disease, 40, 41
low-risk disease, 42
metastatic disease, 42
molecular classification, 42
patient presentation, 39
PSA testing, 35, 37, 39
regional disease, 40, 41
stages, 39–40
survival rate, 39, 40
treatment, 43
tumor characteristics, 37
Prostate-specific antigen (PSA), 35
Proton beam therapy, 49–50, 57–58

R

Radiation/proton beam therapy
early-stage (I–II) disease, 53–54
image-guided techniques, 53
stages IIIA–IIIB
chemotherapy, 54
full-dose induction chemotherapy, 55

IMRT, 55
N1/N2 disease, 56
postoperative radiation therapy, 55–56
toxicity, 54
Radiation Therapy Oncology Group (RTOG), 277
Radical prostatectomy, 38
Radiotherapeutic techniques, 38, 86
RCC. *See* Renal cell carcinoma (RCC)
Regional nodal treatment, 26–27
Renal cell carcinoma (RCC), 133–135
Revolutionary technique, 155–156
Richter syndrome, 212
Romaguera, J.E., 258
Rosenberg, S., 227
Rosen, G., 325
Rothmund–Thomson syndrome, 324
Rutledge, F.N., 98, 100, 104, 107

S

Salvage therapy, 53
Sample algorithm, 2, 3
Second intergroup Ewing's sarcoma study (IESS-II), 331
Sentinel lymph node (SLN), 26, 27
Sentinel node biopsy (SLNB), 155
Single nucleotide polymorphisms (SNPs), 58
Small cell lung cancer (SCLC)
chemotherapy
alternating/sequential chemotherapy, 67
combination, 66–67
cytotoxic agent, 67
increase dose density/intensity, 67
prolonged administration, 68
systemic disease, 66
clinical presentation, 64–65
first-line chemotherapy, 72
history and prognosis, 65–66
incidence of, 63
irinotecan, 72
PCI, 69–71
second-line treatment, 72
sensitive relapse, 72
stages, 63–64
treatment
extensive-stage, 69–70
limited-stage, 68–69
Small lymphocytic lymphoma (SLL). *See* Chronic lymphocytic leukemia (CLL)
Smith, L., 264
Soft tissue sarcoma
distant, 315, 316
extraskeletal nonepithelial tissue, 311
genomic and proteomic aberrations, 317
heterogeneous nature, 311
imatinib, 317
KIT or *PDGFRA* gene, 318
metastatic disease, risk of, 317
nonmetastatic disease, 312–313
phase 2 randomized study, 313
regional, 315, 316
survival data, 313–315
SWOG trial, 313
targeted drug identification, 317
Specialized Program of Research Excellence (SPORE), 42
Spitzer, G., 259
Statistical methods
follow-up section, 14–15
long-term progress, 13
patient selection criteria, 13–14
potential biases
detection and screening, 15
diagnostic criteria and procedure, 15–16
prognostic profile, 16
supportive and palliative care, 16
regional tumors, 14
SEER staging system, 14
survival analyses, 15
Stem cell transplantation (SCT), 212, 219, 259–260
Stereotactic ablative radiation therapy (SABR), 49
Stereotactic body radiation therapy (SBRT), 49
Suit, H., 100
Surgery, HNC
clinical presentation, 275
endoscopic approach, 277
goal of, 275
intracranial/extracranial approach, 276
mandible and maxilla, 276
nasal cavity tumors, 274, 276
outcomes of, 275
soft tissue defects, 276
surgical management of, 276
vascularized bone flaps, 276
Surgical technique, 102, 113, 123, 186, 333
Surveillance Epidemiology, and End Results (SEER), 14, 295
Syndrome of inappropriate antidiuretic hormone (SIADH), 65
Systemic chemotherapy, 51–53
Systemic disease, 141

T
Tamoxifen-alone therapy, 23
Third intergroup Ewing's sarcoma study (IESS-III), 331
Thomas, E.D., 230
Three-dimensional conformal radiation therapy, 49
Thyroid cancer
  AJCC-TNM staging, 296–297
  asymptomatic stability, 308
  cross-sectional image, 307
  distant metastatic disease, 300–301
  histologic subtypes, 299–300
  historical perspective, 298–299
  incidence of, 295
  Kaplan–Meier survival, 301–303
  locoregional disease, 307
  outcomes of, DTC patient, 304
  patient outcomes, 308
  remnant ablation, 307
  SEER data, 295, 298
  survival rates, DTC, 304–306
  TSH level, 308
Topotecan, 72
Transgenic mouse models, 130
Transurethral resection (TUR), 144
Tumor registry, 2, 265
Tumor registry methodology, 91, 112, 158
Tyrosine kinase inhibitors (TKIs), 52

U
U.S. Food and Drug Administration, 220

V
Velasquez, W., 259
Vincristine, doxorubicin (adriamycin), and dexamethasone (VAD), 264

W
Wallace, S., 103
Walters, R., 281
Weber, R., 281
Werner syndrome, 324
Wilson's disease, 167

Y
Yang, J.C., 312